MONEY, POWER, and HEALTH CARE

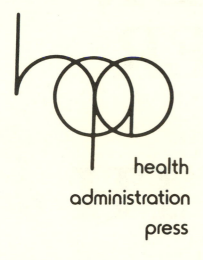

health
administration
press

MONEY, POWER, and HEALTH CARE

Evan M. Melhado
Walter Feinberg
Harold M. Swartz
Editors

Health Administration Press
Ann Arbor, Michigan   1988

Library of Congress Cataloging-in-Publication Data
Money, power, and health care.
  Includes index.
  1. Medical economics—United States. 2. Medical
care—United States. 3. Medical policy—United States.
I. Melhado, Evan Marc, 1946–   . II. Feinberg,
Walter, 1937–   . III. Swartz, Harold M.
[DNLM: 1. Delivery of Health Care—United States.
2. Economics, Medical—United States. 3. Health
Policy—United States. W 84 AA1 M7]
RA407.3.M66   1987   333.4'33621'0973   87-27665
ISBN 0-910701-26-1

Health Administration Press
A Division of the Foundation of the
  American College of Healthcare Executives
1021 East Huron Street
Ann Arbor, Michigan 48104-9990
(313) 764-1380

Table of Contents

List of Tables

List of Figures

Contributors

RICHARD J. ARNOULD is Professor of Economics and was formerly Associate Dean of the College of Commerce and Business Administration at the University of Illinois at Urbana-Champaign. He received his Ph.D. in economics from Iowa State University. He has extensive experience in various areas of industrial organization, public policy, and health economics. He has served as a consultant for state and federal agencies investigating regulatory policy, and is currently a trustee for Carle Foundation, a diversified health care provider in Urbana, Illinois.

PAMELA K. BARTELS obtained her M.D. and M.S.W. degrees through the Medical Scholars Program at the University of Illinois at Urbana-Champaign in 1987 and is now in a residency in family practice at the Mountain Area Health Education Center in Asheville, North Carolina.

JAMES E. BLACK is a fifth-year student in the Medical Scholars Program, pursuing the M.D. jointly with the Ph.D. in the Neural and Behavioral Biology Program at the University of Illinois at Urbana-Champaign. He has special interests in the history of pediatrics, pediatric communication, and women in medicine.

WALTER FEINBERG was formerly director of the Medicine and Society Faculty Development Seminar in the University of Illinois College of Medicine at Urbana and is Professor of Educational Policy Studies at the University of Illinois at Urbana-Champaign. He also holds a joint appointment in the Unit for Criticism and Interpretive Theory. He obtained a Ph.D. in philosophy from Boston University. His research interests include issues of equity and professional education as related to the growth and distribution of knowledge and authority.

ANN BARRY FLOOD holds a Ph.D. from Stanford University. She is Associate Professor in the Department of Health and Safety Studies at the University of Illinois at Urbana-Champaign and in the College of Medicine at Urbana. She also holds concurrent appointments in the Department of Sociology and the Institute of Government and Public Affairs. In the College of Medicine, she directs the sociomedical seminar series and coordinates a segment of the summer medicine and society course. Her research is on organizational aspects of health care and effectiveness of therapeutic procedures. Most of her work deals with inpatient surgical care, but she also is studying compliance behavior among outpatient cancer patients.

SUZANNE R. LANGNER is Adult Nurse Practitioner and Clinical Nurse Researcher at the Graduate Hospital in Philadelphia. She received her M.S. in nursing at the University of Pennsylvania and her Ph.D. in nursing from the University of Illinois at Chicago. Her primary research focus is on the process of family caregiving to dependent elderly relatives. Her primary interests are to replicate family caregiving research with different populations and in different settings, and to develop existing programs to older adults and their families as part of the mission of a teaching hospital.

WALTER W. MCMAHON is Professor of Economics at the University of Illinois at Urbana-Champaign with a concurrent appointment in the University of Illinois College of Medicine at Urbana. His fields are human capital, health economics, and macroeconomics. His current research and recent publications concern the effects of education, health, and research and development on productivity. He is currently working on a book that explores the contributions of these factors to a growing economy.

EVAN M. MELHADO is Associate Professor in the Departments of History and Chemistry and a member of the Program on Science, Technology, and Society at the University of Illinois at Urbana-Champaign. He also holds a concurrent appointment in the University of Illinois College of Medicine at Urbana. He obtained his Ph.D. in history from Princeton University, and he has specialized in the history of science and medicine. He has helped design and teach the summer medicine and society course in the College of Medicine at Urbana and has long been involved in the governance of the Medical Scholars Program. His research interests include the history of the physical sciences in the 18th and 19th centuries and of medicine and health care in the 19th and 20th centuries.

THOMAS W. O'ROURKE is Professor in the Department of Health and Safety Studies at the University of Illinois at Urbana-Champaign and in the College of Medicine at Urbana. He holds M.P.H. and Ph.D. degrees, and his research is in two areas. The first is directed toward the integration of a social science perspective into health education. He is coauthor of the U.S. Surgeon General's Report, *Smoking and Health* (1979). His second research area encompasses health planning, health policy formulation, and consumer participation in health care, and in these areas he takes an active role in shaping policy at national, state, and local levels.

JOHN W. POLLARD received his M.D. from the University of Minnesota in 1957 and his M.B.A. from the University of Illinois in 1977. He is Chief Executive Officer of Carle Clinic Association, a large multispecialty group practice in Urbana, Illinois, and is Chairman of the Board of CarleCare, a health maintenance organization. Recently he became president of the American Group Practice Association. His principal interest is in the socio-economics of health care.

DANA RUBIN obtained her M.D. and M.S.W. degrees through the Medical Scholars Program at the University of Illinois at Urbana-Champaign in 1987 and is now in a pediatrics residency at Boston City Hospital.

HAROLD M. SWARTZ is Professor of Medicine at the University of Illinois College of Medicine at Urbana, and Professor of Physiology and Biophysics in the School of Life Sciences and an Affiliate of the Institute of Environmental Studies at the University of Illinois at Urbana-Champaign. He holds M.P.H., M.D., and Ph.D. degrees. His professional expertise is in radiation biology and biophysics, fields in which he has published extensively and continues an active program of laboratory research. He was a principal investigator for the project sponsored by the University of Illinois College of Medicine and the National Institutes of Health on Curriculum Development in Environmental Health and principal investigator for the Cost-Containment Project at the University of Illinois College of Medicine sponsored by the National Fund for Medical Education. He has been extensively involved in the design, development, and guidance of the Medical Scholars Program.

CHARLES B. VAN VORST received his M.B.A. from George Washington University. He has served as Vice President of Operations of Methodist Hospital in Indianapolis and now serves as President of Carle Foundation, a diversified health care provider in Urbana, Illinois. He has consulted with a number of health care providers on a variety of health care issues and is currently a member of the Illinois Health Care Cost Containment Council. He also serves on the board and the executive committee of the Illinois Hospital Association.

PAUL A. WILSON is Associate Professor in the School of Social Work and Associate Research Scientist in the School of Public Health at the University of Michigan. He received his M.S.W. and Ph.D. degrees from Washington University, St. Louis. His major research interest is effective social service and health care delivery systems; specifically, the relation of formal and informal sources of caregiving, coordination of services for community-based care of the chronically ill, and client-oriented program development processes.

Introduction

Evan M. Melhado, Walter Feinberg, and Harold M. Swartz

THE ONGOING TRANSFORMATION
OF THE HEALTH CARE SECTOR

American health services are in the midst of profound changes. Whereas the development of the health sector in this century long consisted of the gradual elaboration of basic structural features, since the 1960s the health services have been perceived as out of control, and reform proposals have proliferated (Anderson 1985, pts. 4, 5). The system has recently undergone many changes, and still others seem imminent. In the 1970s, calls for reform were outpaced by the effects of economic forces that were reshaping the system even as policy makers struggled to understand the health sector, to articulate the ends it should be made to subserve, and to institute measures that would bring facilities and services into accord with the goals of policy (Gray 1983, 1986). The outcome of these changes can scarcely be predicted, but some of the forces at work, both within the health sector itself and within health policy circles, as well as their potential implications, can be elucidated.

The basic pattern for provision of services was set into place in the period from approximately 1875 to 1914 (Starr 1982; Anderson 1985). Physicians, as private, entrepreneurial practitioners, operated on a solo, fee-for-service basis. Entry into the profession was limited by high barriers, chief among which was prolonged, expensive, and recondite training. Practice was increasingly linked to privileges in a new institution—the voluntary, acute care general hospital—which did not employ physicians but served their interests so as to gain their patients (Vogel 1980). Within the hospital, nursing assumed its familiar form as overwhelmingly a women's job, one lacking professional status and subordinate to the medical profession (Melosh 1982). Specialization began to mark the practice of medicine, arousing some fears among general practitioners, but general practice long

remained predominant (Stevens 1971). Health insurance was, for all practical purposes, absent, but physicians and hospitals provided some gratis
or low-priced care for the poor (though the extent of these services was
likely inadequate to the needs of a large and heavily exploited industrial
working class) (Lubove 1968; Anderson 1985, chap. 6).

The earliest battle for compulsory health insurance, which occurred
in the 1910s, served chiefly to ratify existing arrangements and solidify the
opposition of organized medicine to governmental interference in medical care (Anderson 1968; Lubove 1968; Numbers 1982; Starr 1982). Not
only within the sphere of professional judgment in diagnosis and therapy,
but also in the social and economic dimensions of health services, organized medicine claimed the right to dictate the character and conditions
of medical practice, and other interests found little cause to contest the
claims of physicians.

In the depression, middle-class demands for insurance and declining
incomes of physicians and hospitals inaugurated the rise of voluntary
insurance. Responding in 1932 to proposals by the Committee on the Costs
of Medical Care, physicians conceded the propriety of voluntary insurance
for physician services, provided that the insurance mechanism lay under
the control of the profession. This concession was grudgingly transformed
into action only a decade later, as medical societies, seeking to stave off
governmental programs, began to offer insurance, known as Blue Shield
plans, for physician services. Hospital insurance, by contrast, emerged
much more quickly in the form of Blue Cross plans, which met the middle-
class desire for insurance and stabilized the incomes of hospitals (Anderson 1975; Anderson 1985, chap. 10).

Like the hospitals themselves, the Blues assumed the form of voluntary, nonprofit entities and drew over themselves the mantle of public service long enjoyed by the hospital industry. Though commercial insurers
began to compete for the health insurance market, the Blues remained
dominant. They served the middle class, and modest welfare programs on
the state level began to complement both traditional local welfare programs and the charity offered by providers to the poor. In all cases, insurance mechanisms did not disturb the basic patterns of medical practice and
hospital organization. Insurers did not seek to reorganize the health services, attempted little in the way of utilization controls, and confined themselves to retrospective reimbursement of providers' charges. Voluntary
insurance spread more rapidly than many observers predicted. The nation
was satisfied with its progress in the 1950s, willing to allow its natural
growth to fill gaps in coverage of the population, and accepting of the usual
welfare measures for the poor (Anderson 1985, pt. 3). At the same time, the
growing prestige of medicine fostered increasing support for medical education and medical research, which contributed gradually to the techno-

logical powers of medicine, its differentiation into specialties, and the costliness of its services (Starr 1982, book 2, chap. 3).

Specialization and technical expertise induced the fragmentation of medical services and institutions. Patients lacked a clear sense of which providers to seek and when, while general practitioners, who might have provided guidance, were a vanishing breed (for example, Kennedy 1972). This fragmentation and the cost escalation resulting from the combination of retrospective reimbursement and technologically advanced practice combined to foster the perception that the health services system was out of control.

Concern about cost escalation emerged in the early 1950s, but it became a major theme only a decade later. It grew intense largely in reaction to rapidly escalating rates demanded by the Blues, and it resulted in changing the orientation of health planning efforts. The federal-state Hill-Burton program, enacted in 1946, invoked planning to guide the subsidized growth of hospital facilities in underserved, largely rural areas; but state and federal planning and regulatory laws passed in the 1960s expected planning to constrain growth in well-served, metropolitan areas (Starr 1982, book 2, chap. 3; Payton and Powsner 1980; Anderson 1985, pt. 4). These new measures, predicted in part on "Roemer's Law" (the existence of beds results in their utilization), aimed to restrict utilization by restricting the supply of beds (Havighurst 1973; Payton and Powsner 1980). Most observers agree that planning and regulation failed to achieve these goals and instead permitted the generation of excess capacity in the hospital industry supported by third-party reimbursement of hospital expenses (for example, Enthoven 1980, 44 and chap. 6; see also Brown 1983). The fragmentation of the health sector became prominent as it was perceived to impede the access of middle-class beneficiaries of voluntary insurance to health care. Simultaneously, the 1960s were marked by increased demands to improve the access of the poor to health services. Cost escalation, middle-class dissatisfaction, and equity concerns combined to bring planning and regulation to the federal level, and equity concerns led to the passage of Medicare (a federal entitlement program providing health benefits to the elderly) and Medicaid (a federal-state revenue-sharing program providing services for the poor). However, these new programs consciously preserved the prerogatives of the medical profession and, like the earlier growth of voluntary insurance for the middle class, did nothing to disturb the basic patterns of the health sector. The consequences of these programs included the socialization of enormous and intensely escalating costs, the emergence of government as a profoundly interested party to the organization and financing of health services, and the growth of a climate in which the prerogatives of medicine and the long-standing structural features of the health sector were no longer held sacrosanct (Hodgson 1973).

The immediate outcome of these developments was a reform agenda that aimed to rationalize the health sector by subordinating it to intensified regulation and by using the anticipated efficiency gains to expand entitlement to the entire population under a system of national health insurance (for example, Falk 1970; Davis 1975). Among the circumstances inhibiting the success of this agenda in the 1970s was the end, by 1974, of the long postwar period of economic growth, an event that called into question the feasibility of financing expanded entitlement (Starr 1982, book 2, chap. 4; Klein 1981, especially p. 199). Moreover, declining faith in the utility of high-technology medicine to effect improvements in health at the margin cast doubt on the wisdom of expanding entitlement to a standard of care long enjoyed by the middle class (for example, Havighurst 1977, 318). Because regulation was increasingly perceived as having failed to solve the problems of the health sector, the long push for direct, governmental control of health services was losing legitimacy (Havighurst 1974; Noll 1975). Government would have to bring the health services under control by indirect methods. Advocacy of market strengthening and competition grew accordingly (Ellwood 1975; Enthoven 1980; Pauly 1980).

As it did, economic forces began to affect the health sector independently of thought about policy. The end of economic expansion, the maturation of the hospital industry in the 1970s, tighter reimbursement, and the appearance of competitors combined to make excess capacity and overbedding onerous burdens. The inevitable "shakeout" began, leading to closures, mergers, growth of proprietary hospitals, and gradual disintegration of the public service mantle that had long clothed the hospital industry (Feldstein 1983, 311–20; Starkweather 1981, chap. 1; Arnould and Van Vorst 1985; Gray 1986). Competition among hospitals and institutional providers led these organizations to think of patients more as consumers, to compete with physicians for consumers rather than depend on physicians to bring them in, to exploit traditional marketing methods, to rearrange packages of services, and to modify standards of care so as to reduce costs.

Thus, economic forces, largely unaided by policy, brought on many of the changes sought by advocates of market-oriented reforms. Federal policy intensified the emergence of a traditional market (as opposed to a public service sector) less by fostering particular competitive arrangements (as some competitive theorists hoped it would) than by instituting, in the 1980s, a system of prospective reimbursement under Medicare. State policy contributed by devising new, competitive methods for the delivery of services to beneficiaries of Medicaid (Davis 1983; Gibson 1983). Though the new order remains ill-defined, its emergence is accompanied by profound changes in expectations about the nature and utility of health care, in perceptions about the responsibility of society to the poor, and in professional roles, powers, and responsibilities.

As for the role of health care in American society, the pressure for equity in access to health services has lessened as faith has declined in the healing powers of medical care and as concern about financing has risen with costs. The nation seems prepared to acquiesce in a two- or multi-tiered system of care, in which beneficiaries of public programs receive, at most, basic benefits while others exercise the right to purchase any amount of care they can afford. In this environment, the poor have contended with tightened eligibility requirements and reduced benefits.

Many supporters of health services for the poor believe that a market-oriented system of health services is fundamentally hostile to redistributive concerns (for example, Rosenblatt 1981, 1109–14). This hostility is not inherent in competitive theory, however, and the dominant lines of market-oriented policy have explicitly envisioned ways to accommodate the interests of the poor (though not to the extent of providing them with all of the services used by the middle class) (Enthoven 1980). However, in the current political environment, the nation has been content to allow competitive pressures to operate with little regard to their consequences for the poor, and government has diminished the benefits and scope of public programs. The perception that these policies increase medical indigency, reduce the health status of the poor, and increase the pressure that the poor exert on municipal and other public providers may compel renewed attention to the provision of services to the poor (Hadley, Mullner, and Feder 1983). For the present, however, the interests of the poor have been profoundly eclipsed by the desire to cut costs.

The power of physicians to define the nature of practice and to determine financing is being severely eroded. Under competition, utilization controls and prospective reimbursement are constraining the reach of professional judgment in the provision of services and are violating the long-asserted right of the medical profession to escape control by government or industry (Starr 1982, book 2, chap. 5; Luft 1981, chap. 12, especially pp. 312–13). Women, spurred by the feminist movement and by a conviction that caring as well as curing is a legitimate part of health services, have contested the gender biases they perceive in medicine (for example, Ruzek 1978; Rodriguez-Trias 1984). In nursing, the activism of women appears as an effort to achieve professional status and assume service roles more nearly coequal with those of physicians than subservient to them, and in medicine it appears in the vastly enhanced recruitment of female students (Fawcett 1984; American Nurses' Association 1965; Eisenberg 1983; Iglehart 1986). Primary care is beginning to acquire renewed emphasis at the expense of technologically advanced specialties (Miller 1983). Some medical schools are fostering awareness of the social and cultural dimensions of medicine among their students, and the students are proving more receptive to extraprofessional influences on their socialization (Petersdorf and Feinstein 1981; Freiman and Marder 1984). New interests have therefore arisen, seeking to dissipate the overarching authority and influence of the medical profession and to acquire the power to define the character of health services.

A competitive environment, prospective reimbursement, utilization controls, diminished concern for the poor, and centrifugal dissipation of professional power are the hallmarks of the present era. Money and power are the themes of current changes in American health care; this volume attempts a preliminary description and assessment of the nature and consequences of those changes.

A MULTIDISCIPLINARY PERSPECTIVE ON HEALTH CARE

The essays in this volume provide a multidisciplinary analysis of recent upheavals in the health sector and their implications for consumers, professionals, and organizations in health care. We take a multidisciplinary approach out of the conviction that innovations in health policy often founder on unintended consequences that might have been foreseen but for the limited perspectives of policy makers. We discuss money because, at least since the Second World War, the economics of health has been a principal motive force in the evolution of health policy and health services. We speak of power because of the influence exerted by social forces on the distribution of power and authority in health care. We look at consumers, professionals, and organizations, for we seek to understand how changes in the economics and politics of health affect the roles and behavior of patients and providers and therefore the overall performance of the health system, and we hope to enable the actors in the system to respond constructively.

Sound thinking about health services demands a multidisciplinary analysis of the changes taking place in the health sector. Too often, health policies have focused narrowly on single problems and have been instituted without analysis of their likely influence beyond their immediate targets (cf. Luft 1985). The expanded access to health services achieved by Medicare and Medicaid, for example, entailed largely unforeseen economic consequences that now fuel the push toward competition and prospective reimbursement. As attention has shifted to cost containment, the goal of fiscal accountability now drives policy without adequate attention to its impact on equity, access, and the quality of care. Identifying the unintended consequences and analyzing their implications for policy formulation demand a breadth of knowledge and expertise that only a multidisciplinary perspective can provide.

The essays in this volume exemplify such a perspective. They are the outcome of studies and discussions conducted over several years by the

Faculty Seminar in Medicine and Society at the University of Illinois at Urbana-Champaign. The seminar draws its members from university faculty, health care professionals in academic departments and in the community, and students in the Medical Scholars Program, an M.D./Ph.D. program conducted by the Graduate College and the College of Medicine. Represented in the seminar are disciplines in the humanities and social sciences as well as in the biomedical sciences, health education, social work, nursing, and medicine. This diverse group has taken an active role in conceiving and revising each essay, so that each reflects more than the disciplinary specialties of its authors. The essays aim to identify fundamental issues, to define them more broadly than the specialists' perspective allows, and to suggest by example the kinds of multidisciplinary analyses demanded by the formulation of health policy. The resultant collection, though not fully comprehensive, nevertheless provides a broad perspective on the political economy of American health care.

Introducing the volume are two essays that analyze the new competitive approach to health care delivery and pose many of the issues treated in the later papers. The opening essay, by Evan M. Melhado, a historian of science and medicine, provides an intellectual history of competitive theory as a candidate for a national health policy and attempts to exhibit the relations of competitive theory with broader changes in thought about the role of government in American society. Identifying two clusters of competitive policies, Melhado links one of them with changes in the discipline of economics and the increasing application of dispassionate analysis (instead of advocacy) to the health sector; he associates the other with new perceptions of the propriety and efficacy of governmental programs generally, and of health care and previous health policy in particular. Proponents of both clusters shared a lowered estimate of the significance and utility of health care, a willingness to regard it as only one among many consumption goods, and a belief that traditional health policy, by holding market forces at bay, perpetuated the well-cataloged deficiencies of the health sector. The remedy proposed by competitive theorists was therefore to introduce market forces, dismantle regulation, and confine the role of government to that of guarantor of competitive conditions and provider of subsidies for the purchase of health insurance by the poor. Patients would therefore become sovereign consumers, seeking satisfaction of their wants in a market of competing sellers of services (or of insurance packages that pay for services). Providers of services would increasingly bend to the will of a managerial hierarchy and to the efficiency exacted by management in meeting consumer demand in a competitive market. Among the issues raised by this account and pursued by other authors in this volume are the relative virtues of governmental and individual responsibility for health care, the implications for equity of a shift from regulation to competition, the nature of consumer sovereignty in a competitive market, and the diminution of professional prerogatives in the provision of health services.

If Melhado assesses the theory of competition in health care, Walter W. McMahon, an economist of education and health, juxtaposes theory with practice. He identifies the forces pressing for the introduction of competition on both federal and state levels, argues that perverse incentives institutionalized under regulation have fostered intense cost escalation, isolates the forms taken by new competitive arrangements, and describes the theoretical basis for the operation of these arrangements. In his perspective, the central novelties of the health sector in the 1980s are deregulation, negotiation in advance of prices for stipulated services (as opposed to the largely unlimited retrospective reimbursement typical of past practice), and the reduction of barriers to entry. He provides a typology of the forms in which these novelties appear (for example, health maintenance organizations and preferred provider organizations) and articulates the basic theory on which their operation depends. Though favorably disposed toward competition, McMahon finds that policy makers, while fostering the growth of competition, have paid minimal attention to the needs of the poor; and he points out that competitive arrangements imply the need for new ways of training providers of health services. These consquences of the new competition are pursued in later essays.

The second group of essays treats the effects of competition on three major participants in the market for health services: providers (the supply side) and (on the demand side) consumers generally and the poor particularly. Richard C. Arnould, an economist, Charles B. Van Vorst, president of Carle Foundation Hospital in Urbana, Illinois, and John W. Pollard, a cardiologist and chief executive of Carle Clinic Association (a large, multispecialty group practice in Urbana), discuss actual and anticipated responses of providers to the growth of competition within their traditional markets. They share McMahon's conviction that retrospective third-party reimbursement is largely responsible for inefficiency in the provision of health services; and they argue that more formal economic coordination is needed among the participants in the market for health services so that payment mechanisms will reliably impose the appropriate financial risks on providers and consumers.

The authors maintain that fuller coordination can result from more complete contractual arrangements among health care providers, but that integration seems to offer the greatest possibilities for efficiency. Though acknowledging the emergence of several forms of integration, the authors concentrate on what they regard as the likely advantages of vertical integration among providers at different stages in production (such as hospitals, nursing homes, providers of ambulatory care, and insurers). Integrated organizations will alter the traditional fiduciary or agency role of the physician and introduce a new "agent-coordinator" role, in which the physician or other professional will assume responsibility for the efficient provision of services. The precise nature of the new role will depend on the extent of integration of the provider organization. The authors suggest several models of integration and explore the efficiency gains that may be anticipated from them.

With his eye on the demand side of the market, Thomas W. O'Rourke, a health educator and consumer activist in health care, asks whether competitive policy genuinely fosters consumer sovereignty. Consumerism in health care, he points out, antedated the rise of competitive theory in health policy circles. Consumerism rested on expanded conceptions of rights and on the perception that health care providers had organized the health sector to serve not consumers' interests, but their own. In challenging the prerogatives of providers and calling for new kinds of providers and services, consumerism prefigured the challenge to professional autonomy raised by the new competition. Accordingly, O'Rourke's essay shows that in principle many complaints lodged against American health care by its more radical critics are resolved in a competitive market. It also reveals, however, that consumerism has aspired to broader changes than those likely to emerge from the competitive marketplace and that many consumer activists find public ownership of the health sector a more appealing means to achieve their goals. O'Rourke concludes that, within a limited realm, competition may bring benefits, but that it is unlikely to meet the needs of the poor and cannot realize a vision of health care that transcends the market.

The accessibility of health services to the poor under the impact of competition, budget cutting, and the shift of social policy from federal to state levels is the topic pursued by Paul A. Wilson, a professor of social work, and Pamela K. Bartels and Dana Rubin, students in the Medical Scholars Program who are pursuing degrees in social work jointly with medicine. Concentrating on Medicaid, they argue that, despite its many problems, it has been a major force for improving the health of the poor and that current economic and political conditions threaten its viability. Cuts in federal funding and transfer to the states of discretionary powers over many social programs have compromised the aspiration to provide the poor with high-quality, dignified, and accessible care and to include them within the mainstream of American medicine. Tightened eligibility requirements and reduced benefits have adversely affected the health and well-being of the poor. However, the authors take encouragement from the congressional commitment to preserve Medicaid and from the positive features of state-level efforts to restructure it. They conclude by identifying the central issues that will have to be addressed as Medicaid is reorganized.

These issues include the extent to which the poor can be accorded freedom of choice as buyers in the health care market (that is, enjoy consumer sovereignty); the geographical accessibility of health services to the poor and the likely need for supply subsidies such as neighborhood health centers; and the need to determine the differing responsibilities of state and federal governments in meeting the goals of Medicaid.

The final group of essays concerns the effects of a changing political and economic environment on the status and authority of health care professionals. However unpredictable these effects may be, a dispassionate examination of earlier episodes can suggest the kinds of conflict they may precipitate. James E. Black, a student in the Medical Scholars Program, provides an example. Black looks at the emergence, early in the present century, of pediatrics as a specialty in the United States. Before any physicians had successfully claimed child health services as their preserve, social forces had emerged, largely from outside of medicine, to define the sphere of child health, to identify the health care needs of children and the services necessary to meet those needs, and to claim control over the delivery of the services demanded. Pediatricians, initially indifferent, eventually perceived these developments as threats to both their prestige and their economic interests. They responded to this perception by attempting to dominate child health care and therefore found themselves in competition with rival groups of potential providers. The combination, characteristic of modern pediatrics, of progressive social and political values with a high esteem for science and research, can be understood only by exploring the mechanisms by which pediatricians successfully eliminated their competitors. The case differs from the present in that the competition among providers emerged simultaneously with efforts to define the market that lay at the center of their contest, whereas now providers are losing their once-tight grip on an already established market. Nevertheless, the 1910s prefigured the consumerism and expanded conceptions of rights in the 1960s and 1970s and presaged the kinds of competition currently appearing among groups of health care professionals, and between professionals and extramedical pretenders to control over health services. In addition, the episode suggests the sorts of social and political justification offered by the contenders in pursuit of their goals.

A recent example of interprofessional competition for the right to define and control certain kinds of services is explored by Walter Feinberg, an educational philosopher, and Suzanne Langner, a nurse practitioner and nursing educator. They identify within nursing an argument for the increased professionalization and autonomy of nursing, for a reduction in the emphasis of the health system on crisis intervention and specialized services (spheres of the physician), and for increased attention to prevention, nurturing, coping, primary care, and expansion of access to care (spheres of the professionalized nurse). This argument rests on the belief that the social and behavioral sciences can provide a knowledge base for the professional practice of nursing, just as the biomedical sciences underlie the practice of medicine. The authors argue that both medicine and nursing seek to legitimate their authority by claiming to meet the requirements of an effective health care system, but that many students in these fields tend to link their future professional status to personal characteristics rather than to the requirements of health care. This individual focus renders these students unable to perceive the justification for the established authority of physicians or the potential utility of establishing professional standards in nursing. The authors conclude by suggesting that more explicit attention to the status of professions and the aims of professionalization must form part of professional education; by arguing that, through the creation and marketing of new institutions and services, nursing may be able to exploit the current competitive environment to realize an autonomous form of practice; and by warning that, despite its merits, the professionalization of nursing must proceed without undermining the nurturing role that is essential to effective health care.

Professionalization and professional education are also central to the concluding essay. Harold M. Swartz, a physician, medical educator, and biomedical scientist, and Ann B. Flood, a medical sociologist, review the profound changes that have taken place in medical education, medical practice, and the broad social and economic environment of medical care over the past three decades. They argue that changes in the recruitment of medical students, altered expectations among them, differences in their clinical experiences during training and in the career opportunities open to them, the declining autonomy of medical practice, and the persistent intrusion of social and economic forces into the formerly insulated world of medical care have created a generation gap within the medical profession. Those trained 30 years ago differ profoundly from new graduates in their views of physicians' roles and professional obligations and in their ability to adapt to change. The authors argue that efforts to analyze the medical care system and plan for its development must take into account these differences, and they hold that medical education must prepare students to understand and respond constructively to the continued pressure exerted on medicine by changing social and economic circumstances. To meet this educational need, the authors offer proposals based on their experiences at the University of Illinois College of Medicine at Urbana. These proposals include a program of sociomedical education conducted apart from the usual basic medical curriculum; a faculty development program, drawing heavily on the humanities and social sciences, to train the faculty needed to support the sociomedical component of medical education; and a joint degree program to produce leaders in medical education who can be expected to organize and staff similar programs of instruction and research at other institutions.

Despite the variety of topics these essays address, they revolve around several central themes: escalating costs; measures to contain costs and rationalize service delivery; the emergence and effects of market institutions and procedures; declining autonomy of physicians and rival claims to provide services or control their provision; professional education; the rights and responsibilities of providers, consumers, and the poor; and the roles of government in health care. No single discipline can dominate this multitude of issues or the numerous contexts in which the issues emerge, and a narrow disciplinary perspective cannot grasp their complex relations. The many disciplines represented by the authors of these essays and the light the essays shed on one another, by contrast, clearly evoke the complexity and gravity of current changes. To the extent that this is so, this volume may help the actors in the health sector to respond thoughtfully and constructively to current changes and may aid policy makers in proceeding with clarity and deliberation.

REFERENCES

American Nurses' Association, Committee on Education. 1965. "American Nurses' Association's First Position on Education for Nursing." *American Journal of Nursing* 65 (December): 106–11.

Anderson, Odin W. 1968. *The Uneasy Equilibrium: Private and Public Financing of Health Services in the United States, 1875–1965.* New Haven: College and University Press.

———. 1975. *Blue Cross Since 1929: Accountability and the Public Trust.* Cambridge, MA: Ballinger.

———. 1985. *Health Services in the United States: A Growth Enterprise Since 1875.* Ann Arbor, MI: Health Administration Press.

Arnould, Richard J., and Charles B. Van Vorst. 1985. "Supply Responses to Market and Regulatory Forces in Health Care." In *Incentives vs. Controls in Health Policy: Broadening the Debate,* ed. by Jack A. Meyer, 107–31. Washington, DC: American Enterprise Institute.

Brown, Lawrence D. 1983. "Common Sense Meets Implementation: Certificate-of-Need Regulation in the States." *Journal of Health Politics, Policy and Law* 8: 480–94.

Controls on Health Care. 1975. Papers of the Conference on Regulation of the Health Industry, January 7–9, 1974. Washington, DC: National Academy of Sciences.

Davis, Carolyne K. 1983. "The Federal Role in Changing Health Care Financing." *Nursing Economics* 1 (July/August): 223–38.

Davis, Karen. 1975. *National Health Insurance: Benefits, Costs, and Consequences.* Washington, DC: Brookings Institution.

Eisenberg, C. A. 1983. "Women as Physicians." *Journal of Medical Education* 58: 534–41.

Ellwood, Paul M., Jr. 1975. "Alternatives to Regulation: Improving the Market." In *Controls on Health Care,* Papers of the Conference on Regulation of the Health Industry, January 7–9, 1974, 49–72. Washington, DC: National Academy of Sciences.

Enthoven, Alain C. 1980. *Health Plan: The Only Practical Solution to the Soaring Cost of Medical Care.* Reading, MA: Addison-Wesley.

Falk, I. S. 1970. "National Health Insurance: A Review of Policies and Proposals." *Law and Contemporary Problems* 35: 669–96.

Fawcett, Jacqueline. 1984. *Analysis and Evaluation of Conceptual Models of Nursing.* Philadelphia: F. A. David.

Feldstein, Paul J. 1983. *Health Care Economics.* 2d ed. New York: Wiley.

Freiman, M. P., and W. D. Marder. 1984. "Changes in the Hours Worked by Physicians, 1970–1980." *American Journal of Public Health* 74: 1348–52.

Gibson, Rosemary. 1983. "Quiet Revolutions in Medicaid." In *Market Reforms in Health Care: Current Issues, New Directions, Strategic Decisions,* ed. by Jack A. Meyer, 75–102. Washington, DC: American Enterprise Institute.

Gray, Bradford H., ed. 1983. *The New Health Care for Profit: Doctors and Hospitals in a Competitive Environment.* Washington, DC: National Academy Press.

———, ed. 1986. *For-Profit Enterprise in Health Care.* Washington, DC: National Academy Press.

Hadley, Jack, Ross Mullner, and Judith Feder. 1982. "The Financially Distressed Hospital." *New England Journal of Medicine* 307: 1283–87.

Havighurst, Clark C., ed. 1974. *Regulating Health Facilities Construction.* Proceedings of a Conference on Health Planning, Certificates of Need, and Market Entry. Washington, DC: American Enterprise Institute.

———. 1977. "Health Care Cost Containment Regulation: Prospects and an Alternative." *American Journal of Law and Medicine* 3: 309–22.

Hodgson, Godfrey. 1973. "The Politics of American Health Care: What Is It Costing You?" *Atlantic Monthly* 282: 45–61.

Iglehart, J. K. 1986. "Federal Support of Health Manpower Education." *New England Journal of Medicine* 314: 324–28.

Kennedy, Edward M. 1972. *In Critical Condition: The Crisis in America's Health Care.* New York: Simon & Schuster.

Klein, Rudolf. 1981. "Reflections on the American Health Care Condition." *Journal of Health Politics, Policy and Law* 6: 188–204.

Lubove, Roy. 1968. *The Struggle for Social Security, 1900–1935.* Cambridge, MA: Harvard University Press.

Luft, Harold S. 1981. *Health Maintenance Organizations: Dimensions of Performance.* New York: Wiley.

———. 1985. "Competition and Regulation." *Medical Care* 23: 383–400.

Melosh, Barbara. 1982. *The Physician's Hand.* Philadelphia: Temple University Press.

Meyer, Jack A., ed. 1983. *Market Reforms in Health Care: Current Issues, New Directions, Strategic Decisions.* Washington, DC: American Enterprise Institute.

———, ed. 1985. *Incentives vs. Controls in Health Policy: Broadening the Debate.* Washington, DC: American Enterprise Institute.

Miller, Rosalind S., ed. 1983. *Primary Health Care: More than Medicine.* Englewood Cliffs, NJ: Prentice-Hall.

Noll, Roger G. 1975. "The Consequences of Public Utility Regulation of Hospitals." In *Controls on Health Care,* Papers of the Conference on Regulation of the Health Industry, January 7–9, 1974, 25–48. Washington, DC: National Academy of Sciences.

Numbers, Ronald L. 1982. "The Spectre of Socialized Medicine: American Physicians and Compulsory Health Insurance." In *Compulsory Health Insurance: The Continuing Debate,* ed. by Ronald L. Numbers, 3–24. Contributions in Medical History, No. 11. Westport, CT: Greenwood Press.

Pauly, Mark V., ed. 1980. *National Health Insurance: What Now, What Later, What Never?* Washington, DC: American Enterprise Institute.

Payton, Sallyanne, and Rhoda Powsner. 1980. "Regulation through the Looking Glass: Hospitals, Blue Cross, and Certificate-of-Need." *Michigan Law Review* 77: 203–77.

Petersdorf, R. G., and A. R. Feinstein. 1981. "An Informal Appraisal of the Current Status of 'Medical Sociology.'" *Journal of the American Medical Association* 245: 943–50.

Rodriguez-Trias, Helen. 1984. "The Women's Health Movement: Women Take Power." In *Reforming Medicine: Lessons of the Last Quarter Century,* ed. by Victor W. Sidel and Ruth Sidel, 107–26. New York: Pantheon.

Rosenblatt, Rand E. 1986. "Health Care, Markets, and Democratic Values." *Vanderbilt Law Review* 34: 1067–1115.

Ruzek, Sheryl Burt. 1978. *The Women's Health Movement: Feminist Alternatives to Medical Control.* New York: Praeger.

Starkweather, David B. 1981. *Hospital Mergers in the Making.* Ann Arbor, MI: Health Administration Press.

Starr, Paul. 1982. *The Social Transformation of American Medicine: The Rise of a Sovereign Profession and the Making of a Vast Industry.* New York: Basic Books.

Stevens, Rosemary. 1971. *American Medicine and the Public Interest.* New Haven: Yale University Press.

Vogel, Morris J. 1980. *The Invention of the Modern Hospital: Boston, 1870–1930.* Chicago: University of Chicago Press.

2

Competition versus Regulation in American Health Policy

Evan M. Melhado

In the history of federal health policy in the United States, the 1970s appear to mark a major turning point. The decade opened with widespread cries of "crisis" in American health care delivery and with a twofold agenda of reform: subjecting the delivery of health services to intensified planning and regulation and entitling the entire population of the country to comprehensive health benefits under a system of national health insurance (NHI). As the decade ended, that reform agenda stood in disarray. Instead, the leading themes among formulators of American health policy were competition and market strengthening, dismantling of regulatory apparatus, and acquiescence in a lesser conception of entitlement. This study, a preliminary attempt to characterize and explain this shift, briefly summarizes methods, assumptions, and main themes and then develops its points in detail.

METHODS, PRESUPPOSITIONS, AND MAIN LINES OF THE ARGUMENT

The approach taken here presents the shift as an episode in the intellectual history of policy formulation (cf. Fox 1979). The focus is less on detailed policy prescriptions than on their underlying, fundamental principles. These principles are exhibited through characterizing the ideas shared by exponents of each of the various policy positions (although the differences among advocates of any given position are necessarily understated). The characterizations are not used to assess or judge the relative merits or viability of either the fundamental ideas or the particular proposals derived from them; instead, they serve as the reference points for an analysis of policy shift. The analysis attempts to identify a novel alternative to antecedent health care policies, exhibit its motives, and explain its rise to dominance within policy circles.

In acknowledging the dominant position of competitive health policy, the study does not assume that the procompetitive agenda lacks critics or that proponents of older traditions are silent. Both critics of the new and advocates of the old are easy to find,[1] but this study rests on the perception that they are now minor players on the health policy stage. It is true that competitive theory has led to few concrete policy initiatives, especially on the federal level. However, its partisans have gained a wide hearing and have gone far to establish the plausibility and perceived utility of their opinions. They have become the leading interpreters of recent developments in the health sector, they have contributed to the perception within policy-making circles and among political decision makers that the emergence of competition in the health sector is at least acceptable if not indeed positively desirable, and they have constituted the chief source of ideas for those charged with guiding the evolution of competitive market arrangements within the health sector. In this dominant position, competitive theory has successfully eclipsed the aspiration toward universal entitlement to comprehensive benefits, and it has lacked even minimally articulated competitors as candidates for a new national health policy (cf. Marmor, Boyer, and Greenberg 1981; chap. 1 of this text).

In explaining the rise of competition, the study assumes that shifts in the status of national policy agendas do not simply reflect the political balance of power as conventionally understood.[2] A traditional political perspective on competitive policy may suggest that emphasis on the market implies a conservative pedigree; as a corollary, that competition is inhospitable to the expansion of entitlement to health services; and that proof of these assertions lies in the eclipse of national health insurance by the concern for cost containment among competitive theorists. However, a large literature on public policy in both the United States and other western countries suggests the relatively minor significance of the typical political dichotomies of left and right or progressive and conservative or of partisan affiliation to the formulation of social policy and even to its implementation.[3] By contrast, this study identifies two distinct but related clusters of competitive policies that it traces to forces outside of conventional politics, and it argues that these forces have dictated the evolution of thought about national health care policy independently of shifts in the political balance of power.

Two Clusters of Competitive Proposals

Economists put forth one cluster of competitive proposals, "consumer cost sharing."[4] Cost sharing would impose on consumers an increased share of the costs of health care by including heavy copayments and deductibles in health insurance policies, and it would meet the needs of the poor by providing income-graduated governmental subsidies for the purchase of insurance. Cost sharing would operate under prevailing fee-for-service (FFS) arrangements. It anticipates that consumers, facing a higher cost burden, would press providers to accept a fiduciary responsibility for patients' financial as well as medical interests, thereby inducing providers to enter into price competition with one another.

Cost-sharing proposals emerged from lines of economic thought elicited after the Second World War by novel public programs that involved unprecedented levels of expenditure and investment. Economists increasingly devoted themselves to devising the principles that should underlie these public expenditures. In health policy, they gradually departed from an earlier pattern of simply advocating increases in health facilities and manpower, and they began to apply instead a more dispassionate form of analysis to optimizing public provision. Though initially concentrating on investments, economists gradually turned to redistributive programs such as publicly funded insurance. In the 1970s, this kind of analysis was exploited to find more efficient means for the expansion of entitlement to health services than the means anticipated by advocates of comprehensive NHI. Income-graduated consumer cost sharing was the outcome.

Cost sharing therefore reflected not opposition to entitlement programs, but a desire to optimize the use of public resources (M. Feldstein 1963; Pauly 1971a). It was predicated upon the perception that governmental investment decisions and the regulatory apparatus they implied should be jettisoned in favor of subsidizing the purchasing power of those whose spending on health care society wants to increase. Accordingly, advocates of cost sharing envision a reform of the demand side of the market and a consequent evolution of the supply side with minimal governmental intervention. Equating the public interest with the aggregation of individual preferences, advocates of cost sharing aim to bring resource allocation into conformity with the unobstructed expression of consumer demand, to bring prices into line with this closer approximation to an optimal allocation, and to respond to equity concerns by enhancing the purchasing power of lower-income groups. Cost sharing therefore seeks to separate efficiency (resource allocation) from equity (entitlement), and it regards entitlement as the aggregate expression of the willingness of some individuals to pay for enhanced consumption by others. If proponents of cost sharing advocated a lesser standard of entitlement than advocates of comprehensive NHI, their position rested not on antipathy to entitlement but on three other convictions: that the efficacy of health care, at the margin, was uncertain; that this uncertainty removes whatever justification may have existed for depriving consumers, including those whose purchasing power is publicly subsidized, of the power to decide for themselves what health services are desirable; and that the sovereign consumer—traditionally at the focus of welfare economics—not the professional expert, should dictate the allocation of resources. Health care was viewed as only one among many individual consumption goods.

The other cluster of competitive policies, "competitive health plans," is more widely known than cost sharing. As articulated by Paul M. Ellwood, Jr., Walter McClure, Clark C. Havighurst, and Alain C. Enthoven, this cluster largely shares the focus of cost sharing on resource allocation in the market and the underlying conviction that health care is merely a consumption good, and one of doubtful marginal value; however, it also calls for reorganizing the supply side of the market for health services so that both services and insurance would be sold by large bureaucratic organizations (health plans).[5] The two principal advantages claimed for competitive health plans result from two fundamental characteristics: the plans would offer packages of health services in exchange for a prepaid capitation fee; and they would compete with one another for consumers, who would become the clients of the plans (that is, be insured by them). Capitation constitutes an incentive structure operating within the plans; competition for consumers constitutes an incentive structure operating among the plans. Capitation implies that the plans bear the costs of inefficiency in the production and delivery of health services and that they reap the rewards of efficiency. Competition for consumers further intensifies the cost consciousness of the plans, for consumers will be attracted to competing plans that offer services at lower price; it also assures that the plans will strive to tailor various combinations of price and quality to suit consumer demand. Competition among plans would also foster consumer protection, for consumers would leave providers known to cut corners. Additional safeguards to consumers could include public provision of information about plans, minimum quality regulation, and policing of the market by employers, unions, and government. The needs of the poor could be met by a system of income-graduated vouchers that could be used to buy a package of benefits from a plan. The most prominent example of the competitive health plan (and long the only one under discussion) is the health maintenance organization (HMO), which exists in several forms, but theorists of health plans increasingly envision a variety of other arrangements (see chaps. 3 and 4 of this text).

Like advocates of NHI, theorists of plans aspired to remedy the widely acknowledged problems of the health sector, but they differed profoundly in their choice of means. Both groups agreed on the need to break a pattern of intense cost escalation in the health sector and to impose order on what was widely perceived as its fragmented and incoherent structure. Supporters of NHI expected that planning and regulation could impose order on the health system and render it efficient, and they hoped that these gains could finance an expansion of entitlement. Moreover, they assumed that entitlement expressed not the willingness of some to pay for increased consumption by others but higher social values that transcended individual preferences. To realize these values, they aimed to improve and expand public provision, while significantly diminishing the scope for private markets. By contrast, theorists of plans saw in planning and regulation mechanisms that had served the interests of the providers of health services. Having argued that all the well-known shortcomings of the health system flowed from provider dominance and that regulation of any industry inevitably serves the regulated interests, they feared that NHI would complete the imposition of provider control over health care, grant it the durability typically conferred by regulatory laws, and thus worsen all the problems that it had been advanced to remedy. They therefore rejected governmental controls and aimed instead to reorganize the supply side of the market. By capturing the benefits of modern market organization and subjecting providers to incentives that would make them responsive to consumers, the health sector could be harnessed to the public interest (understood in the same terms as used by advocates of cost sharing), not the private interests of providers. Though entitlement was not the chief concern of the theorists of plans, they argued that a socially optimal level of entitlement (again, defined along lines like those used by advocates of cost sharing) could be achieved by a system of income-graduated subsidy for the purchase of insurance from competitive plans. Improving the performance of the private health sector was their aim; public provision could continue to be accommodated into a largely private system of health care.

If cost-sharing proposals issued from the needs of the welfare state to make optimal use of resources, the theory of competitive plans emerged from a second characteristic mechanism of policy change: the perception of failure in the operation of past policy (Heclo 1974; cf. Fox 1985, 353–55 and n. 13; and Ehrenreich and Ehrenreich 1970, 233–34). The perception of policy failure that grew during the 1960s among observers of the new, postwar governmental programs elicited two kinds of proposal for change: either adjustment of existing policy mechanisms or radical break with past practices. In the case of health care, traditional efforts to plan health facilities and manpower needs had persistently failed to bring the coherence and achieve the cost control desired by its advocates. The elusiveness of these goals led advocates of regulation to seek increases in the authority of planners (that is, to give them "teeth" or regulatory powers) and adjustments in their methods. From the mid 1960s, planning therefore gave way to controls over capital investment in the hospital industry (and therefore over market entry) by certification of need, a mechanism borrowed from public utility regulation. Advocates of competitive plans, by contrast, believing that past policy was wholly discredited, joined advocates of cost sharing in calling for an end to regulatory methods, but they also went further and demanded the dismantling of previously instituted regulatory mechanisms. Reform of the demand side of the market could succeed only if the supply side was reconstructed.

Policy Failure and Policy Shift

In calling for a sharp break with past practices, competitive theorists instanced a conviction, increasingly disseminated among policy makers and social scientists, that government had failed in fulfilling its obligations and in meeting the expectations that it had created among citizens that governmental intervention would bring enhanced welfare and social progress. Social scientists, who had previously been employed to identify the legitimate occasions for governmental intervention and to design programs to meet perceived needs, turned instead to diagnosing policy failure. Issuing from several sources, these diagnoses conspired to suggest that policy failure resulted either from choice of inappropriate means of intervention or from the fundamentally political character of governmental administrative and regulatory institutions. These conclusions created a climate for policy change by fostering the perception that the customary forms of governmental intervention seemed not merely inadequate for achieving public goals, but positively detrimental to the public interest; and, in several instances, they provided intellectual tools for the antiregulatory campaign conducted by competitive theorists.

For example, Charles Schultze (1977, 2–4) and Theodore Lowi (1969, 68–72) both argue that governmental programs had failed to satisfy expectations raised by postwar affluence, and they both find the favored instruments of governmental programs and regulatory and administrative agencies to be ill suited to realizing the public interest (cf. L. Brown 1983, 3–11; Klein 1981, especially p. 191; and Wolf 1979). Ignoring the political economy of regulation, Schultze simply asserted that regulation was ill suited to the complex tasks faced by government. Accordingly, he suggested incentives as a way to bring private decision making into conformity with public goals.

Unlike Schultze, Lowi found in the political economy of regulation and administration the causes of political failure. Regulation was not ill suited to the tasks entrusted to it; rather, Lowi held, government had abdicated responsibility to articulate the goals of public policy, substituted bargaining among private interests for the pursuit of clear goals, and consequently permitted the private beneficiaries of bargaining to thwart the public interest. The change in the role of government reflected the rise of pluralism within social science and the rise of its broader public counterpart, interest-group liberalism. Supposing that society consists of a diversity of interests competing within the context of a broad consensus, the interest-group liberal supposes that social justice will flow from bargaining among the interests and believes that government should do no more than sponsor and facilitate bargaining. The recasting of government in this mold, according to Lowi, resulted in the exploitation of governmental regulatory and administrative agencies by narrow, private interests. His remedy was to reestablish the responsibility of government to articulate public goals and to express these goals clearly in the legislated mandates of governmental institutions.

Also emphasizing the dominance of the interests in regulatory settings (but denying Lowi's claim that older forms of regulation differed from the newer) was a literature from economics, particularly as developed by the Chicago School. The school adopted the concern of the political scientists for interest groups and portrayed regulation as a form of competitive bidding among the interests for the redistributive favors of government. The outcome enhanced the well-being of small groups with concentrated interests at the expense of a broader but more diffuse public interest, and it reflected not the usual political divisions of left and right but the effectiveness of interest groups in buying power and the effectiveness of the regulators in broadening support and minimizing opposition.

In the 1970s, the spread of such analyses led students of policy to reject earlier forms of collective intervention and demand less invasive and, it was hoped, more efficacious means of advancing public ends. In health policy, competitive theorists clamored to extricate government from its extensive involvement in health care. Advocates of cost sharing, though not given to analyzing regulatory institutions, nevertheless urged that government withdraw immediately and confine itself to subsidizing the purchasing power of the poor; advocates of plans, mindful of the political economy of regulation, demanded that government first sponsor a reconstruction of the health sector and thereafter assume responsibility both for the purchasing power of the poor and for establishing the appropriate incentives and guaranteeing the conditions necessary for competition.

Once articulated, these or any other novelties in public policy could achieve a dominant position only after their main lines had been sufficiently reiterated to become familiar and plausible to the old school, their principles had matured sufficiently to support the full weight of the social problems to which they were addressed (cf. Polsby 1984, 126–28, 153–54), and the problems themselves continued to resist traditional solutions. In this case, the central themes of competitive policy had been articulated early in the 1970s, and efforts to press competitive theory on the Nixon administration and Congress led to passage of the Health Maintenance Act of 1973. However, even as amended subsequently in the 1970s, that act did not serve as the foundation for a new national health policy. Advocates of competition realized that the act was narrowly circumscribed, and most observers recognized that opposing interests would diminish its efficacy. Little more than another imperfect demonstration project, the act was preceded the year before by major regulator legislation (the Social Security Amendments that instituted, among other things, medical oversight of utilization under professional standards review organizations) and was dramatically overshadowed the very next year by another major regulatory bill, the National Health Planning and Resources Development Act (PL 93-641). Only from the late 1970s, especially following 1979, when amendments to the 1974 law mandated regulators to foster competition, did competitive theorists express a full awareness of the responsibility to work out their position in detail and to confront it with the impediments to implementation (Havighurst 1982; cf. Ginsburg 1981, 40; Ginzberg 1983, 1859; and Klein 1981, 198–99). As old problems persisted and worsened, advocates of competition increasingly gained a hearing. As they did, market forces began to bring the health sector into conformity with their policy prescriptions. Though they cannot take credit for this development, their efforts helped make the realities of competition palatable and their language provided policy makers and decision makers with the tools for analyzing current changes in health care and devising responses to them.

THE COMPLEXITY OF REFORM AND THE
MATURATION OF COMPETITIVE THEORY

The mid 1960s brought to advocates of NHI their first significant victory in their otherwise frustrated half-century of activism—Medicare.[6] As Robert and Rosemary Stevens (1974, chaps. 2, 3) argue, Medicare was a result of the aging of the population and the rejection by the middle-class elderly of the Kerr-Mills program of 1960. As a supplement to antecedent forms of public assistance, Kerr-Mills provided means-tested medical benefits tainted by the poor-law stigma. Like the original Social Security law of 1935, Medicare doubtless also reflected the fear of the working generation that shouldering the growing dependency (in this case medically induced) of the older generation would drain the resources it hoped to devote to the younger (Patterson 1981, 75; Lubove 1968, 133–35; Marmor 1970, 18; Anderson 1985, 165 and n. 24). Consistent with the entire tradition of public provision in this country (Patterson 1981; cf. Marmor 1970, 123–25), social insurance (Medicare) responded to middle-class demands, while the poor were left with the welfare tradition, in this case Medicaid, established by Congress in 1965 along with Medicare.

The Origins of the Health Care "Crisis"

Despite their underlying philosophical and political differences, both Medicare and Medicaid bore the character of open-ended reimbursement schemes that invited cost escalation. To appease organized medicine these programs explicitly disclaimed federal control over the practice of medicine or the organization of medical care. Procedures for reimbursing hospitals were generous and remote from scrutiny. The providers of health services (that is, physicians and hospitals), constrained only by traditional professional ethics, enjoyed a virtually unlimited draft on public resources.[7] Though cost escalation in the health sector antedated 1965 considerably and had indeed lain behind much of the pressure that led to Kerr-Mills and to Medicare and Medicaid, the explosive cost increases in the health sector and the socialization of high costs entailed by these two public programs had two major effects: they broke the back of governmental deference to provider interests, fostering inquiry into the extension of governmental controls into the health care sector; and they highlighted other deficiencies in the health sector, including inefficiencies in the market for private insurance as well as broader problems with equity and access (Stevens and Stevens 1970 and 1974; Sundquist 1968, 287–321; Hodgson 1973; Roemer 1970, especially p. 301; Falk 1970; Mechanic 1970; Anderson 1985, 194–96). Maldistribution of manpower and institutions, gaps in insurance coverage, fragmentation of insurance mechanisms and provider organizations, overspecialization, inability of the middle class (as well as the poor) to obtain appropriate and timely care are a few of the many failings laid at the feet of what increasingly came to be called the "nonsystem."[8]

That the middle class as well as the poor suffered from these failures likely explains why Medicare and Medicaid did not meet but intensified demand for expanded application of social insurance principles to the health sector. In addition, increasingly broadened notions of the rights of citizenship legitimized the claim that society had failed by denying a right to health care to all its members.[9] NHI would not only rectify the deficiencies of the health care system but also meet growing demands for distributive justice.

Alternative Remedies

Thus, by the late 1970s, expanding criticism of the health sector simultaneously exposed the need for profound reforms and seemed to create a political climate that would make reform possible. Proponents of NHI supposed that, at a single stroke, a suitably designed program would solve major issues of cost, access, and equity.[10]

However, the need for reforms seemed far clearer to advocates of NHI than did the principles that should underlie the reforms. The very magnitude and diversity of the criticism that had been heaped upon the health system deprived NHI advocates of coherence and focus in their efforts to design policy measures. I. S. Falk, long a leading figure in the traditions of compulsory health insurance and an architect of the Kennedy-Griffiths Health Security plan for NHI, provides a good example (1970, 674–75) of this unfocused approach:

> Broad consideration of the major causes of crisis in medical care begins with the fiscal difficulties, the relatively high costs and comparatively steep annual escalations, but the list of causes goes on to include areas which present even more complex and more perplexing questions than does the issue of finances. A hundred problems could be enumerated, but upon inspection they can be subsumed in the following four categories . . . :

> (1)   national shortages in various categories, both old and new, of health manpower and facilities;

> (2)   steeply rising costs and their financing;

> (3)   inadequacies in the system for assuring availability and delivery of needed services; and

> (4)   lack of sufficient and effective controls for the assurance of quality of care.

> These causes of crisis are not discrete. On the contrary, they are interlocked one with another, and, indeed, the difficulties of dealing with the interrelations among them might be fairly regarded as a fifth major cause.

In a similar vein, David Mechanic (1970, 251) observed:

> As we look toward the future of health organization in America, there is much that lacks focus. Many of the issues at stake are intricately linked, and their piecemeal discussion is by its very nature deficient. Without some clear concept of the overall system and its priorities, it is difficult to specify the necessary manpower needs, the way in which different forms of manpower will interrelate, the kinds of physical facilities necessary, the types of new paraprofessionals that can fill gaps, and many other items of importance.

Proponents of NHI shared a belief in the "intricacy" of the problems faced by policy makers and in the need to gather the appropriate data that would permit planners and regulators to specify and provide the requisite human and material resources. Though they remained persuaded that the task could be accomplished, they hesitated in the face of its magnitude and complexity.

By contrast, unencumbered by the weight of past policy, competitive theory—particularly the theory of competitive plans—was marked by boldness and confidence. For example, Ellwood and his collaborators at what is now InterStudy in Minneapolis asserted in their classic summary of the "health maintenance strategy" that "[t]he health system is performing poorly because its structure and incentives do not encourage self-regulation" and that "[m]arket mechanisms, such as competition and informed consumer demand, which might provide a check on the provision of unnecessary services, inflation, and inequitable distribution, do not exist in the health industry" (Ellwood et al. 1971a, 292). Their conclusion (ibid., 298) was as simple as it was bold:

> The emergence of a free-market economy could stimulate a course of change in the health industry that would have some of the classical aspects of the industrial revolution—conversion to larger units of production, techno-logical innovation, division of labor, substitution of capital for labor, vigorous competition, and profitability as the mandatory condition of survival. Under these conditions, HMOs would have a vested interest in regulating output, performance, and costs in the public interest, with minimal intervention by the federal government.

No hesitation before the complexities of the system marks this statement. Instead, competition was touted as the blade to cut the Gordian knot that gave pause to advocates of NHI.[11]

Advocates of competition thus early enjoyed two great advantages over partisans of NHI: By linking all issues to the structure and perfor-mance of an anticipated competitive market, their theory exhibited con-ceptual coherence and economy. By invoking the discipline of the competitive market that would force providers to identify demand and meet it efficiently, competitive theory obviated the need to gather data, determine the desirable distribution of resources, and devise methods to realize the goals of planners. Instead, governmental intervention and the professional expertise on which it supposedly relied could simply be left out of the picture.[12]

The Recent Shift to Competitive Theory

Despite these claimed advantages, competitive theory began its rise to dominance only at the end of the 1970s. An index of how recent has been the shift in health policy is provided by the introduction to a collection of essays on NHI published in 1980 by the American Enterprise Institute (AEI), a policy research organization that has been prominent in the analy-sis of health care delivery. Entitled *National Health Insurance: What Now, What Later, What Never?* (Pauly 1980a), the volume exhibits the eclipse of an NHI agenda aimed at comprehensive benefits and constrained by federal regulation. In his foreword to the volume, William J. Baroody, Jr., then president of the AEI, remarked (Baroody 1980) that his organization nearly a decade earlier had published an analysis of various proposals for NHI, and he noted that they seemed to revolve around the twin and conflicting problems of gaps in access and increases in cost. By contrast, the newer volume

> illustrates that the character of the debate has changed since 1971. As a result of a decade of policy-related research, there now appears to be a greater will-ingness to question the basic concept of NHI as a grand solution to all the per-ceived problems in health. . . .

> With the growth of skepticism about the ability of national health insurance to solve the real problems, . . . health policy research has turned to the design of policies that might reduce the growth in public and private expenditures without reducing the high quality of care and the freedom of individual choice that we value in our present system.

Two subsequent volumes of the AEI, *A New Approach to the Economics of Health Care* (Olson 1981) and *Market Reforms in Health Care* (Meyer 1983), suggest the full dimensions of the shift. In the former, Baroody observed (1981, xvi–xvii) that

> [h]ealth policy analysts are beginning to think of the health care sector more as an economic system. The focus of the health policy debate is on changing the incentives in medical care delivery and financing to encourage a more efficient allocation of resources, reflecting cost-conscious consumer and provider choices. It is becoming evident that fundamental structural changes in medical care delivery and financing can lower the cost of health care for both public beneficiaries and private insurance enrollees.

Public programs were not to be dismantled or forgotten. Rather, structural reform of the health sector in the interest of efficiency had become a central objective of public policy. As for the more recent tome, he claimed that it carried the "transition [in health policy] a step further by obtaining practical and detailed information on the consequences of implementing competitive policies and on the pitfalls lying between proposed changes in legislation and a world in which true competition is actualized (Baroody 1983, xi–xiii; cf. also Havighurst 1982, 5; 1981, 1118–20). While other voices have not been so sanguine,[13] the growing perception among competitive theorists of the need for detailed analysis of their policy prescriptions characterizes current competitive literature.[14]

Boldness and clarity of vision were therefore insufficient to propel competition to its dominant position. Also undergirding its rise were a decade of research and discussion; a persistent criticism of the aspiration toward entitlement to universal, comprehensive benefits under NHI and of the regulatory principles it invoked; and a willingness to address the complex legal, ethical, economic, and social issues posed by a major shift to competition. As noticed below, competitive theory found an increasingly receptive audience as long-standing problems persisted despite major efforts to control them and as the perception grew that regulation sufficiently strong to solve them was politically unacceptable. As more nearly competitive arrangements developed in the 1980s, competitive theory made them comprehensible and palatable and provided the language and concepts for understanding them.

THE HEALTH PLANNING AGENDA

The regulatory approach invoked by advocates of NHI and criticized by competitive theorists was the outcome of a health planning tradition or, more accurately, one of two streams of thought about health planning. The older stream, issuing from Progressive-era reformers, advocated planning in conjunction with public provision of health services or health insurance; the other linked planning with voluntary provision. Though the two streams possessed much in common, they differed fundamentally in their assumptions about the relations between public and private interests. Advocates of public provision anticipated that public planning agencies would articulate the public interest, and they expected that providers could be compelled to pursue the public interest only through public control over health services. By contrast, advocates of voluntary control supposed that goals of public service could be achieved jointly with pursuit of the private interest, particularly that of the nonprofit voluntary hospitals.

The Origins of Health Planning

The older, public model of planning emerged in the United States from the famous Committee on the Costs of Medical Care (CCMC). During its five years of activity (1927–32), the CCMC produced pioneering and broadly influential socioeconomic studies of the American health care system.[15] The committee began work when the nation's small hospital bed capacity was growing rapidly in response to the infusion of funds that came largely from private philanthropy.[16] Its aim was to rationalize this expansion by identifying unmet needs for health care, advocating a regionalized system of health care delivery as most suited to meeting needs efficiently, and placing the regionalized system on a foundation provided by planning.[17] Interest in regionalization was prompted by the British Dawson Report of 1920 (Ministry of Health 1920), which recommended a regional organization aimed at integrating preventive and curative medicine. The CCMC built on this scheme by recommending a coordinated, decentralized system facilitating a two-way flow of patient care through the regional hierarchy. Corresponding to the regionalized hierarchy of delivery institutions was to be a hierarchy of planning institutions, based in the local communities and culminating in state agencies. The agencies were to take responsibility for both planning and coordination.

Like its British predecessor, the CCMC model of regionalized health care reflected its authors' predilection for social insurance. The model leaned in the direction of public insurance programs, tended to link public provision with public (as opposed to voluntary) control, and demanded broad community representation in planning and policy making. This direct-service or direct-patient-care model, as Pearson (1976, 44–48) calls it, was overshadowed in America by a voluntary or planning-and-coordination model that providers advocated. Though incorporating many features of the direct-patient-care model, the voluntary model, as the label suggests, reflected the interests of what Payton and Powsner (1980) characterize as the elite leadership of the voluntary hospital industry and the closely allied public health establishment. Leadership in the health planning tradition issued from this group.[18]

Though both models of planning aspired toward efficiency, neither was fundamentally dedicated to cost control. Each reflected the supposition that an objective criterion of need could be established as the chief determinant of utilization of health services. This emphasis on planning for unmet need was itself largely a legacy of the Progressive-era movement for social insurance. In its battle against continued reliance on voluntary institutions, that movement had claimed that the dimensions of need exceeded the capacity of voluntary resources, and it had routinely supported this claim with elaborate studies predicated on the methods of the then newly flourishing social sciences. The same viewpoint underlay the work of the CCMC, which published as its Report No. 22 *The Fundamentals of Good Medical Care* (Lee and Jones 1932; Rosen 1976; Fox 1979; Lubove 1968; Klarman 1977, 27, 29). As the voluntary hospital industry took over leadership in pressing the case for health insurance, its focus changed from public provision in the service of the working class to private provision in the service of the middle class. Nevertheless, the voluntary hospital industry appropriated the notion of planning for unmet need, and its work both reflected and fostered the expansionism that marked American health care from the end of the First World War to the "crisis" following the establishment of Medicare and Medicaid (cf. Starr 1982b, 128–30).

Blue Cross and the Voluntary Hospital Industry

Planning and CON are thus chapters in the history of voluntary health insurance for the middle class, that is, of Blue Cross. From its inception in the 1930s, Blue Cross has been marked by tension between its role as the major financing system for the hospital industry and its capacity as a fiduciary for its subscribers or for their agents (unions, employers, governments). This tension finds its counterpart in the literature of the health services. Odin W. Anderson (1975; 1985, chap. 10), a long-standing student of health insurance and health services, emphasizes the sincerity of dedication to public service evident in the founding generation of Blue Cross and the enduring effort of its promoters to reduce the dissonance between these conflicting roles; and he stresses the magnitude of the voluntary, non-profit sector in American health care and the consistency of its growth with the social and economic characteristics of the country (cf. Somers and Somers 1961, 294–97, 413–21). Others argue that the public service mantle of Blue Cross and of the voluntary hospital industry is a screen obscuring the straightforward pursuit of private interest and the subordination of public to private goals.[19] In this view, the nonprofit status conferred by society in exchange for the provision of highly valued public services amounts to unjustified advantages exploitable in a competitive market (Havighurst 1970c, 752, 757–59; 1981, 1133–34; 1982, 363–75; Russell 1980, 278); and reliance on voluntary institutions that pursue their own interests has deprived the nation of accountability in the execution of public policy. Blue Cross, for example, has served not merely as a fiscal intermediary in Medicare and Medicaid, but also as the policy-making body in the administration of these programs, and it has largely avoided close scrutiny of its operations and deflected such demands for reform as have arisen.[20]

As noticed below, these hostile perceptions of Blue Cross and of the hospital industry figured in the emergence of competitive theory. Regarded as the outcome of hospital interests, planning and regulation seemed to competitive theorists no more than a later stage in a process that granted private interests excessive power and influence over a major sphere of public concern. To pursue regulatory policy was to perpetuate the problems in American health care.

From the critical perspective, the tension between the two roles reached an early denouement in the formulation of reimbursement policy. Blue Cross could either press hospitals to hold down rates, thus serving subscribers, or take sufficient revenues from subscribers to pay for any service at any price, thus serving the hospitals. By choosing the policy of retrospective, full-cost and (eventually cost-plus) reimbursement, Blue Cross permitted hospitals to improve the quality and expense of services in line with developing standards of practice. The result was rising costs and the inability of Blue Cross to exercise control over hospitals.

Planning and Regionalization

Hospital interests began to press for planning and regionalization in the boom years of the 1950s. Among the many factors that fostered a sense of the need for planning, two were paramount. Cost escalation led to repeated premium increases followed by public outcry from the middle-class clientele of Blue Cross and threats by state insurance commissioners to institute cost controls over the hospital industry. At the same time, suburbanization, a prominent postwar phenomenon, was bleeding middle-class patients away from the large urban hospitals, threatening their pre-eminence and their functioning as centers of medical education and research. Should competition materialize from smaller institutions just when cost controls threatened to limit resource flows into the hospital industry, the leading role of the largest institutions would be seriously threatened. Moreover, unrestrained cost escalation that lacked justification could lead not merely to governmental cost controls but to public control of insurance. Regionalization and health planning seem to have been proffered by the hospital industry to ward off these eventualities (Payton and Powsner 1980, 238, 241 n. 63, 243; cf. Ehrenreich and Ehrenreich 1970, 193, 201, 221).

The planning agenda was also consistent with the interests of physicians. The unmet "need" that planners aimed to meet was defined in part on the basis of informed medical judgment and in part by analyzing manifest demand (e.g., pressure on bed supply), itself a function of physicians' practices (though long thought by health planners and economists of health to be a function of the incidence of illness). The supposition that medical matters could be analyzed only by specialists enhanced the power of physicians over planning; indeed, physicians were the leading professionals in the field of hospital planning. Moreover, the rise of third-party payment insulated the physician from constraints imposed by patients' ability to pay and freed practitioners to follow the dictates of the "technological imperative," as Fuchs (1968, 1974) calls it, the desire to practice the most technically advanced medicine without regard to costs.[22]

In pressing for planning, the hospital industry did not credit the public conviction that cost escalation was the central problem. It argued that high-quality medical services were expensive and that cost escalation only reflected the success of the hospital industry in providing them.[23] The hospital industry found not its finances at stake so much as its legitimacy. Planning would enable the industry to persuade the public to accept this expensive system, because it provided a needed service. To eliminate small hospitals was to foster efficient management, and to plan was to demonstrate the willingness of hospitals to subordinate their own interests to those of the community. Planning would bring the public to focus not on costs but on the structure of the system as a whole. Planning agencies, resting on broad community representation, would thus legitimate the traditional focus on high-quality services, give their high costs community sanction, and protect the industry from competition (Payton and Powsner 1980, 244–47).

Planning would therefore have to limit the growth of small and middling institutions and confine the expansion of the industry within limits justifiable by notions of need. To accomplish these effects, proponents of planning refashioned the concept of regionalization. Originally, it was designed to extend services to underserved, particularly rural areas and link them via small towns to the urban centers, as in the Hill-Burton program.[24] However, suburbanization presented the opposite problem of rapid and uncoordinated growth that hospital interests wanted to curb. The solution was "areawide planning" aimed at rationalizing hospital growth in metropolitan areas. All the hospitals in such an area were to be large, only one would be a tertiary care institution, and the others would be community general hospitals. Areawide planning would substitute control of beds for control of costs. The concentration of the industry that would follow, the demand for highest-quality services in all institutions, the use of cross-subsidization to pay with the income from lucrative services for additional high-quality services that were not self-supporting, and the elimination of cream-skimming competitors—all inevitably conspired to drive up costs. As Payton and Powsner (1980, 243) put it, "[a]ny 'cost savings' attributable to regional planning would be due to the avoidance of 'unnecessary' costs within an increasingly costly system (cf. Havighurst 1973, 1184–85).

The hospital industry was successful in exploiting planning to achieve public legitimacy largely because planning was consistent with two broader cultural themes: the high valuation and prestige enjoyed through the 1960s by technologically advanced medical care; and the political climate of the country in the 1960s and early 1970s, which sanctioned the focus of federal social policy on the local level and fostered "maximum feasible participation" in decision making by the full spectrum of local interests (Lowi 1969, 79–85; Havighurst 1973, 1180, 1196–99; Bice and Kerwin 1976; Gottlieb 1974, 16, 20; Grosse 1974, 28; L. Brown 1982, 4, 21–36; Weiner 1978, 18–20, 27). Since there was as yet no need to legitimate the value of high-quality care, the hospital industry could readily argue its case that communities would have to pay for the sorts of service they demanded. At the same time, the rise of interest-group liberalism and its legitimation of a spectrum of interests, the support of local (as opposed to state) interests by federal policy makers, and the belief that bargaining among local interests would bring social justice in the allocation of resources meshed nicely with the aspirations embodied in the planning tradition. A regionalized system, reflecting local and regional interests and guided by a hierarchy of planning institutions resting on community representation, was a mold virtually tailored to the political themes of the 1960s. The Comprehensive Health Planning program of 1966 was perhaps the fullest reflection of this conjunction of forces before the rise of certification-of-need laws; the last expression of that conjunction, the National Health Planning and Resources Development Act of 1974, invoked CON to enforce the outcomes in the health sector of interest-group bargaining on the local level.[25]

Certification of Need

Certificate-of-need (CON) laws attempt to control capital investments and market entry into the hospital industry by requiring "a prior administrative determination that a public need for additional facilities or services exists (Havighurst 1973, 1143–44). Calls for adoption of supply regulation in the hospital industry began in the late 1950s and continued into the 1970s. An early example is Ray E. Brown, who in 1959 began popularizing the notion that hospitals should be franchised by a state agency to provide planners with leverage to enforce control over the supply of beds. A decade later Anne Somers (1969a; 1969b; and cf. 1971) pursued the need for regulation in a landmark study of the subject, and shortly thereafter an expert in public utility regulation (Priest 1970) enunciated the foundations for its application to hospitals.[26]

The emergence of CON is the sequel to the rise of planning.[27] Like planning, CON was fostered by the leadership of the voluntary hospital industry. It, too, was not aimed at containing costs, though cost containment was indeed offered as its principal justification. Payton and Powsner (1980) suggest that CON was the extension of planning in states where the industry could not succeed in limiting construction of new facilities (particularly of small and often proprietary suburban hospitals) without the aid of government. Governmental licensing (or franchising) of hospital construction would put teeth, as the saying went, into voluntary regional planning. According to this interpretation, cost escalation did pose a threat to the legitimacy of the voluntary hospital industry, and the industry responded by putting forth CON as a remedy. The acceptance of this proposal by legislators reduced the criticism directed at the hospital industry for its rising costs and granted the industry cartellike controls over the supply side. In essence, the hospital industry advanced its own interests (by obtaining control over the supply of beds) by misrepresenting CON as a cost-control measure.[28]

The first CON law appeared in New York in 1964 (Payton and Powsner 1980, 250–61; Somers 1969a, 143–48, 166–70). It rested on recommendations of a study commissioned by the state superintendent of insurance and the state commissioner of health following confusing testimony in hearings about rate increases for Blue Cross in 1958. Known as the Trussell Report (Columbia University School of Public Health and Administrative Medicine 1961), the study explicitly "did not accept cost containment as a legitimate foundation of public policy towards hospitals, did not focus on measures to reduce costs, and did not suggest that controls on hospital construction, which it recommended, were to be considered a method of cost control" (Payton and Powsner 1980, 249). Instead, the report held (ibid., 250) that reimbursement provided by Blue

Cross was insufficient to permit hospitals "to supply optimum services to the public." The report therefore recommended vesting control over supply in industry-dominated regional planning councils.

Nevertheless, the partisans of CON presented it as a mechanism of cost control. In justifying this claim, they cited the recent discovery, by Milton Roemer of the Cornell School of Hospital Administration, of what became known as "Roemer's Law." Simply stated, the law holds that hospital utilization will increase to fill the supply of beds (Shain and Roemer 1959; Roemer 1961; cf. Klarman 1977, 31). That supply creates its own demand was invoked as a lever for cost control: limiting supply would limit utilization. Though Roemer denied this interpretation in testimony before the New York Joint Legislative Committee on Health Insurance Plans, arguing that higher quality of services, not excessive utilization, was responsible for cost escalation, proponents of CON persisted in their interpretation (Payton and Powsner 1980, 255, 268–77; cf. also Klarman 1977, 31–32; and Havighurst 1982, 278–81). Legislators, faced with rising demand for a solution to cost escalation in the hospital sector, accepted this interpretation and enacted CON into law.

The New York law, known as the Metcalf-McClosky Act of 1964, was the model for state CON statutes. In the growing atmosphere of crisis that followed the establishment of Medicare and Medicaid, these laws spread, having been passed in some 23 states by 1973 (Payton and Powsner 1980, 260–64; Havighurst 1973, 1141–48; Curran 1974). Meanwhile, the federal government had developed an intense interest in limiting costs. Since experts widely regarded areawide planning and CON as ways to limit costs and to bring order and efficiency to an inchoate system, the federal government began promoting passage of state planning and CON laws.[29]

On the federal level, CON first appeared in 1967, as the government started encouraging the states to use planning agencies in regulating hospital construction. Legislation submitted in 1967 but passed only in 1972 as part of the Social Security Amendments of that year (which, inter alia, inaugurated PSROs) allowed (but did not compel) the states to enter into agreement with the federal government to withhold reimbursement under Medicare and Medicaid for capital expenses for a facility lacking approval by a state or regional planning agency (section 1122 review) (Gottlieb 1974, 23–24; Somers and Somers 1977, 240; Havighurst 1982, 53; Law 1974, 70 and n. 429). The federal push for planning and CON culminated in the National Health Planning and Resources Development Act of 1974 (PL 93-641).

Some advocates of planning in the late 1960s and early 1970s held that planning should serve only advisory functions, but most began demanding that planning agencies be given powers to realize planning through regulation.[30] The 1974 law was the last major expression of the latter view. It was intended to strengthen planning, deploy CON nationally as part of the gradual drift toward regulation of the health sector, clarify the purposes of both planning and CON, diminish proliferation of federal programs, and remedy defects in earlier planning efforts. If planning had failed in the past, more and better planning, enforced through regulation, would succeed.

Planning and NHI

The legitimacy secured by provider interests in the 1960s and early 1970s and the apparent conformity of their goals with those of NHI advocates fostered the confluence of the planning and NHI agendas. Because health planning emphasized the goal of efficiency and obscured its effects on costs, it could appear to advocates of NHI as the perfect instrument for rationalizing a malfunctioning system. "Simply stated, the goal of regionalized medical care has been seen by its proponents as the improvement of the availability, quality, and efficiency of personal health services (Pearson 1976, 5). Health planning aimed at assuring services adequate to need, and it held that "[c]oordination of activities is likely to help reduce costs (by preventing unnecessary duplication of facilities and services) and to improve efficiency (by providing for movement of patients through the system and by sharing administrative and professional skills) (May 1967, 18). These goals were formulated in response to one of the two major problems, fragmentation of the health sector, that had exercised proponents of NHI. Similarly, the fundamental document that underlay the health planning legislation of the 1960s, the final report of the Joint Committee of the American Hospital Association and the U.S. Public Health Service (1961), recommended areawide planning as a remedy for the same kinds of problem identified by advocates of NHI (deficiencies in access, lack of systematic organization, and inefficiency in provision); and, like them, it also demanded preservation of the prevailing level of quality and rejected a two-class system of care (cf. May 1974, 47).

Accordingly, the National Health Planning and Resources Development Act of 1974 reflected not only the interest of the hospital industry, but the confluence of the long-standing pressure for planning with the more recent push for comprehensive national health insurance. The apparent imminence of NHI legislation intensified concern for rationalizing the system so that new resources would be efficiently exploited.[31] From the late 1960s, the focus of health planning shifted, therefore, from expansion under voluntary insurance for the middle class back to public programs—the preoccupation of many members of the CCMC and their Progressive-era predecessors. Planning would govern the expansion of entitlements beyond the poor and elderly to encompass the entire population. Universal entitlement to high-quality benefits would now be realized through mechanisms that had successfully provided them to the middle class in the great expansionary phase of American health care delivery.

THE PUBLIC SECTOR: LEGITIMATION AND DISILLUSIONMENT

Competitive theory may be traced to two sources of policy change: the need to rationalize expenditures devoted to large-scale governmental programs in the postwar era (cost sharing) and perceived failures of antecedent policy (competitive plans). In both instances, the application of the social sciences, especially economics, to the study of governmental programs played a prominent role. Cost sharing may be traced to the tradition of public expenditures analysis that emerged in response to the postwar legitimation of the public sector and aimed to optimize governmental spending on programs of novel character and dimensions. Competitive plans may be referred to a policy environment characterized by perceptions of governmental failure and informed by the diagnoses of failure provided by social scientists. This section portrays the rise of public expenditure analysis as a consequence of the enhanced legitimacy of the public sector after World War II, and it describes some leading themes in the literature of governmental failure that flourished in the 1970s.

Economics and the Enhanced Legitimacy of the Public Sector

The principal motive for the increased application of economics to public policy after World War II was the expanding role of government as a purveyor of large public programs entailing major expenditures (Prest and Turvey 1965, 684; Lyons 1969, 233–44; Haveman 1969, 2–4; Greenhouse 1966, 272; Chase 1968b, 1–2; Schultze 1977, 7). Whereas earlier expenditure programs had been extensions of the New Deal (Social Security, workers' rights and benefits, Keynesian intervention by government to affect the rate of growth), postwar programs were aimed at allocating national resources, providing social services, and redistributing income. William J. Baumol's *Welfare Economics and the Theory of the State* (1952), though resting on several precedents, is nevertheless commonly taken as the fountainhead of a literature dedicated to applying theoretical welfare economics to the analysis of governmental spending programs. The legitimation of governmental action as a remedy for market failure and the identification of criteria for optimal allocation of public funds among competing uses became major themes for economic analysis.[32] This tradition increasingly challenged "the classical presumption that economic efficiency would be attained with voluntary decision making occurring in free markets by independent buyers and sellers and a public sector with minor economic functions (Haveman 1969, 3). Governmental intervention no longer "represented only a minor aberration from universal private decision making" (ibid.; cf. Steiner 1969, 24). This theoretical tradition possessed an empirical counterpart, antedating the postwar changes, that attempted to analyze the benefits of federal investments in water resource projects. In the postwar world, this tradition provided precedents for empirical work on all aspects of public expenditures on the federal level (Prest and Turvey 1965; Haveman 1969, 3–4; Schick 1966, 255; Wildavsky 1966, 293 n. 1; Krutilla 1969, 277–80).

These developments rested on a new view of the legitimacy and worth of governmental programs. "As long as government was considered a 'necessary evil'," Schick (1966, 249) observes, "and there was little recognition of the social value of public expenditures, the main function of budgeting was to keep spending in check. . . . However, as the work and accomplishments of public agencies came to be regarded as benefits, the task of budgeting was redefined as the effective marshalling of fiscal and organizational resources for the attainment of benefits" (cf. Greenhouse 1966, 272).

The new emphasis on governmental expenditures bore links to the Keynesian economics prominent since the New Deal. The concern of Keynesian theory for the relationship between public expenditures and the state of the economy inaugurated an evolution in the perceived functions of budgeting. In the 1960s a new sort of budgetary thinking issued from the developing analysis of governmental expenditures. The managerial approach to budgeting, emphasizing the management of large programs and the extension of administrative control over them, had succeeded the pre-Keynesian emphasis on constraining spending on inputs; and the Program-Planning-Budgeting (PBB) system, emphasizing not management but program planning in the interest of rationalizing policy, in turn succeeded the management orientation.[33] The PBB system issued from military policy, which, together with the traditional field of tax policy, lay at the focus of early postwar economic analysis of public policy (Baumol 1965, 20; Haveman 1969, 1–2; Lyons 1969, 82–83, 179–80, 189–210). In the 1960s, program budgeting came to represent for the federal government as a whole the application of economic principles to optimizing public expenditures.

The economists who took on these tasks thought of themselves as impartial experts clarifying the policy choices available to the interests. In the United States, the role of disinterested expert was sanctioned largely by the rise of pluralism within the social sciences. As noticed earlier, pluralism supposed that, within a broad consensus, competition and bargaining among diverse interests would bring social progress. Assuming a position of neutrality among the interests, the economist could exploit the professional armamentarium to identify means for achieving any given agenda and to analyze the consequences of various policy choices (Fox 1979, 325–27). In this self-conception, the economist does not formulate the public interest but supplies the means for clarifying policy options; standing outside the fray, the analyst assumes a posture not of Olympian detachment, but of disinterested service as a technical expert (Eckstein 1961, 445–46; Margolis 1977, 210–11; Wildavsky 1966, 297).

In principle this way of applying economics to policy choice was positive, not normative; that is, it aimed to specify the likely consequences of any given policy choices (a descriptive and causal account), rather than to assert what ought to be done. Nevertheless, the role of *applied* scientist, however disinterested, carried normative implications. By considering themselves the servants of decision makers, the experts were accepting responsibility for devising programs with normative intent. Moreover, as noted below, the principal theoretical tradition that was applied to governmental decision making—welfare economics—is by definition a normative enterprise: it seeks to identify and recommend those decisions that would lead to increases in public welfare.[34] The analyst therefore devised programs thought broadly acceptable and recommended them, at least implicitly, to society at large. Moreover, the predication of disinterestedness on the existence of a broad consensus implies that only those programs ought to be considered that are consistent with the prevailing consensus.[35]

Public Expenditures Analysis: Investments and Redistribution

The enhanced legitimacy of the public sector focused economists' attention on the justifications and methods of public policy and thus inaugurated a tradition of public expenditure analysis (for example, Chase 1968a; U.S. Congress 1969; Haveman and Margolis 1970; 1977). Analysts proceeded by identifying instances of market failure that justified public intervention and by exploiting cost-benefit analysis to facilitate design and selection of public programs. This literature is marked by three characteristics relevant to the present study: its authors concentrated on investment (as opposed to consumption) goods as candidates for public provision or production (Bonnen 1969, 428–29); in exploiting cost-benefit analysis they attempted to maximize the economic welfare of society, which they defined as the cumulation of individual welfare;[36] and they concentrated on the efficiency of resource allocation rather than on considerations of distribution or equity.[37] These analysts thus gave little scope for conceptions of a higher social interest transcending individual interests; they largely ignored social mechanisms for decision making; and they

generally declined to provide policy makers with analyses of the distributional issues that, apart from efficiency considerations, commonly decided
the political fate of proposed governmental interventions.[38]

These characteristics of expenditure analysis diminished its useful-
ness to policy makers and deprived it of relevance to the central redistributive issues prominent in the 1960s. Nevertheless, some practitioners
of expenditure analysis were concerned about this problem of irrelevance,
and two of their proposed solutions are presented here. Both of them
revolve about the difficulty of discriminating issues of allocational efficiency (remedying market failure) from issues of equity (determining who
gains or loses as a result of public interventions).

The first solution proceeds from the impossibility of a clear separation and seeks recourse in an appropriate revision of cost-benefit analysis
to include the redistributional effects that lay at the center of political
decision making. It gives principled emphasis to the politics of redistribution by seeking evidence for the values underlying political decisions
not in any simple accumulation of individual utilities but in the history
of political decision making. The other solution supposes that, at least
for some programs, a clear separation of efficiency from equity is possible.
This approach adheres to the individualistic basis of cost-benefit analysis
by including in individual utility functions the willingness to pay shown
by some consumers for enhanced consumption by others. This point of
view underlay the theory of cost sharing in health care.

Responding to the political urgency acquired by redistributive issues
in the 1960s and aiming to render the economist's analyses more useful
to the policy maker, analysts such as James Bonnen (1969) and Burton
Weisbrod (1968; 1969) aspired to include the distributional effects of
public programs within the purview of expenditure analysis. Weisbrod
suggested the possibility, in principle, of including distributional effects
in the cost-benefit calculus through a "grand utility" approach. However,
the difficulty of this method—discriminating the distributional effects and
weighting them by criteria that could command assent—encouraged him
to try as an expedient the "separate presentation" of distributional effects
in juxtaposition with the typical cost-benefit analysis.[39]

Weisbrod's proposal had the merit of linking cost-benefit analysis
with the politics of decision making, but it occasioned no fundamental
progress with the long-standing issue of separating equity from efficiency
(Blaug 1968, 593–97, 602–3). Analysts of public expenditures in general
did not succeed where their predecessors had failed. As late as 1977,
Charles Schultze was still emphasizing what he considered the virtual
impossibility of separating efficiency and equity and the resultant difficulties for the design of rational policy. Like Weisbrod, he emphasized
the redistributive politics that determine the fate of programs, and he

called for increased efforts to identify the *losers* in proposed interventions so that, by compensating them, government could neutralize their opposition to promising reforms (Schultze 1977, 22–25, 67–76; cf. Joskow and Noll 1981, 8–9).

However, the means Weisbrod rejected for separating efficiency from equity seemed promising to other analysts. Its appeal emerged less from consideration of the political relevance of cost-benefit analysis in application to decisions about public expenditures than from a narrower and more practical issue: whether and how to price the goods and services provided or produced in public programs. Implicitly, this question shifted the emphasis in expenditure analysis from investment in bricks and mortar to consumption decisions by the beneficiaries of investments and to redistribution as an enhancement to consumption. Viewed from the demand side rather than the supply side, public programs offered goods to be purchased, and the possibility of separating redistributional effects from allocational effects emerged in the theory of pricing public goods. That possibility also underlay the theory of cost sharing.

This approach nevertheless issued from concern with allocational efficiency. In the 1960s, three traditions of economics converged on the allocational effects of the pricing structure for public goods: public finance, public utilities, and the marginal-cost pricing literature of welfare economics.[40] Economists expected that zero pricing of public or partially public goods provided through governmental investments would cause them to be regarded as costless by their beneficiaries, whose decisions would therefore lead to inefficiencies in the allocation of resources; and they recognized that the pricing structure faced by users of regulated goods and services—because it reflected historical costs of capital investments rather than current opportunity costs—likewise fostered allocational inefficiency. The three traditions (public finance, public utilities, and marginal-cost pricing theory) conspired to suggest the imposition of user charges on the beneficiaries of public investments. Such charges would discipline the use of public services just as price disciplines the use of private ones; they would serve the goal of efficiency in the short run by bringing price into line with marginal cost and constraining effective demand and in the long run by inhibiting excess investment that might be required to meet excess demand fueled by artificially lowered or zero prices.[41]

Redistribution emerged from considering the potential utility of pricing as a mechanism for making the beneficiaries of public programs bear some of the costs incurred by the programs. Since the benefits of governmental programs could be construed as externalities that impose on some citizens the costs of benefits received by others, user charges were seen as advantageous in redirecting some of these costs onto the beneficiaries of the programs (for example, Milliman 1969, 294–97, 308–9).

If broader redistributive concerns were met by some general mechanism, such as the negative income tax widely discussed in the 1960s, imposition of user charges on the beneficiaries of public programs would provide a relatively clear separation of the redistributional consequences of public intervention from the anticipated improvements in resource allocation.[42]

However, the propriety of a broad redistribution that could allow the recipients of redistribution to pay for services with user charges was subject to debate. Those in favor of it tended to depart from the individualistic mainstream of welfare economists in holding that there exists a general, social interest in redistribution (or indeed other forms of collective action) (Weisbrod 1969; Bonnen 1969; Steiner 1969, 29–41; Feldman 1971, 509 and n. 2). In this view, society benefits from granting at least a minimal purchasing power to all; in doing so, it elevates the poor to the status of sovereign consumers who, like other citizens, enjoy discretion over the disposal of their income (Weisbrod 1969, 189–90).

The opposing view, resting on fuller fidelity to the individualistic perspective, maintained that redistributive programs should reflect the desires of those paying for them and should therefore freely exploit transfers in kind rather than in cash; and that not society, but the taxpayers financing the programs should be understood as their beneficiaries. In this view, society does not enhance the autonomy of consumers otherwise priced out of various markets; rather, taxpayers express their sovereignty by dictating the expenditure patterns of those receiving the transfers. Redistribution creates not sovereign consumers, but dependent recipients of welfare. This view underlay the redistributive programs of the 1960s and 1970s. Instead of a negative income tax, Congress authorized specific programs in support of nutrition, housing, education, and health care. As Weisbrod (1969, 196 and cf. 189–90) put it, "taxpayers appear to be saying that they should decide not simply to whom income will be transferred but how the funds will be spent by (or for) the recipients" (cf. also Havighurst and Blumstein 1975, 24–25).

Economists largely shared the congressional preference for taxpayer sovereignty, and the preference for in-kind transfers gradually found justification in economic theory.[43] In 1971 Paul Feldman argued, in a general overview of debates about redistributive measures, that desire for income redistribution should be regarded as a cumulated or aggregated expression of the individual utility functions of taxpayers, that redistribution should be financed by taxing those willing to pay for it, and that the programs thus financed should reflect the utilities of the donors.[44]

As noted below, the health economists who advocated cost sharing adopted a position midway between these two positions by combining aspects of each. They linked the growing preference for transfers in kind with the apparent consensus among economists for the propriety of user charges (and for their underlying supposition that social programs should enhance the economic autonomy of their beneficiaries). Taxpayer sovereignty could be honored by dictating the services provided, in this instance, health services (as subsidized by insurance), and the populations receiving the subsidies; consumer sovereignty could be honored to a limited extent by making the recipients of the subsidies autonomous purchasers within the market for the subsidized services; allocational efficiency could be enhanced by levying user charges on the benefits provided. National health insurance could take the form not of universal entitlement to comprehensive benefits, but of subsidized purchase by specific groups of citizens of basic services carrying user charges.

Incentives and Public Policy: Schultze

The shortcomings of public expenditure analysis acknowledged by some of its practitioners became acute as disillusionment with governmental programs increased in the 1960s and 1970s. In the work of Charles Schultze, a leading practitioner of expenditure analysis and Budget Director in the late 1960s, the failures of governmental interventions resulted in a broad indictment of public policy generally and a call to replace regulatory and administrative agencies with private markets operating under suitably devised incentives. The remedy found a responsive chord among competitive theorists.

Schultze's belief in the inadequacy of prevailing means of governmental intervention first emerged in a paper of 1969 in connection with the PBB system and public expenditure analysis; and his ideas broadened to encompass not only public investments but also regulation. This enlarged view was the subject of the Godkin lectures he delivered in 1976 and revised for publication the next year under the title *The Public Use of Private Interest.*

Schultze's initial views (1969) rested on two convictions about the traditional approach to public investments: as ex post responses to the sequelae of economic growth in the private sector, public programs were not designed to prevent the problems themselves; and, once in place, they aimed at palliating symptoms, not eliminating their source. Drawing on examples from flood protection projects and water treatment plants, Schultze argued that investments in these facilities did not constrain irrational use of flood plain lands or suppress production of pollutants. They concentrated resources in the public sector to clean up messes after their creation in the private sector. Proper remediation demanded not just measures ex post facto, but also ex ante facto.

Preventive policy demanded intervention in several categories of decision making. Unlike the production of purely public goods, like

defense, Schultze observed, most recent forms of governmental intervention involved the private sphere, in which large numbers of dispersed and
independent decision makers affected outcomes. The decision makers
included the private economic actors whose behavior produced the
problems selected for public action and the administrators charged with
realizing the aims of public programs. Even in purely public programs, in
which private decisions played no role, federal action often entailed joint
operations with lower levels of government, many of them geographically
dispersed. Preventive programs could succeed only by affecting the diversity of actors involved and bringing their diverse actions into conformity
with central goals.[45]

The instrument Schultze (1969, 203) recommended for achieving this
effect was incentives:

> For two reasons . . . the problem of incentives deserves particular attention
> in the formulation of public expenditure policy: *first,* because national
> objectives increasingly depend for their realization on the joint action of
> many independent decisionmakers, private as well as public; and *second,*
> because the growing complexity and geographical diversity of public pro-
> grams requires decentralized decisionmaking within the public sector itself.

In the case of private decision making, Schultze argued not merely
that incentives are lacking to bring private action into conformity with
public goals, but that existing incentives encourage actions precisely counter to the stipulated goals of public programs. To exemplify such negative
incentives, as he then called them, he cited favorable tax treatment for
speculation in urban land (which counteracts the objectives of urban
development plans) and prevailing methods of hospital reimbursement
(which served only to raise costs). In his book of 1977 (54 n. 26, 63–64),
Schultze relied on much the same examples but succeeded in attracting
greater attention to the idea by replacing the term "negative" with "perverse." As replacements for perverse incentives, Schultze recommended
primarily prices and user charges that would impose on decision makers
the costs resulting from decisions that do not conform to public goals.

In regard to decision making within the public sphere, Schultze's
book of 1977 dropped his idea of 1969 that public programs could be
improved by confronting public decision makers with marketlike incentives. Instead, he now juxtaposed a discussion of regulation with his earlier
emphasis on investments and the perverse incentives governing them.[46]
Though regulation had not been prominent in the literature of public
expenditure analysis, Schultze found in studies of environmental regulation precedents for the superiority of market incentives over regulation,
and he called for replacement of regulation with markets in which suitably
designed incentives could impose on decision makers the costs of socially
undesirable actions (for example, Kneese and d'Arge 1969, 96–97, 100; cf.
Kneese and Schultze 1975; and Schultze 1977, 53–54).

With this argument, Schultze no longer implied (as he had in 1969) that the incentives faced by regulators induced them to depart from the public interest, but that the new kinds of task facing government had made regulation an outmoded instrument of public policy. Regulatory failure could be traced to the novel dimensions and complexity of public problems, which rendered impossible the detailed specification of inputs and outputs on which regulation and other centralized interventions depended. Though older governmental programs had been successfully organized along simple bureaucratic lines, regulatory institutions could no longer be expected to transmit what Schultze characterized as "commands and controls" from a central decision-making instance to diverse actors.[47] From this perspective, remedying regulatory failure did not require a theory of regulation (as other opponents of regulation believed), but simply followed from the perception that publicly defined objectives are more likely to be achieved when government confines itself to setting the ground rules for decision making and imposing constraints on behavior (Schultze 1977, 6-13).

Schultze's book proved broadly appealing. Its inclusion of regulation together with investment under a single analytical framework; its consistency with the traditional reluctance to diminish voluntary prerogatives;[48] its recognition that national goals could be met only through numerous, decentralized actions; and its depiction of centralized institutions and large investments as ineffective in achieving public goals together constituted a broad and compelling brief against past policy and a path to bold recommendations for reform of governmental interventions (ibid., 9-15). His book affirmed the novel responsibilities of government in the postwar world, but it spurned replacement of private with public institutions; it invoked the economist's long-standing professional concern for the role of incentives in the organization of markets, but it now applied them to public programs; it rejected the conservative's supposedly reflexive aversion to governmental intervention, but it did not endorse the liberal's ostensible readiness to institute regulation or other forms of direct control. Schultze thus endeavored to advance social policy in a way transcending the typical political labels and shibboleths.[49]

For Schultze, this de minimis approach to public policy seemed an apt remedy for disillusionment with governmental programs. Faulty instruments of public intervention had disappointed rising expectations (ibid., 2-4). Policy makers nevertheless continued to exploit old methods in great measure because mobilization of public support for action entails demand for quick results, and both speed and certainty are widely taken to be achievable only by administration, not by construction and evolution of markets (ibid., 76-83, 87-89; cf. Enthoven 1980, 101; Wolf 1979; Klein 1981). The problem was to recognize the complexity of policy problems and devise means that could function without requiring detailed specifications. The job could be done by markets operating under suitable incentives.

Despite the apparent breadth and persuasiveness of Schultze's ideas, his indictment of public policy and his incentives-based remedy focused on only one side of public policy: the technical adequacy of its means. As noticed above, he did pay some attention to the politics of decision making, but only to the extent of calling for clearer identification of those expected to suffer losses from proposed interventions (so that their opposition could be diminished by compensating them). However, the political mechanisms that selected the ends of policy were not among his concerns. Rather, he seemed to accept the public interest rationale typically invoked to justify public intervention and to suppose that the problems selected for intervention could be identified with one or another of the usual forms of market failure.[50] For Schultze, the problem was to isolate cases of market failure clearly and to devise suitable remedies. That regulatory failure might have resulted from political considerations obscured by the language of the public interest was not one of Schultze's themes.

However, the deregulatory movement of the 1970s and the disillusionment with collective intervention that underlay it derived in great measure from the conviction that regulatory and administrative agencies operated in a political environment that made any simple public interest rationale for regulation beside the point. That conviction is indebted to the attention accorded interest groups by political scientists inspired by the pluralist conception. The history of this conception within political science lies outside the scope of this study,[51] but it is important to note that pluralism did not immediately inspire a critical assessment of governmental institutions. On the contrary, it inspired the idea that the proper role of government was to sponsor interest-group bargaining. Only as policies predicated on this view came to be seen as dissatisfactory did political scientists question the abdication of a more positive role by the state. Lowi provided a leading example of such questioning in 1969.

Interest-Group Liberalism: Lowi

Like Schultze's book of 1977, Lowi's volume of 1969 was an indictment of government by administration and regulation. However, Lowi did not trace policy failure to persistent and unquestioned use of an outmoded mechanism. Instead, he emphasized an intended abdication of governmental responsibility to define the public interest and realize it. These tasks had been recast in the mold of interest-group liberalism, a vulgarized version of the pluralism that flourished within political science.

From the supposition that politics amounts to the mutual bargaining, adjustment, and agreement among organized interest groups and from the notion that government is an epiphenomenon of politics thus conceived, exponents of interest-group liberalism concluded that the very process by which the goals and methods of public authority are formulated is self-justifying. Supposing that social justice would follow from bargaining and mutual adjustment among interests, government deprived agencies of their regulatory tasks and transformed them into sponsors of interest-group bargaining.

Interest-group liberalism rendered irrelevant the old distinctions between traditional liberals and conservatives. What separated them now, according to Lowi, was merely the interests with which they affiliated themselves. President Eisenhower, no less than his successor, was an interest-group liberal, though Lowi (1969, 77) conceded that "explicit and systematic expression of interest-group liberalism is much more the contribution of Democrats," and Lowi found in the programs they devised in the 1960s the best examples of this doctrine in action and of its costs. In sphere after sphere of public policy, Lowi described how popular control had decayed as all portions of the public not specifically organized to affect the policies in question were shut out of administrative and regulatory proceedings; how existing structures of privilege were strengthened and new ones were created (as organized interests were coopted into the formulation and execution of policy); and how the weakening of popular government, the support of privilege, and resistance to change characteristic of this kind of governing typically produced conservative decisions.[52]

Lowi thus attributed the failure of public policy to different causes from those cited by Schultze, and he proposed a different sort of remedy. Like Schultze, he held that earlier forms of regulation were relatively effective, but he traced their virtues not (as Schultze had) to the relative simplicity of their tasks, but to the clarity with which their objectives had been formulated and enacted into law. In the past, and in some cases in the present, delegations of power from Congress to agencies were accompanied by clearly articulated standards. If government would once again assume responsibility for taking positive stands and articulating its decisions in the statutes governing administrative and regulatory agencies, then planning and evaluation would become possible, responsibility and accountability could be fixed and assessed, and justice might be attained in the execution of policy. Regulation was in principle possible and indeed desirable, provided it was predicated on clear goals. Once the public interest was clearly articulated, disinterested experts could once again become its servants.

The Antiregulatory Literature

Lowi's conviction that regulation had undergone a demonstrable secular change from a functioning public interest model to a dysfunctional pluralist model was not shared by other analysts of regulation. Among some economists, the conviction grew that the public interest model of regulation had never been realized in practice and that recent programs were no different in kind from their predecessors. Opinions varied about the prospects for regulatory reform, but these analysts agreed that the failures of regulation to advance the public interest resulted from features inherent in the political economy of regulation.[53]

Leading the new economic approach to regulation was the Chicago School of economics (Reder 1982). Particularly as it grew under the leadership of Milton Friedman, Chicago differed from the Keynesian mainstream of economics inter alia in preferring positive analysis to normative assumptions. Though this positive emphasis did not initially inhibit Chicago from espousing conservative policy measures and opposing intervention by the state for normative (as well as positive reasons), as the school evolved, especially under the influence of George Stigler, its positive aspect gradually eclipsed the normative (ibid., 25–32, 35–36). This change occurred as "the interaction between political and economic variables increasingly intruded upon the *positive* explanation of observed behavior . . ." (ibid., 25). While reducing the taste of Chicago for advocacy, this attention to politics induced members of the school to apply their standard tools of economic analysis beyond the realm of ordinary economic phenomena to clearly political phenomena such as legislation and regulation and to the interest-group contests that had attracted political scientists.[54] The normative question of how to maximize the public welfare was thus not a prime concern of Chicago; instead, primacy was accorded the explanation of political-economic behavior on the assumption that actors behave rationally.[55] From the perspective of Chicago, the study of regulation was less a matter of normative (if dispassionate) applied science than (much more nearly) positive pure science.

The normative mantle which had typically cloaked regulation through the 1960s invited the skepticism of Chicago.[56] Though more a set of typically implicit assumptions than a theory (Posner 1974a, 335 n. 1), its opponents invested the public interest view with the status of a theory, and, as they developed their opposition to it, they gradually succeeded in isolating its foundations from antecedent literature (for example, ibid.; Noll 1985c, 18–24). The "theory" descended from Progressive-era traditions that aimed to rectify the shortcomings of the unfettered market and to protect consumers from monopoly pricing. It supposed that regulation could compensate for the absence of competitive conditions in markets that lacked them and that apolitical experts, as opposed to corrupt politicians or monopolizing businessmen, could successfully devise measures to uphold the public interest (cf. Noll 1971, 33–34). Upholders of this view generally supposed that the announced goals of regulation could be accepted at face value; that a clear separation could be maintained between the making of policy and its application in practice; that governmental agencies charged with remediating market failure were costless and efficient; and that regulatory failure had to be explained either by failure to implement regulation adequately[57] or by corruption, decay, or superannuation of regulatory institutions and methods.[58]

Accepting such normative assumptions and identifying sources of their perversion or perturbation were uncongenial to the Chicago School. Instead it inquired into the actual effects of regulation and sought to explain them with reference not to errors, corruption, or shortcomings, but to the rational behavior of the protagonists in regulatory settings.[59] Stigler's initial finding, in the case of electricity—that regulation possessed no effects (Stigler and Friedland 1962)—helped launch inquiries both within and outside Chicago into the effects of regulation. Over the subsequent decade, economists discredited the public interest theory of regulation, provided foundations for a positive account of regulation, and developed the materials for a comprehensive indictment of regulatory practice.[60]

The central thread in this development was the attention increasingly paid to the redistributive politics of regulation. A major form of redistribution, the internal subsidy, appears when regulators compel regulated firms to charge monopoly prices for some services (while preventing erosion of these prices by entry control) and to use the excess revenues thus obtained to subsidize other services (Posner 1971; Comanor and Mitchell 1972). Awareness of this redistributive mechanism did not inevitably force abandonment of the public interest theory, for it could be preserved by the supposition that regulators substituted their own conception of the public interest for consumers' interests and exploited internal subsidies to finance "good works."[61] Nevertheless, redistribution seemed to many to call for an alternative approach. Posner, for example, found the internal subsidy sufficient grounds to reject the public interest theory, for it was incompatible with consumer protection and it was too common to be regarded as merely aberrant (Posner 1971, especially pp. 27–28; cf. Jordan 1972, 153–54). Instead, Posner (1971) argued, the subsidy is an indirect form of taxation that serves the interests of certain customers of regulated firms. However, the main consequence of the perception that redistribution is a major outcome of regulation was neither the planning nor the taxation hypothesis, but the producer-protection hypothesis, which held that the regulated firms were the principal beneficiaries of regulation.

The producer-protection hypothesis, like the planning and taxation hypotheses, resembles in some respects one of the older explanations of regulatory failure, the "capture theory." Devised by political scientists, the capture theory explained regulatory failure as a gradual decline in the respect accorded by regulators to their legal mandate and a corresponding willingness to compromise with the interests.[62] The capture theory focuses on the regulated firms as an interest group that manages to dominate the regulatory agencies and transform them into protectors of the regulated. It thus accepts the public interest view of regulation at face value and refers regulatory failure to subversion by the interests. The producer-protection and taxation hypotheses shared this concern with the competition of interests for the redistributive fruits of regulation, but producer-protection differs in supposing that exploitation of regulation by producers is more than an infrequent perturbation from the public interest model. Instead, producer-protection considers redistribution the principal effect of regulation and finds that producers were its most frequent beneficiaries. Regulation was not the occasional victim of the regulated, but an instrument for their enrichment.

In an influential paper, William H. Jordan (1972) argued for the producer-protection hypothesis by proceeding from Stigler's initial finding that regulatory activity lacked effects. He held that the extent to which regulation has effects depends upon the prior structure of the market in which it was instituted and that, where effects could be discerned, they were inconsistent with consumer protection and highly consistent with producer protection. In natural-monopoly industries, scanty evidence of regulatory effects is consistent with producer protection not consumer protection, for the latter implies that monopolistic practices would be constrained not preserved. In oligopolistic or competitive industries, by contrast, regulation permits cartelization, thus benefitting the regulated firms at the expense of consumers. This empirical study was highly suggestive, and it gave much credence to the major theoretical exposition that Stigler provided in 1971.

In part, Stigler's study both "crystallized" the revisionism just described and transcended it.[63] Though it suggested that producer protection was the most common outcome of regulation, it was a broad theory of political coalition building that in principle accommodated other outcomes. In particular, Stigler's research program of applying economics to other than ordinary economic goods suggested that regulation and the benefits it confers are goods typically demanded by industries or occupations and supplied by government; and that regulatory phenomena must be understood with reference to the political tasks faced by those demanding regulation. The theory therefore departed from the supposition of the public interest model that regulation is provided without cost. Costs include the votes or resources expended to buy regulatory benefits from political parties and to neutralize opposition and the benefits foregone by resort to regulation instead of private cartelization (for regulation, unlike cartelization, redistributes control of an industry among its member firms, grants some control to powerful outsiders, and imposes the costs of the procedural safeguards required of public processes). Finally, the theory identifies small groups with a large stake in regulatory politics as the most likely victors in regulatory politics. Large groups with diffuse interests and high costs of organization are unlikely to work to mobilize votes or pay to obtain support or neutralize opposition. As Peltzman (1976, 212) put it,

> in Stigler's model, unlike most market models, there are many bidders [for the benefits of regulation], but only one is successful. There is essentially a political auction in which the high bidder receives the right to tax the wealth of everyone else, and the theory seeks to discover why the successful bidder is a numerically compact group.

Peltzman generalized this theory by examining regulation from the standpoint of the regulators themselves. The inspiration was consumer choice theory, which invoked tastes as shaping the consumer's utility function. Making the regulators analogous to consumers and the power relationships analogous to tastes, Peltzman followed the "highly rewarding research strategy" of consumer-choice theorists "to beg questions of taste formation and concentrate instead on the behavioral effects of changes in constraints in a regime of stable tastes." Thus, leaving aside political power relations, the theorist of regulation could examine the behavior of regulators under changing constraints (for example, changes in productivity and growth, shifts in demand, changes in per capita wealth among the groups benefitting from regulation). Moreover, by invoking only the most familiar sorts of constraint and treating them with the most familiar supply-demand apparatus, Peltzman obtained "refutable implications about a wide range of regulatory behavior" (ibid., 240).

The result was to identify the outcomes of regulation with the results of the rational political calculus of the regulators. Sticking first to Stigler's model, which assumes one winner of the political auction, Peltzman examined the "crucial decision" that the regulator must make, the size of the favored group and that of the group taxed. The argument showed that even if one interest captures all the benefits of regulation, "these must be less than a perfect broker for the group would obtain." With regulation, outsiders to an industry gain some control over it. This conclusion, which Peltzman labeled an "ad hoc" detail of the capture literature, proved to be an integral result of regulation. Moreover, the "taxation by regulation" described by Posner need not imply anything more than that "a rational regulator will still tax cartel profits to secure his own position" (ibid., 214, 217).

Peltzman then argued that a rational regulator will exploit differences within the beneficiary group and devise a suitable structure of benefits and costs. The result is that some other interests (besides the principal beneficiary group) may be benefitted and some producers may be taxed even if most of them are beneficiaries (ibid., 218–19). Moreover, in analyzing the impact of economic forces on the structure of prices under regulation, Peltzman argued that the regulator will seek to maximize support by substituting political for economic criteria in setting prices (ibid., 219, 231–39). The approach suggested that the internal subsidy characteristic of regulation is a tax that the regulator levies on the profits resulting from price discrimination. Operating on the principle that the opposition of all groups must be equated at the margin, the regulator uses the revenues thus obtained to spread the costs of high-cost customers among all customer groups. Peltzman saw no need to point out that his analysis explains the subsidy without reference to the public interest (for example, in the planning-by-regulation hypothesis); but he did note that it explained the subsidy with reference to neither "taxation by regulation" nor ad hoc pacification of opposition; instead, it portrayed the subsidy as an outcome of the political economy of regulation (ibid., 236, 239).

With the economic theory of regulation, the Chicago School aimed to deduce all the observed features of regulation without reference to normative considerations and with reliance solely on the rationality of protagonists in the regulatory arena. However, by eschewing the normative, Chicago abandoned concerns of reform. Those students of regulation who aspired to rationalize public policy, however, hoped to combine the positive picture with normative proposals. The most prominent instance of this approach is Roger Noll, who retains an element of the public interest in his views but also obtains a very general view of regulation by referring its characteristics, much as Peltzman had, to the rationality of the regulators.

Labeling this approach the political-economic theory,[64] Noll (1975, 29) suggested

> that regulators try to serve some concept of the general public interest, rather than act as conduits for the interests of the regulated firms. The problem regulators face is to identify this general public interest in a milieu in which information is uncertain, expensive, and biased, and in a society which contains numerous groups whose interests are conflicting rather than harmonious.

The theory was not opposed to the economic theory, but Noll claimed it was "more complex and dynamic" (ibid.). It argued that to gauge their success in satisfying the public interest, regulators look to external indicators. These indicators include the extent to which the courts override regulatory decisions, the reactions of legislative decisions to agency behavior, and the performance of the regulated industry. Agencies will seek either to maximize indicators of approval or minimize indicators of disapproval.

Like the economic theory, Noll's political-economic theory argues that representation before agencies is a costly political process favoring small groups with concentrated interests. If the interests of the general public are diffuse, they will not affect regulatory proceedings. Rather, decisions favor the regulated firms and other well-represented interests. Also working to reduce the effects of a broad public interest is the influence of legislative subcommittee members over regulatory proceedings. Unlike the passage of legislation, oversight by subcommittees produces a minimal public record and permits legislators to be more responsive to the interests.

The economists' theories of regulation thus coincided in their conclusions with those of Lowi: regulation is dominated by the interests. Though Lowi advocated a return to what had appeared to him a genuine form of public interest regulation, the Chicago School and those inspired by it argued that the public interest model did not describe the behavior of any regulatory regime or the outcomes of its actions. Noll's example shows that the new analysis of regulation need not exclude the public interest as a relevant factor, but he nevertheless concludes that the political environment in which regulators try to pursue the public interest induces them to favor the regulated.

At the end of the 1970s, Charles Wolf (1979) achieved a synthesis of much antecedent literature on governmental failure. Wolf argued that governmental interventions to remedy market failure are themselves subject to failure and that any decision to institute public intervention must compare the likely nonmarket failures with the known market failures. Nonmarket failures result from the absence of mechanisms "for reconciling calculations by decision makers of their private and organizational costs and benefits with total costs and benefits." Decision makers therefore substitute private goals, or internalities, which correspond to the externalities of market failure. Internalities include budget growth ("more is better"), technological advance ("new and complex is better"—or perhaps worse), and information acquisition and control ("knowing what others don't know is better"). Wolf's summary (ibid., 123) of the differences between externalities and internalities succinctly captures many of the features of policy failure developed by its various earlier diagnosticians:

> Whereas externalities in the market sector are costs and benefits realized by the public but not collectible from or by producers, the internalities associated with nonmarket output are usually *benefits* perceived as such by producers and paid for by the public as part of the costs of producing nonmarket output. Consequently, internalities tend to raise costs and supply functions. These shifts, moreover, are likely to increase over time as nonmarket agencies succeed in building special constituencies within Congress and the public that are more immediately concerned than is the broader taxpaying public over whom the costs are spread.

Though Wolf presented this argument as part of a framework for "implementation analysis," that is, a method for anticipating nonmarket failures, he nevertheless conceded that clear criteria for a decision to intervene are lacking (ibid., 118). Accordingly, Wolf's study, though inspired by the normative impulse toward rationalizing public interventions, could well have been read by skeptics of regulation as confirming their conviction that no adequate regulatory or administrative interventions could be devised. Though incentives-based approaches have been little realized in practice (Joskow and Noll 1981, 21–24), those who found them appealing may well have read analysts like Wolf as confirming their conviction that deregulation and reconstruction of markets with suitably designed incentives were the only rational approaches to public policy.

Certainly, for advocates of competitive plans, working in an environment of disillusionment with governmental programs generally and persuaded of the shortcomings of health sector regulation, the incentives-based approach seemed the only sensible alternative. Some of them were mindful of the importance of incentives even before Schultze published, but Schultze gave them a rallying point.[65] The emphasis on incentives, in combination with a knowledge of the political economy of regulation, induced advocates of plans to claim that regulation was a fatally flawed instrument of public policy. In the health sector, regulation would leave the causes of problems intact, it would institutionalize perverse incentives, and it would perpetuate the subordination of public to private interest.[66] Advocates of competitive health plans called for deregulation to the maximal extent and replacement of regulation by private decision making under suitably devised incentives.[67]

THE ECONOMICS OF HEALTH AND
THE THEORY OF COST SHARING

If planning and regulation reflected the expansionary traditions of the hospital industry, competition aimed to curb the flow of resources into the health sector and to subdue cost escalation by invoking the discipline of market competition. Both approaches to health care policy exploited economics, and the shift from planning to competition entailed a shift in the applications of economics to health care. The earliest significant applications of economics to health care were sponsored by the planning tradition and reflected its expansionary biases (cf. Anderson 1966, 27), whereas competitive theory relied on the still normative but more nearly dispassionate approach of public expenditure analysis.

Illustrative of changes in the 1960s is a comparison of Seymour E. Harris's *The Economics of American Medicine* of 1964, a work pervaded with notions of need, with Herbert E. Klarman's book of 1965, *The Economics of Health*, a book reflecting the public expenditures approach. In the former, Harris (1964, xi) allowed that

> My major interest is to exploit financial institutions in such a manner as to increase resources going into medicine, making the most effective use of the resultant inputs, and in particular to bring about an improvement in the distribution of medicine. . . . Adequacy of medical services depends not only on the flow of cash into medical markets but also on that of manpower, drugs, hospital beds, and the like. Incentives must be adequate to yield the needed flow of doctors, dentists, nurses, drugs, and so on, of the required quality. . . .

By contrast, Klarman maintained that the "economist's contribution [to the problem of allocating resources] is to state the costs (or, what is the same, the consequences in terms of opportunities foregone) of alternative courses of action"; and he asserted that "A particular health program is justified not because it is necessary or good, but because it constitutes a better use of resources than some alternative program."[68]

Though the application of public expenditures analysis to health care gradually fostered the differentiation of health economics from the broad mainstream of public expenditures analysis, the evolution of cost-benefit studies of health care followed much the same path as that taken by public expenditure analysis generally: from a preoccupation with rationalizing federal investment programs to a concern for redistribution of consumption goods. In health care, redistribution meant entitlement programs. Proposals for consumer cost sharing in health care emerged from the effort to optimize public financing of entitlements, understood as publicly provided enhancements to consumption. Cost sharing represents therefore the second of two stages in the history of economics as applied to health: first, a shift from simple advocacy of expansion as a response to unmet need (in the planning tradition) to the rationalization of federal investment programs (in the public expenditures tradition); then (within the public expenditures tradition), a shift from investments to consumption.

The first stage, the eclipse of advocacy by analysis, was facilitated by two factors. One was the ascendancy within American social sciences of pluralism, which, as noted earlier, supposed that within a broadly defined consensus, competition and bargaining among the diversity of interests constituting society would bring social progress. Assuming a position of neutrality among the interests, the economist could exploit the professional armamentarium to identify means for achieving any given agenda and to analyze the consequences of various policy choices.[69] Also promoting a disinterested approach to health programs was the theory of human capital in application to health programs. As exploited by Selma Mushkin, the theory "made the application of economic analysis to health issues less controversial because it subsumed the controversial issue of how to finance medical care under the larger question of the benefits of improved health" (Fox 1969, 321).

Health Care as an Investment

Mushkin's use of the theory of human capital did more than enhance the disinterestedness of health economics, however. The theory of human capital made possible the treatment of health programs as investments and their early subordination to the techniques of public expenditure analysis. Her approach was very like that of others in the field of expenditure analysis: she employed theoretical welfare economics together with the practical precedents from the literature on water resource projects. However, the investments she analyzed with these tools were not in bricks and mortar, but in health: "The origin of recent economic research on the value of human capital created by health care lies in the development of public expenditure theory and the emphasis given to cost-benefit analysis" (Mushkin 1962, 153; cf. Klarman 1982, 590).

Mushkin (1962, 131) recognized that "[h]ealth services are similar to education . . . in that they are partly investment and partly consumption, and the separation of the two elements is difficult." Other economists also recognized the lack of complete analogy between the more ordinary sorts of investment and health and education (for example, Prest and Turvey 1965, 731). Nevertheless, the theory of human capital provided a bridge that allowed the treatment of social service programs in the same terms as investments in bricks and mortar. The basic point of departure was in principle quite simple:

> The concept of human capital formation through both education and health services rests on the twin notions that people as productive agents are improved by investment in these services and that the outlays made yield a continuing return in the future. Health services, like education, become a part of the individual, a part of his effectiveness in the field and factory. The future increase in labor productivity resulting from education or from health programs can be quantified to an extent useful for programming purposes. (Mushkin 1962, 130)

From this perspective, the resources devoted to health care are an investment producing a yield, the "labor product created by [health] care and savings in health expenditures in the future, if any, as a consequence of reduction in disease" (ibid., 136). The yield may be measured in various ways: on a cost basis, as "the present value of the future earnings generated through health programs," or as the "present value of the future labor product." The central problem was therefore measurement of the labor product added as a result of health care (ibid., 136–37). The effort to accomplish that measurement clarified the nature of the yield from health programs:

> It is, essentially, an estimate of the money value of the labor product lost as a result of death, disability, and debility. The prevention or cure of these pro-

> vides a labor product that is added and gives an estimate of added income flow, or it can be converted into an estimate of capital formation through health programs by capitalizing this annual added labor product attributable to health care. (Ibid., 143)

Once classified as investments, health programs could be treated consistently with the mainstream of cost-benefit analysis in application to public investment programs (Klarman 1982, 585–86).

Mushkin's work was marked by several other assumptions. It supposed that the results of health programs could be determined quantitatively and that the economic benefits could be assessed accordingly. It further supposed that the absence of the ordinary sort of market in the health sector inhibited expression of consumer desires and that therefore the computation of benefits as added earnings and savings in expenditures on health care was the only means to evaluate candidates for public provision (Mushkin 1962, 153–54). This justification of her own enterprise tacitly sanctioned the absence of ordinary market arrangements in the health sector and implied the first supposition that experts could and did know the results of various interventions. As for the propriety of enhanced earnings as the measure of benefits, she did notice that some analysts had rejected a strict accounting of earnings and demanded treatment of social value judgments that confer value on economically unproductive lives (children, the aged, and the disabled) and that others demanded account of the noneconomic costs and benefits (affective losses and reduced quality of life) (ibid., 154–56); but she largely confined herself to measurements of labor product and enhanced national income. Moreover, as Klarman (1982, 592–93) reports, the earnings approach was highly influential among the program planners in the Department of Health, Education, and Welfare who were trying to carry out the promulgation of the PBB system in the 1960s. As major backers of Mushkin's methods, they reinforced the preoccupation of economists with the economically active segments of the population.

However, subsequent events diminished this preoccupation. Despite Mushkin's confidence, doubt was increasingly cast on the significance of earnings as an appropriate measure of value because of its neglect of economically unproductive individuals and of intangible benefits. At the same time, willingness to pay for a given improvement in health status seemed conceptually preferable but extraordinarily difficult to assess in practice (ibid., 587–89). The difficulty stemmed not only from the free-rider problem, which leads potential beneficiaries of programs to understate their willingness to pay in hope that they will benefit from the willingness of others, but also from the inability of consumers to appreciate the intended improvements in health and to determine their significance. In consequence, Klarman reports, economists increasingly abandoned their efforts to put a monetary value on the benefits. An analysis that falls short of this final step is called cost-effectiveness analysis. Because it lacks an estimate of the monetary value of benefits, the comparisons it permits are more limited than those resting on cost-benefit analysis. Thus, cost-effectiveness analysis permits comparisons of alternative programs designed to reach the same goals (for example, additions to life expectancy from alternative therapies for a given disease), but not among programs intended for different purposes. Economists of health care increasingly reconciled themselves to comparing only those programs aiming at similar results.

Leading in the same direction is the difficulty of identifying the outcomes of health programs. Mushkin's approach clearly rested on her conviction that the improvements in health status resulting from a given health program could be identified with reasonable accuracy and that the resultant economic benefits of increased participation in the labor force could be calculated. However, Klarman (ibid., 592) points out that though the promulgation of the PBB system put a premium on efforts to evaluate the economic benefits of programs, analysts were compelled to stop short, because "the health care experts did not always have the requisite knowledge about program effects or outcomes." Accordingly, economists and planners had to rest content with cost-effectiveness analysis.

For Klarman, these developments since Mushkin's pioneering work intensified the differences between the usual sorts of investment and social program. Because intangible benefits had come to seem vastly more important than originally assumed, education and even more so health care seemed like consumer goods, not investment goods.[70] In the light of these developments, Klarman (1982, 592, 598) offered two recommendations for research: health services research aimed at specifying the outcomes of interventions and studies of "people's preferences for and rankings of diverse changes in health status, . . . an activity that Mushkin encouraged and sponsored." An alternative approach, one taken by advocates of cost sharing, is based on the supposition that expert determination of the value of care is difficult or perhaps impossible in principle. Out of this conviction, advocates of cost sharing argued that people's preferences are appropriately measured as manifest demand in the market. They dropped the idea of health as an investment and focused on consumption.

These divergent responses suggest that Mushkin's approach was closer to the traditions of planning than to the position taken by advocates of cost sharing. Though the supposition of vast unmet need and the simple advocacy of broad expansion of health services were gone, the investment approach nevertheless supposed that major improvements in health and expert determination of the outcomes and benefits of health care programs were possible. Advocates of cost sharing, by contrast, had come to doubt the efficacy of health care at the margin and denied the possibility of expert determination of need for care or expert evaluation of health-improving interventions. The shift from the investments approach to cost sharing is illustrated below.

Need versus Demand, Planning versus Consumer Sovereignty

As shown above (by the juxtaposition of Harris and Klarman), the needs-based approach to the allocation of health resources was an early casualty of the public expenditures approach. Martin Feldstein, whom Klarman cited approvingly, had argued (1963, 25–26) that thinking "in terms of 'need' or 'best possible care' is misleading," since any additional care that may be provided, though possibly useful, is the denial of resources to other uses. In other words, the economist's goal of optimization explicitly exhibits the resource costs of need-based planning. In his econometric study of the British National Health Service (NHS), Feldstein made his point in more concrete terms. His analysis of hospital utilization had revealed something akin to Roemer's Law, the dependence of the demand for beds on the supply, while he noted that analysts of need had predicated their calculations on manifest demand, as if it were an independent variable. Such studies provided the misleading but reassuring conclusion that "the current number of beds in an area is the correct number for the current period" (M. Feldstein 1967, 193). Planning for need merely ratified the existing supply and therefore all the forces promoting expansion of supply.

Planning for need, like need itself, was therefore a casualty of the new approach to the economics of health programs. Planning for need was rapidly supplanted by planning to preserve or improve health or health status and that, in turn, was succeeded by consumer sovereignty. These developments issued from the standard concern of the public expenditures tradition, the identification of market failure and the justification of collective intervention to remedy failure. Concern for market failure in the health sector focused attention on the lack of measures of the outcomes of health care and indeed raised the possibility that outcome measures were unattainable. Without such measures, expert determination of need was ruled out and so was any justification for continuing to deprive consumers of the power to allocate resources by expressing demand in the market. The fountainhead for much of this discussion was Kenneth Arrow's classic paper of 1963, "Uncertainty and the Welfare Economics of Medical Care."

Arrow held that the absence of insurance against certain kinds of risk to health was a prima facie case of market failure that justified governmental intervention; that, in general, the institutional arrangements distinguishing the health sector from other sectors amount to compensations for market failure; that all the well-known peculiarities of the medical care market, including arrangements that allowed providers to shape and control the health sector, either resulted from uncompetitive conditions or had appeared as compensations for them; and that these deviations fore-closed the possibility of separating matters of equity from the aim of alloca-tional efficiency. Arrow thus shared the view common among practitioners of public expenditures analysis that allocational and equity effects could not be disentangled in public programs.

Though Arrow had portrayed the overall structure of the market in the health sector as largely noncompetitive, the cost-sharing proposals ultimately inspired by his paper dealt only with the demand side of the market. For Arrow, the major problem on the demand side was consumer ignorance. Because medical care is technical and specialized, the consumer grew reliant on providers, providers had acquired their extensive control over the supply side, and government had found cause for regulation of the health sector. In essence, Arrow believed providers' control over health care was justified by the technical complexity of their knowledge and skills, and he similarly believed in a public interest model of regulation that entrusted public policy to disinterested specialists. Moreover, Arrow evidently thought there was no escape from provider dominance of health care and no recourse from additional public intervention to correct the remaining failures of the market. These views would become targets for criticism by advocates of competitive plans, but Arrow's paper, except to the extent that it helped disseminate the standard list of departures from competitive conditions in health care and reflected commonly held views about market failure in health care and the role of government, did not inspire their criticisms. His paper induced not so much a demand for deregulation (reform of the supply side) but for cost sharing (reform of the demand side). Proponents of cost sharing argued that consumer ignorance was not so serious an obstacle to informed consumer choice as had been thought, but they did little to enquire whether the supply side as currently constituted could be made to provide the necessary information even if consumers in principle could evaluate it.

Though Arrow's critics later claimed that many of his arguments amounted to little more than assumptions, for the analysis of the demand for health care and health insurance his paper was of fundamental sig-nificance. One recent analyst of health services research noted that the paper "connected the economics of health to mathematical analysis and the most sophisticated welfare economics" (Fox 1979, 322). Moreover, it was an enduring achievement. As late as 1971, Pauly could still describe Arrow's paper as "the only extended treatment of the economics of medi-cal care and the economics of medical insurance" (Pauly 1971a, 155; cf. 1978, where Arrow's "classic" article still looms large). The analysis of governmental expenditures on health care largely depended on the effort to separate what Arrow's readers regarded as his advocacy of public intervention from his analytical methods. Proposals for consumer cost sharing resulted from this effort.

Early criticisms of Arrow included a commentary by Dennis Lees, a British economist. In discussions of the British National Health Service, Lees (1960; 1961; and cf. 1962), along with John and Sylvia Jewkes (1961), had denied any differences in kind between the health sector and other sectors and accordingly demanded return of British health care to the market. Collaborating with Robert G. Rice, Lees argued (Lees and Rice 1965, 141) that Arrow's supposed market failures were merely consequences of transaction costs that made the absent services prohibitively expensive to produce or buy and pressed the case for voluntary insurance in meeting insurable risks.[71]

Martin Feldstein, then engaged in analyzing the NHS, rejected these demands to return health care to the market, and he attempted to articulate the goals of governmental expenditures on health care. He agreed with the critics' contention that the determination of social costs and benefits of various allocation decisions was difficult in the absence of the market, but he accused the critics of finding in this difficulty "an excuse for returning health care to the market place." Feldstein (1963, 23) thought such proposals not only unhelpful, given the likely permanence of the well-established British NHS, but also misguided: "[S]hould not health care be allocated to maximize the level of health of the nation instead of the satisfaction which consumers derive as they use medical services?" The goal of providing decision makers with the tools to optimize the expenditure of public funds called for specifying the objectives of public policy and identifying the most efficient route to achieving them. Since consumer satisfaction in consumption decisions would not necessarily improve health and since health was the ostensible reason for allocating resources to health care, the specification of objective standards was necessary. The characteristic position of Mushkin and her successors is evident here, as is the relative proximity of their position to that of the planners: opportunity costs of various programs demanded comparison, the precondition of which was the determination of the anticipated improvements in health. Planning was possible and necessary to meet the goals of public policy, but it should invoke health not need and it should rest on the optimization procedures of expenditures analysis.

However, Feldstein soon began to realize that the specification of outcomes demanded by this approach was difficult. In his econometric study of the NHS, he pointed out, among numerous practical obstacles to a full-scale optimization, that there was no agreement on how to measure the health of a community and that there were no "cardinal measures of the efficacy of alternative methods of care" (Feldstein 1967, 188–89). However, his reaction to lack of information was to temporize pending development of suitable concepts and acquisition of the relevant data. He therefore offered a provisional method for comparing the utilization/cost mix of alternative programs.

In the United States, Mark Pauly, though mindful of Feldstein's views, sided with the critics and unhesitatingly embraced consumer sovereignty instead of planning. Following some comments on the exchanges between Arrow and Lees (Pauly 1968), Pauly (1971a) took up the general question of optimizing public provision of insurance. In this effort, he resembled Feldstein in urging, as a matter of principle, that resource allocations must be based not on supposed need for services that might prove only minimally beneficial, but on optimizing the distribution of resources among competing claimants (ibid., chap. 1). However, unlike Feldstein, he supposed that, given a suitable structure for the insurance market, allocation of resources could be accomplished—but only by permitting consumers to express effective demand, rather than empowering planners to meet some goal (whether need or health). Pauly proceeded by identifying Arrow's assumptions and isolating the conditions that permit an optimally organized market for insurance.[72]

While Arrow (1963, 967) held that it "is the general social consensus that the *laissez-faire* solution for medicine is intolerable," and therefore accepted restrictions on quality from the supply side, Pauly began by assuming the possibility of consumer sovereignty and inquiring into the justifications for limiting it. Mindful of Martin Feldstein's "penetrating critique of the needs approach" (Pauly 1971a, 6) and Feldstein's suggestion that the health of the nation serve as the criterion for distribution of health care resources, Pauly argued that the benefits derived from medical care in the form of health are not measurable or even definable and that, at the margin, the consumption of health care may be more satisfying to some than health per se.[73] Having started from the question of optimizing public provision rather than from Feldstein's problem of planning public production, Pauly was willing to let the absence of outcome measures justify reliance on consumer choice. Health care was not an investment good but a consumption good. The variable value of health care, at the margin, to its individual consumers was here laid out as the foundation of consumer sovereignty.

The viability of consumer sovereignty, however, depended also on rejecting other supposed peculiarities that, as noticed earlier, were routinely taken as indicating market failure and therefore justifying collective intervention. The existence of consumer ignorance, one of the major market failures cited by Arrow and numerous other students of the health care market (cf. Mechanic 1978, chap. 12; Langwell and Moore 1982, 5–7), for Pauly justified only provision of information, not of insurance (Pauly 1971a, 11–12). He argued that ignorance may lead not only to underconsumption of care, as widely assumed, but also to excessive consumption, and he supposed that judgments of the appropriate quantity of care reflect paternalistic interference, which "is outside the scope of welfare economics" (cf. Pauly 1978, 17). If the solution to ignorance were public provision of information, then the extent of ignorance would be a result of the degree to which consumers valued available information or took the trouble to obtain it; any lack of information would therefore "not necessarily be an indication of a nonoptimal situation." Remedying ignorance by quality regulation has some merits, according to Pauly, but suffers from the lack of a "meaningful way to measure quality." Moreover, "it is doubtful that the current situation of stringent licensing [of practitioners] and actual legal barriers to information flow is an efficient one" (Pauly 1971a, 12–13; cf. Pauly 1978, 21–27).

Pauly's views about consumer sovereignty and ignorance reveal a major paradox of competitive theory. He justified consumer sovereignty by the lack of information to serve the expert determination of either the extent of need or the degree of quality; nevertheless, he recommended public provision of information "about the results of physicians' work, about the quality of hospitals, and about the effectiveness of courses of treatment, and about the prices physicians and hospitals charge" (Pauly 1971a, 12). In making a consumption decision, consumers should possess whatever information could be made available, but significant use could not be expected of it.[74] Characteristic features of the theory of cost sharing are the view of health care as only one of many commodities offered to consumers in the market place and the supposition that the worth of health care is measured above all else by the sovereign judgment of the consumer.[75]

The Theory of the Demand for Health Insurance and Cost Sharing

Having argued that Arrow had overestimated the extent of market failure and unnecessarily limited consumer choice, Pauly claimed himself able to isolate only one economically justifiable foundation for public provision: externalities in consumption (in particular, the benefit derived by some individuals from the consumption of a good or service by others). The equity claim that the prevailing distribution of income is inappropriate and should be improved by governmental provision reduces, for Pauly, to the same argument that Paul Feldman developed for the analysis of any publicly provided enhancements to consumption: Those who desire public programs to increase the consumption of goods or services by others should be considered the beneficiaries of the programs and taxed to pay for them. Pauly therefore endorsed taxpayer sovereignty. His task then reduced to optimizing the tax-supported subsidy.

However, his analysis of optimization also introduced an element of consumer sovereignty, for it also recognized individual diversity in demand for insurance (Pauly 1971a). In supposing that health care is a normal good (that is, that the consumer buys more of it with increasing income) and that individual demand depends solely on income, Pauly showed that providing additional care, reflecting the externality in consumption, could be achieved by a cut in price per unit (that is, insurance) that varies with income (that is, that the effective price of care should rise with income). In addition, since individuals differ in their demand for medical care, the total subsidy would vary with income. Here, Pauly established the fundamental principle of income-graduated subsidy as the foundation for efficient public provision. Not universal entitlement to comprehensive benefits, but unequal public provision is optimal. Moreover, by noting that individuals would be willing to pay a charge for the privilege of buying subsidized care, he pointed out that coinsurance could be invoked to encourage conservation of care. Cost sharing, that is, a user charge, could constrain utilization.

On the basis of this analysis, Pauly proposed a system of "variable subsidy insurance" (VSI), which would provide virtually comprehensive coverage for the poorest, impose deductibles or coinsurance that increase with income for those of somewhat higher incomes, and for others supply a "catastrophic" policy (ibid., 58–64; Pauly 1971b, 33–48). Simultaneously, Martin Feldstein (1971) proposed an essentially similar scheme, under the name "major risk insurance" (MRI), which, like VSI, rested on considerations about the impossibility of expert determination of need, consumer sovereignty, and taxpayer sovereignty.

Income-graduated consumer cost sharing respected consumer sovereignty (because it rested on acknowledging individual variation in the demand for health insurance) and taxpayer sovereignty (because it responded to the externality in consumption). It presaged efficiency, moreover, both because it rested on the optimization principles of welfare economics and because it provided an explicit mechanism to conserve costs. The possibility of separating optimal resource allocation from distributional equity, which Arrow denied, thus issued from pursuit of the analytical model Arrow first proposed.

Cost Sharing, the Supply Side of the Market, and Equity

In offering these proposals, both Pauly and Feldstein explicitly rejected any direct efforts to reorganize the delivery of health services (that is, restructure the supply side of the market for health care) and called for minimizing the role of government in the market. For example, Pauly remarked (1971b, 36; cf. M. Feldstein 1971, 103, 105; and Seidman 1980, 319) that VSI does not entail any measures that would directly alter the delivery system itself. . . . [t]here is really no substantive empirical knowledge about what are, and what are not, efficient ways to deliver care. Since the need for change has not been conclusively established, the approach that would be followed in VSI would be to design incentives that would induce the system to arrange itself in appropriate ways rather than to use direct public intervention to produce change.

Though both Pauly (1971a, 63) and Martin Feldstein (1971, 105) recognized the possibility that their proposals were compatible with prepaid group practice (that is, competitive plans), their aim was to avoid direct structural reform (cf. Seidman 1980, 319).

The unwillingness to tamper with the supply side resulted only in part from the perceived lack of the knowledge that might authorize structural reform. In part, it also resulted from the same sorts of conviction that motivated the growing interest in incentives. Government, particularly to the degree that it undertakes direct intervention in the economy, does a poor job. Controls are ineffective or counterproductive (Pauly 1971b, 33, 41). By contrast, an incentives-based approach could allow government to achieve its ends without meddling (Pauly 1971a, 63; 1971b, 41; M. Feldstein 1971, 98, 103, 105). Desire to avoid structural reform also rested on the desire to avoid antagonizing the interests. Feldstein, for example, expressed concern (1971, 98, 103) that controls "would certainly require a large number of arbitrary policy decisions and engender the hostility of the basic providers," and he argued that under MRI the "current freedom of physicians and hospitals would be preserved." Incentives, that is, could preserve the goodwill of providers by shielding them from arbitrary controls. Advocates of competitive plans were confronted with the same problem, and they invoked a similar solution. However, they differed from advocates of cost sharing in demanding reform on the supply side of the market to place the incentives directly on the providers.

Advocates of cost sharing also argued that expansion of entitlement demanded lowering the standard of care. They took up this theme in the late 1970s when, despite a decade of discussion, no NHI proposal had yet been enacted. In Pauly's volume on NHI, for example, Pauly himself observed (1980b, 2) that advocates of comprehensive benefits under NHI, in refusing to accept anything less, had permitted the poor and those suffering from catastrophic illness to be "held hostage for comprehensive NHI"; Bernard Friedman proposed (1980, 101–2) a replacement for Medicaid that would permit increased protection of the poor through enhanced availability of lower-quality services; and Thomas W. Grannemann observed (1980, 116) that "federal subsidies apply only to high-cost forms of care, making it difficult for states to deliver care [under Medicaid] to many recipients," and he suggested that expansion of eligibility for benefits may rest on abandoning care of high cost and low marginal value.

Advocates of cost sharing thus argued that proponents of NHI had frustrated the achievement of their own equity goals. Expansion of entitlement could not be accomplished by entitling all to a standard of care previously enjoyed only by the middle class, but by subsidizing demand such that lower-income recipients of funds could purchase less than the middle-class standard. Proponents of competitive plans offered a similar argument, as shown below, but they applied it to the supply side of the market under regulation.

THE EMERGENCE OF HEALTH CARE PLANS: COMPETITION VERSUS REGULATION

Advocates of competitive health care plans were moved by many of the same concerns that motivated proponents of comprehensive NHI, but they diverged from NHI proponents in their analysis of the reasons for the shortcomings of the health sector and in their proposed remedy. Advocates of NHI accepted the public interest model of regulation that justified regulation as a remedy for market failure; like Arrow, they traced market failure to the peculiarities of medical care; and, persuaded that those peculiarities rendered medical care inherently different from other commodities, they supposed that structural reform was ruled out and regulation was the sole recourse. Advocates of competitive plans, by contrast, believed that the organization of the health sector reflected the interests of the providers of health services (as opposed to the interests of consumers and therefore the public interest); that the well-catalogued shortcomings of American health care could be traced to provider dominance, not to the peculiarities of medical care; that regulatory mechanisms proposed or already in place served only to enhance provider dominance and intensify its effects; and, like the exponents of cost sharing, that medical care was not inherently unsuited to the market. They could therefore contemplate thoroughgoing structural reform of the health sector. The aim was not to compel providers to behave against their interests, but to restructure their institutions with suitable incentives that would bring their interests into conformity with the public interest.

Promoting Structural Reform

One simple expedient toward the goal of structural reform was the new term, health maintenance organization or HMO, introduced by Ellwood early in the 1970s. Though the idea of the HMO was heavily indebted to antecedent traditions in prepaid group practice (PGP), Ellwood preferred the new coinage. Because it lacked the traditional connotations of PGP, an HMO might escape the traditional criticisms leveled at PGPs by the med-

ical profession; and because it offered flexibility in organizing the delivery of stipulated services under prospective reimbursement, an HMO
might attract providers interested in designing arrangements suited to
their own tastes.[76]

A second and more profound way to enhance the prospects for structural reform against established interests was the incentives-based
approach. As Ellwood and his colleagues put it in 1971 (1971a, 293; cf.
Enthoven 1980, 118),

> Only the physician can determine what care is necessary, and, therefore, only
> he can eliminate unneeded expense. The physician cannot be policed to do
> so but must be motivated by professional ethics and by organizational
> arrangements which align his economic incentives with those of the
> consumer.

The role of physicians as experts was unavoidable. The point was not to
deprive them of that role but to exploit it; the means would not be to control practice, but to constrain it by devising suitable incentives. Because it
left decision making about treatment in the hands of providers and
abjured controlling providers' behavior, the incentives-based approach
seemed less likely than direct controls to antagonize providers and more
likely than intensified regulation to preserve their autonomy (cf. Enthoven
1980, 141; Schultze 1977; Meyer 1985).

Advocates of competitive plans therefore joined advocates of cost
sharing in espousing incentives as a means to achieve reforms without
unduly antagonizing providers. However, advocates of plans differed from
advocates of cost sharing in supposing that incentives had to be applied
directly to the providers (by reorganization of their institutions), not
indirectly (by changing the economic incentives of consumers). Cost
sharing seeks to reform the demand side of the market; competitive plans,
the supply side.

Regulation, because it was imposed directly upon the unrecon-
structed health sector, ruled out structural reform. Ellwood and his
colleagues pressed this point early (1971b, III-1; and cf. III-5), asserting,
"Reinforcing existing professional controls in any new programs aimed at
regulating the cost and quality of health care will assure the continuance
of the existing delivery system." They also urged the same point about planning: "Preserving provider involvement in planning and allocating critical
health resources minimizes the possibility that planners will make drastic
structural and organizational changes in the health delivery system."
Therefore, advocates of competitive plans sought to undermine the case
for regulation and simultaneously sustain the case for a competitive
market. They have therefore persistently posed the alternatives that give
this chapter its title: competition versus regulation. Havighurst, for
example, observed in 1970 (1970a, 229) that

the overriding choice that has to be made is between a market-oriented delivery system and a system in which the financing of care is taken over by the Federal government; adoption of the latter expedient would necessitate extensive regulatory measures to perform the allocative and cost-controlling service normally rendered by market forces.

Similarly, in their classic enunciation of the "health maintenance strategy," Ellwood and his associates proposed (1971a, 291)

a shift from the present Federal regulatory, investment-planning strategy to a strategy that would promote a health maintenance industry.
   The health maintenance strategy envisions a series of government and private actions designed to promote a highly diversified, pluralistic, and competitive industry. . . .

(Cf. also Enthoven 1980, 71, 110–13; P. Feldstein 1983, 248–49; and Havighurst 1982, chap. 1.)

Competition: Incentives Harnessed to the Public Interest

This section focuses on the first term in the dichotomy "competition and regulation"; it describes the advantages of competitive plans that rendered them attractive to their advocates as a candidate for a new national health policy. Advocates have typically described these advantages in the briefest compass, concentrating instead on criticism and analysis of the major alternatives based on regulation. As noted earlier, only from the late 1970s did advocates of plans find themselves prepared to translate their principles into detailed proposals. The principles are the subject of this section; the campaign against regulation waged by theorists of plans follows; advocates' use of empirical evidence about regulation in the health sector,[77] their ideas about how to realize their principles, and their detailed proposals are not treated here.[78]

    Advocates of plans saw a series of benefits deriving from the incentive structures within plans and the market incentives governing competition among plans. As large, integrated firms, competitive plans would reduce the fragmented structure (or cottage-industry character) of the health sector, diminishing the number and increasing the size of providers.[79] The maze of providers and services now confronting consumers would be simplified. Buying comprehensive services from plans, consumers would obtain from the plans themselves a contractual guarantee of obtaining a stipulated package of services as well as guidance to their availability and use. Consumers would thus no longer need to identify and compare large numbers of alternatives. Because they would be financed by capitation, plans would share with consumers the financial risks of con-

sumers' illnesses and therefore have an incentive to apply resources efficiently in providing therapy and preventive services. Among the
efficiencies anticipated from this sharing of risk were declines in the exploitation of high technology and in the use of specialists' services and corresponding increases in primary care and out-of-hospital care. Risk sharing
would thus remedy many of the widely acknowledged problems of the
health sector.[80] As Havighurst (1974, 255) put it:

> The competition provided by HMOs would in due course, in my judgment,
> generate spontaneous utilization and cost controls that would go very far
> toward solving not only the cost and overutilization problems associated with
> overbedding but other problems as well.

Large organized providers would enjoy the advantages offered by
economies of scale and could offer packages of services geared to a variety
of consumer preferences. Large organizations could also devote resources
to establishing markets in relatively underserved areas, contributing to
solving the generally lamented geographical maldistribution of providers
(though a solution to geographical maldistribution would also require
expansion of entitlement so that purchasing power would attract
providers).[81]

Competition among plans for consumers would induce plans to offer
various combinations of quality and cost, thus enhancing the likelihood
that a variety of consumer preferences could be satisfied in the market; and
competition among plans for cost-efficient providers would reward efficient production of health services.[82] By imposing minimal limits on entry
into the market and permitting maximal flexibility in organizational and
managerial forms, policy makers could anticipate the appearance of new
and more efficient technologies for the supply, bundling, and delivery of
health services.[83]

Competition among plans along dimensions of quality and cost
could further meet varieties of preferences and simultaneously exert downward pressure on prices. Finally, sufficient growth in the share of the
market dominated by competitive plans would place them into genuine
competition with the FFS sector, which could therefore be expected to
evolve in socially desirable ways.[84]

These bold and straightforward assertions possessed great appeal to
the Nixon administration, which needed some novel way to intervene in
the growing "health care crisis." Under the sponsorship of the administration, Ellwood's ideas entered the public debate about health policy. The
theory of competitive plans had been launched (though neither the
administration nor Congress proved ready to realize the health maintenance strategy in any form more ambitious than a demonstration
project) (Falkson 1980; L Brown 1983).

Provider Dominance and Regulation as Instruments of Cartelization

The case for structural reform, at least in its main principles, was thus simple and brief. However, reform implied a halt to the advance of regulation and the reversal of its prior progress. Moreover, advocates of plans regarded regulation as more than an obstacle to reform; they also believed that it gave further legal sanction to the main causes of disarray in American health care. In view of growing pressure for regulation of the health sector and the historical durability of regulatory institutions, once installed, they believed the argument against regulation of the health sector was urgent.[85]

Advocates of plans argued that regulation only further fortified provider interests that were already well-entrenched in the health sector. While Ellwood was satisfied simply to assert this claim (for example, Ellwood 1972a; Ellwood et al. 1971b; InterStudy 1970a), Havighurst assumed the task of arguing for it. He began from an antitrust perspective and later coupled his own indictment with themes drawn from the antiregulatory literature. He concluded that the market failures widely taken to justify regulation were owing to provider dominance, that providers had prevented a genuine market from coming into existence, and that regulation gave providers additional protection from the discipline of a competitive market.

He began in 1970 by confronting the widespread belief that the peculiarities of the health care market were the result of market failure. Instead, in a study of HMOs, he offered the thesis "that a congeries of legislatively and professionally conceived and executed trade restraints have heretofore prevented the market from functioning with close to its potential effectiveness and that restoration of the market regime offers the best hope for solving the nation's health care problem in all of its numerous dimensions." He acknowledged that "my advocacy of a market-oriented system will seem strange to those who believe that the present health care crisis itself reflects a colossal market failure." However, "A combination of [professional] 'ethics,' customs of the trade, and pressures of varying degrees of subtlety have repressed even the vestiges of price competition in the delivery of physicians' services. Under these conditions, the market has never had a chance." For Havighurst, the implication was clear: "Any student of antitrust knows that a self-regulatory regime organized for the prevention of 'unethical business practices' is likely to be a device to suppress competition." Accordingly,

> It cannot be argued that the market's failure accounts for the present state of affairs. In attaching blame, if that is important, it seems unfair to expect the organized medical profession to have acted against its self interest. Rather, the fault lies with well-meaning policy makers who failed to make the profession's trade-restraining activities unlawful and indeed enacted many

trade restraints into positive law. The mystique surrounding medical care and the "physician-patient relation" served to validate the profession's assertions of high ethical and quality standards and led many well-meaning persons into becoming, in Kessel's phrase borrowed from the 1930s, "dupes of the interests."

Havighurst subsequently provided an exhaustive analysis of trade restraints in the market for physicians' services.[86]

In discussing HMOs, it was natural for Havighurst to focus on restraints engineered by the organized profession (rather than by institutional providers), for it had been the chief source of opposition to prepaid group practice. Regulation of capital investment, however, concerned institutional providers (chiefly voluntary hospitals); it was the counterpart in the hospital industry to physicians' long-noticed "professional dominance" in the market for curative services. The progress of CON elicited Havighurst's interest in supply regulation in the hospital industry. To explore the topic, he organized a conference on it in 1972. To develop his own position, he drew inspiration from the radical criticism of health planning in *The American Health Empire* (1970) (which treated planning as an instrument of provider interests), and he predicated his criticism of regulation on themes developed in the antiregulatory literature.[87]

The conference aimed "to provide skeptics [of CON] with a forum in which to confront the issues and the advocates." The motive was the expectation that the demonstrated shortcomings of regulation in other sectors would likewise characterize regulation of health facilities by CON. As Havighurst put it in his introduction (1974, 1):

> economists, who are familiar with experience in . . . regulated industries, find it difficult to share the optimism of many experts in the health world concerning the operation of certificate-of-need laws. In their view, restrictions on growth and new entry in other industries have eliminated important competitive pressures and opportunities for consumer choice, created privileged market positions for certain interests, weakened guarantees of efficiency and high-quality performance, retarded certain kinds of innovation while overstimulating others, raised prices, and generally misallocated resources—all with only debatable public benefits, though clear private ones. Moreover, recent economic literature has purported to document the case that regulation's failures are not mere aberrations . . . but are inherent in the political economy of regulation itself.

In the paper of 1973, Havighurst pursued these contentions. There, he confronted planning and CON with a succession of hypotheses, drawn from the antiregulatory literature, and he argued in extenso that, as in other sectors so also in the health sector, planning and regulation were instruments of the regulated interests.[88] This position was bolstered by Havighurst's argument that the special privileges of nonprofit institutions amounted to unfair competitive advantages (Havighurst 1970c, 752,

757–59; 1981, 1133–34; 1982, 363–75; Russell 1980, 278). From this perspective, the choice between competition and regulation reduced to that
"between a system controlled directly or indirectly by essentially well-
meaning providers who accommodate their public responsibilities with
their own self-interest and a system of social control by impersonal market
forces allowing consumers a larger impact and assigning the government
the less intrusive roles of promoter of the competition and referee
(Havighurst 1973, 1217; cf. Ellwood et al. 1971a, 293; and Enthoven 1980,
94, 112).

Regulation of an Expansionary System: A Conservative Measure

Given their interest in incentives and in structural reform, advocates of
competitive plans suggested that widely acknowledged shortcomings of the
health sector could be analyzed in terms of what Charles Schultze had first
called "negative" and later "perverse incentives" resulting from provider
dominance. Thus, in his detailed analysis of CON (1973, 1155), Havighurst
traced CON to "demonstrable market failures attributable to the manner
in which health care is paid for, the control which providers exert over
demand for health care, and the incentives affecting both consumption
and investment decisions." The "main argument" for CON, he suggested
(ibid., 1159–60), was

> quite powerful. It says that the mechanism of third-party payment based on
> cost reimbursement, when coupled with utilization decisions, results in
> externalization [via higher premiums for private insurance and higher taxes
> for public insurance] of much of the business risk involved in creating excess
> capacity.

Similarly, McClure (1976, 31–39, 55) traced cost escalation and other
leading problems of American health care to incentives toward specialized,
high-cost care and the open-ended financing provided by traditional third-
party reimbursement, and Enthoven devoted an entire chapter (1980,
chap. 2, cf. also p. 10; cf. Enthoven 1978a, 651–53) to "Irrational Incentives
and the Growth of Health Care Spending." The argument covered not only
institutional providers (that is, largely voluntary hospitals) but also physicians, whose "technological imperative" was allowed to operate under
third-party payment in both inpatient and outpatient practice (for example, Havighurst and Blumstein 1975, 20–21, 25–30; McClure 1976, 33, 36;
Enthoven 1980, 23).

The incentives approach suggested that, in principle, regulation
could not remedy the problems of the health sector because under regulation the perverse incentive structure that served provider interests at the
expense of the public interest continued to operate. Regulation was not
merely a remedy applied ex post facto; it institutionalized existing, per-

verse incentives. According to Enthoven (1980, 101, 104, 110), for example, the hospital cost-containment program pushed by the Carter administration "contained nothing to correct the perverse incentives in our dominant financing system"; "the effect [of CON] is to protect existing providers from competition from new cost-reducing innovators and to force the efficient to subsidize the inefficient"; and the PSRO program, "like the other regulatory systems, leaves the cost-increasing incentives of fee for service intact." He also argued (1978a, 656; cf. 1980, 101) that Senator Kennedy's Health Security proposal for NHI cannot work, because "[e]xperience with other regulated industries, and with NHI in other countries, suggests that the government would freeze the system in its existing patterns." Quite generally, "[i]n the regulatory approach government would leave today's cost-increasing incentives in place and then try to stop them from having their natural effect by direct detailed controls . . . intended to substitute for rational economic incentives. In my view, the regulatory approach is like trying to make water run uphill, whereas in the competitive market approach the government is merely trying to channel the stream in its downhill course" (Enthoven 1980, 94; cf. Meyer and Penner 1980, 24, 26).

Havighurst offered similar but more detailed analysis. Mindful of the antiregulatory literature, he argued that the responsiveness of regulatory agencies to the parties at interest reduced regulation to a mechanism for subordination of public goals to the goals of providers; and therefore, he claimed, regulation perpetuated the perverse incentives that had produced the problems of the health sector in the first place.[89] He later argued that limiting capital investment by CON places the job of rationing use of limited resources on providers, though "hardly any thought has been given to whether providers can realistically be expected to serve primarily public needs rather than their own preferences and values in performing this allocative function. Despite the lack of assurance on this score, regulation is being implemented in a way that perpetuates the very provider dominance which has produced excessive emphasis on high-technology acute care rendered in institutional settings. . . ." Therefore, "far from sparing the regulators embarrassment in their efforts to limit the health sector's spending proclivities, providers can be expected to expose the regulators' veiled attempts to erode what providers will characterize as quality of care" (Havighurst 1977a, 314; Enthoven 1980, 50). As wielded by providers within the politics of regulatory institutions, the quality imperative would make cost control under CON impossible.

Regulation made the perverse features of the health sector permanent and rigid, ensuring the perpetuation and intensification of the well-known problems of American health care. Regulation was conservative; restructuring to foster competition, radical. By arguing that regulation perpetuated and exacerbated existing problems, by aligning his own analysis with that of radical critics (such as Health-PAC), and by demanding structural reform of the health sector, Havighurst felt entitled to the radical label, and he clearly relished the irony of stigmatizing regulation as conservative (Havighurst 1970b, 668; 1970c, 742; 1973, 1155–56; cf. P. Feldstein 1983, 282).

The Arbitrariness of Regulation

To theorists of plans, a radicalism rooted in American traditions of private enterprise and market mechanisms seemed vastly superior to the arbitrariness of regulation. The succession of regulatory laws that marked the late 1960s and the 1970s seemed to advocates of competition prima facie evidence that regulatory failures, by eliciting new, more pervasive, and more intrusive forms of regulation, presaged unacceptable levels of governmental interference in private decision making as well as excessive concentration on cost control to the detriment of other needs (for example, McClure 1976, 43–44; cf. also Havighurst 1977a, 314; P. Feldstein 1983, 275, 282–83).

Some advocates of plans supposed that a sufficiently stringent form of regulation could perhaps succeed in containing costs, but that its effectiveness would be costly and its methods unpalatable. Enthoven, for example, remarked that

> A system that is sufficiently tough and comprehensive could do the job [of cost containment]. In effect, the government would be controlling the budget of each hospital. [However,] given our values and our political system as it actually operates, such an effective cost-containment program seems unlikely. But even if such a control program were effective in controlling the aggregate growth of hospital expenditures, it would have done nothing to improve the efficiency of hospitals, the quality of their services, or the equity with which those services are distributed.[90]

From this perspective, advocates of competition interpreted the failure of the Carter administration to obtain passage of a hospital cost-containment bill as evidence that Congress was wary of the arbitrariness entailed by the intensification of regulation (Enthoven 1978a, 654; Havighurst 1977a, 316–17; 1981, 1121–22; 1982, 39–42, 140). Havighurst, in particular, regarded the failure of the Carter proposals as the final confession of failure of the planning and regulatory agenda, as the occasion that made Congress receptive to the alternative possibilities offered by competition, and as the backdrop to the 1979 amendments to PL 93-641 (written in part under Havighurst's influence) that explicitly mandated competition and cost containment as goals to be fostered by regulatory agencies.[91]

The arbitrariness of regulation was more than a practical concern; it also struck at the heart of what advocates of competition believed to be fundamental American values. This perception rested on a preference for consumer sovereignty reminiscent of the one developed by advocates of cost sharing. However, for theorists of plans, the importance of consumer sovereignty was intensified by the perception that expenditures on health services had not produced commensurate improvements in health and by a consequent decline in faith in the efficacy of health care; and it was rendered urgent by a perception of elitism in the conduct of recent forms of governmental regulation.

Enthoven, for example, doubted whether aggregate levels of spending on health care were worth the cost. Introducing his book of 1980, he maintained that "much of the value of medical care relates to the *quality* of life—to the relief of suffering and the restoration of function. And we have no good statistical tools to measure this on an aggregate basis. So we cannot give a clear answer to the question of whether or not we are getting much health improvement for these large increases in spending." Given third-party payment, as opposed to the use of the consumer's own money, he maintained, the value of such services for the money is unclear.[92]

To this degree, Enthoven resembled Pauly; but Enthoven went further, arguing that the usual financing arrangements, by misallocating resources, deprive consumers of clearer health benefits that alternative spending might produce: "People's preferences for risk reductions, compared with the benefits they would receive from other uses of the resources, ought to be considered. Some risk reductions are not worth having at the cost. Even from the point of view of health, at some point dollars are better spent on other things, such as food and housing, rather than on more medical care" (Enthoven 1980, 51; cf. McClure 1976, 24–25).

The importance of consumer sovereignty thus increased in proportion to growing skepticism about the value of medical care.[93] Havighurst gave forceful expression (1977a, 318) to a similar view:

> The new awareness about medicine's uncertain benefits . . . has yet to overcome the tendency of policy makers . . . to disparage private choices between health care and other things. Yet increasing skepticism among commonly recognized authorities about the value of health care at the margin suggests (1) that the range and subjectivity of consumers' preferences with respect to medical care does not necessarily signify consumer ignorance or irrationality and (2) that different people can come rationally to different conclusions about what quantity and quality of services to buy. . . . Moreover, private choices are made with information concerning personal preferences that obviously is not available to anyone except the individuals involved. In a democratic society, private decisions might be viewed as having comparative or even absolute legitimacy on this account alone.

The paternalism of regulation and its increasing arbitrariness seemed to threaten traditional values and pose a burden greater than the practical one of burdensome bureaucracy and misallocated resources, however significant these concerns might have been. Moreover, the regulators themselves seemed given to an unprecedented level of elitism and authoritarian disdain for the diversity of individual preferences (Havighurst 1974, 268–69; 1978a). Regulation increasingly had fallen into the hands of a "new class," active chiefly in the newer forms of regulation (which, unlike the traditional, industry-by-industry approach, cut across industrial lines to impose standards for environmental protection and occupational health). Though CON agencies possessed responsibility solely for the hospital industry, Havighurst nevertheless saw in them the elitism of the new class, whose behavior made intensified regulation an ominous prospect:

> [m]y own view is that the ultimate goal [of cost-containment policies] is not stringency for its own sake but an allocation of resources in accordance with people's revealed preferences and that political processes are incapable of determining, measuring, and giving appropriate effect to those preferences. Indeed, as political processes fall more and more under the control and influence of "the new class," they seem less and less likely to serve pluralistic values that I regard as important, more stifling indeed than mere "bureaucracy" ever was. There is no doubt that "the new class" is highly active in health sector regulation and that important values are at stake. Perhaps it is well to draw these lines explicitly and to let the overriding issue concerning the future scope of health care regulation be seen as, quite simply, whether this is any longer a liberal democracy in which there is a presumption in favor of the individual's right to choose for himself and to have his preferences catered to in the economic marketplace.[94]

A similarly revealing statement appears in Havighurst's book on deregulation. There he conceded that his arguments for competition may not overcome doubt

> that enhanced competition under appropriate incentives will bring about material changes in health care financing and delivery that will actually help in controlling costs. It should be a sufficient answer to such doubts to state that the real issue has nothing at all to do with the validity of such predictions. Instead, the only relevant question should be the feasibility of establishing a process that effectively reveals consumer preferences and induces providers . . . to serve them. If such a process were in place, then it could be powerfully argued that the market's verdict should be accepted as an expression of people's wishes—even if the allocation of resources turned out to be no different than it is today.[95]

Competitive Plans and Consumer Sovereignty

Theorists of plans therefore took consumer sovereignty even more seriously than the proponents of cost sharing. Their enhanced estimate of consumer sovereignty correspondingly enhanced the importance of the problem of consumer ignorance, particularly since plans contained incentives for providers to economize and therefore perhaps to cut corners.[96]

However, except for Ellwood and his colleagues (for example, Ellwood et al. 1973), advocates of plans seemed no more sensitive to the paradox that lack of objective standards of care and declining faith in the marginal utility of medical care foreclosed any definition of quality that was independent of the preferences of individuals and thus rendered impossible any clear determination of what information about quality ought to be made generally available in the market or of how information was to be exploited. As shown by the quotations above regarding consumer sovereignty, advocates of competitive plans shared with proponents of cost sharing the conviction that providers should bend not to professionals' standards of quality, but consumers'.

Plans were nevertheless thought superior to cost sharing in facilitating rational decision making by consumers. Plans remove the decisions from the occasion of service, when a vulnerable patient is unlikely to make cool assessments; they relieve the patient of judging technical matters, leaving such assessments to professionals; and they therefore confine consumers to making the less technically burdensome choice among competing health care plans (for example, Enthoven 1980, 34, 139; and Havighurst 1974, 263–64). Moreover, competition among plans would likely narrow range of choice, simplifying the decisions consumers must make.[97]

However, the extent to which a system of competitive plans could bend to consumer demand and yet do better than cost sharing under fee-for-service in protecting the consumer from the consequences of ignorance was not so simply dispatched. Though enrollment in a plan delegated many technical decisions to providers and though the choice among plans was perhaps less technically demanding than a choice among competitive solo practitioners, choosing *among* plans still implied judgments of quality and cost: evaluating a plan required evaluating the benefits it offered, the claims made for the quality of its services at various prices, and (if a plan is not a new entrant into the market) the past history of its performance. Enthoven's solution to the problem involved several considerations. In part the theory of the competitive plans, because it anticipated more direct exposure of providers to the risk of dissatisfying consumers, suggested that the system would be self-policing; in part, the market could be "policed by a minority of well-informed cost-conscious consumers" (Enthoven 1980, 138); in part, the dangers, as just noticed, were thought to be reduced by the relatively lesser technical complexity of a choice among plans; and, perhaps most important of all, a significant governmental role, involving procompetitive regulation and various quality and performance standards, would protect the consumer (ibid., 94, 126–30).

Meyer (1981, 429–33) strongly criticized Enthoven's reliance on procompetitive regulation as needlessly limiting consumer choice, but a likely more characteristic disagreement among advocates of plans revolved about determining the desirable degree of limitation and the role of government in structuring consumer choice. Thus Havighurst (1982, 396–416) responded to Enthoven by suggesting not merely that government would excessively narrow the range of choice, but also that procompetitive regulation is likely to possess all the disadvantages of regulation generally, including the use of the internal subsidy to finance redistribution. However, he did not join Meyer in leaving the consumer to indulge preferences without technical assistance. Instead, he supposed that employers and unions could be expected to police the market and serve consumer interests provided that tax subsidies to fringe benefits are reduced.[98] Only for individual (as opposed to group) coverage should the government take responsibility for protecting consumers. As for public programs, Havighurst had relatively less to say, despite their potentially immense influence on the evolution of the health care market (ibid., 397, 416–19).

Regulation, Competition, and Entitlement: The Utility of NHI

Advocates of plans were opposed not to the expansion of entitlement under NHI but to the regulatory mechanisms that proponents of NHI aimed to exploit. As Havighurst put it in 1980,

> Market advocates have focused their attention on the private sector and have hoped for its reinvigoration through competition. By contrast, regulation advocates have been primarily concerned with public programs, and have generally envisioned a future involving an expansion of such programs and of direct public payment for health care. With this orientation, they have naturally perceived effective regulation as essential to make public programs, as currently designed, workable and to permit the desired expansion to occur. . . . It may thus be noted that where one comes out in the regulation-versus-competition debate has depended heavily in the past on where one was coming from and was headed.[99]

Competitive theorists did not oppose expansion of entitlement, but sought a new health policy that might serve as an example for public programs:

> Public financing programs, while large and important, are seen [by market advocates] as simply mirroring insurance practices that developed in the private sector under conditions of market failure; the codification of these practices in public programs was inevitable in a political environment in which providers' preferences for the existing system had to be respected. By the same token, market advocates see the private sector as capable of leading public programs out of the wilderness by providing new options and approaches that public programs can either emulate or allow beneficiaries to purchase in the private sector with subsidized buying power.

Ellwood (1984) reports that he too began with concern not for entitlement but for the overall performance of the health sector and that his approach supposed that structural reform of the health sector was a precondition for expansion of entitlement.

However, serious attention to entitlement was scarcely incompatible with advocacy of competitive plans. For example, McClure, as one of Ellwood's colleagues, appears to have begun from the same position as Ellwood, but by 1976 he was plunging directly into the problem of organizing a public program:

> [T]he American medical care system will require significant change under any foreseeable form of [NHI]. Indeed, the medical care system is so central to every issue now pressuring government to intervene in health care that significant change appears unavoidable even in the absence of NHI. . . . [S]o tightly are the delivery and the financing of medical care interwoven that the fate of NHI and the medical care system are inextricably tied; decisions on either will determine the shape and success of both. Therefore, in asking what kind of NHI we want, Americans might best begin by asking what kind of future medical care system we want. They are the same question. (McClure 1976, 22–23)

Similarly, Enthoven's proposals (1980, 114) would create a system of national health insurance predicated on structural reform of the market for health services and cost sharing of subsidized purchases of insurance.

Even if Havighurst did not share the interest of McClure and Enthoven in entitlement programs, in the early 1970s he used the apparently imminent passage of a national health insurance as a weapon in the struggle against regulation. In taking this tack, he provided the counterpart on the supply side of the contention of proponents of cost sharing that advocates of NHI had held equity hostage while insisting on comprehensive benefits. The argument centered on the financing of charity care with the internal subsidy available under regulation and the use of entry controls to prevent cream-skimming competitors from appropriating and ultimately eroding the subsidy.

As noted earlier, regulators typically cross-subsidize unremunerative services by charging monopoly prices for remunerative services. Called by Posner "taxation by regulation" and by Comanor and Mitchell "planning by regulation," the procedure has been criticized on several grounds: it causes allocational inefficiencies and excessive expansion of the regulated industries; it escapes accountability to the public by its removal from the normal legislative contexts; and it inhibits innovation because the entry controls necessary to maintain the subsidy exclude innovators and shield the regulated firms from competitive pressure toward innovation.[100] Cross-subsidization had been justified by the supposition that its practitioners possess an orientation toward public service and a sense of beneficence toward public goods. Given that supposition, the practice requires protection in the form of entry controls, for otherwise competitors will enter the market to benefit from the artificially high prices that generate the subsidies.

Among the forms of beneficence generally regarded as financed by cross-subsidization is the provision of unremunerated or charity care to the poor (Havighurst 1973, 1164–65, 1188–92). With reference to the anti-regulatory literature, Havighurst urged (1970c, 752, 786 n. 217; 1973, 1190 n.; 1974, 252) on grounds of both accountability and efficiency that cross-subsidization for this purpose should be replaced with direct subsidy from tax revenues. The argument amounts to the claim that enactment of NHI (understood to be tax-subsidized purchasing power for the poor) would eliminate the need for cross-subsidization of charity care, therefore for entry restriction, and therefore for the regulatory apparatus that accomplishes these tasks (Havighurst 1970c, 752, 768 n., 786 n.; 1973, 1165; 1974, 251). Indeed, Havighurst followed the argument of Reuben Kessel, suggesting that the advance of public programs had already diminished the need for much charity care and significantly reduced its extent. Havighurst concluded that existing public programs had already diminished the equity justification for cross-subsidization under regulation. NHI would merely complete a job already begun (Havighurst 1970c, 768 n., citing Kessel 1958; cf. also Kessel 1970, 273). Far from opposing expanded entitlement, then, Havighurst invoked it to foster the case against regulation.

In fact, in the early 1970s, the problem Havighurst saw in entitlement was that it might not be expanded sufficiently. He noted (Havighurst 1970c, 764) that "the public has been dependent on hospital monopolies for a long time to generate the funds needed to care for the indigent," and he was concerned (Havighurst 1974) that this method of "enforced charity" by internal cross-subsidization might be preferred to a properly financed system of NHI and thus perpetuate regulation. Paradoxically, the advocates of the poor, according to Havighurst, anticipating their ultimate ability to "impose themselves politically on the management of the health care institutions," have supported entry restrictions, despite the existence of "alternatives that might leave the poor themselves, though perhaps not their representatives, better off, indeed with some access to the so-called mainstream of American medical care" (ibid., 253).

Enthoven's position regarding the financing of public programs largely coincides with Havighurst's. In arguing the fairness of his proposals to the poor, Enthoven asserted that his Consumer-Choice Health Plan "uses the most effective way to redistribute purchasing power for medical care—that is, directly. It takes money from taxpayers and pays it to lower-income people in the form of tax-credits and vouchers. By this method, the amount of redistribution is clearly visible, and one can be sure that the money reaches its intended target. . . ."[101] Moreover, the plan "focuses on raising the quality of care available to the poor by ensuring that they have the money (through vouchers) and the access (through the government-run open enrollment) to the same plans that serve middle-income people." Visible public subsidies and access to mainstream medicine for the indigent were two aspirations of proponents of competitive health care plans. Regulation, though justified by its advocates as fostering entitlement, would only hinder attainment of these goals.

NHI Advocates and Competitive Theorists

To say that competitive theorists and proponents of NHI shared goals but diverged in choice of means is accurate only in part. That no citizen should be denied health services because of inability to pay seems to have drawn the assent of all parties. Distinctions existed, however, on the desired extent of benefits and the purposes to be met by the nature of the benefits chosen.

In part, these divergences have already been characterized here. Traditional advocates of NHI aimed at universal provision of comprehensive benefits, that is, realization for all citizens of the middle-class standards of care enshrined in the planning tradition. Competitive advocates aimed to finance expanded entitlement and foster efficiency by making available to low- and moderate-income consumers a lesser standard of care. Since expert determination of need was not possible and since different income groups, given the opportunity, would purchase different packages of services, both consumer sovereignty and allocational efficiency would be served by permitting a range of levels.

Moreover, advocates of plans doubted the efficacy of health care at the margin, as already noted, and they therefore were unlikely to consider that the cause of social justice could be served by making inefficacious services universally available. The poor in particular doubtless have better uses for their money than to buy marginally efficacious health care; they ought to be permitted discretion in using their funds (Havighurst and Blumstein 1975, 24–25). From this perspective, Havighurst observed (1977a, 318) about the poor:

> many observers who give lip service to the insight that only limited benefits are yielded by much health care remain fervently attached to the symbolic goal of comprehensive benefits and equality of access to high-quality services. Yet [that insight] should suggest placing less emphasis on providing the poor with an ideal standard of health care and more emphasis on providing them with other things. . . .

By contrast, Karen Davis, a proponent of comprehensive NHI, maintained (1975, 11), "Even with substantial increases in income through improved income maintenance programs, the poor are still apt to view medical care as a luxury to be indulged in only after the pressing demands for adequate shelter, clothing, and food have been met." In other words, precisely because the poor have better uses for their money, health care or health insurance should be provided in addition to any other forms of redistribution.

Advocates of plans thus acquiesced in, if not a two-class system of care, long an anathema to NHI advocates, then a multiclass system. Though Havighurst from the first (1970c, 729–32) aimed to avoid creating a system of "second-class medicine," neither he nor other competitive theorists aimed at a single-class system of care. Their goal was rather to ensure the poor the opportunity to make choices among the same providers, institutions, and services enjoyed by the middle class.

The values associated with these divergent aspirations were also divergent, but not completely. Advocates of plans valued health care at the margin less than the market (which they regarded as the fundamental device for registering individual preferences and legitimating individual decisions) and hoped for cost containment and efficiency as byproducts of market mechanisms. Advocates of traditional, comprehensive NHI also aimed primarily at realizing other values than the improvements in health that might flow from improvements in access to care. For some activists, such as Victor and Ruth Sidel, enhanced equity was the paramount goal of the transformation that they anticipated for the health system (a national health service rather than merely NHI). Thus, they maintained (Sidel and Sidel 1983, xxvii), "the health-care and medical-care system must have equity and justice as a primary goal even if equity and justice do not contribute to 'health' as conventionally defined." Similarly, Victor Fuchs (1974, 150; cf. Ball 1978, 20) asserted that

> A national health insurance plan to which all (or nearly all) Americans belonged could have a considerable symbolic value as one step in an effort to forge a link between classes, regions, races, and age groups. It will be more likely to serve that function well if not too much is expected of it—if it is not oversold—particularly with respect to its probable impact on health. If too much is promised, then instead of being of positive symbolic value it may serve as another source of divisiveness.

Because entitlement to comprehensive benefits was to enhance equity more than health, advocates of NHI were unmoved by declining faith in the efficacy of advanced medical care. They acknowledged the point, as Havighurst maintained, and agreed with advocates of plans on the likely greater importance of public health than medical care; but they nevertheless declined to revise their entitlement goals. Instead, they seemed to argue that because some medical care was highly important, comprehensive benefits were justified. The Sidels, for example, remarked (1983, xxx) that

> there are those who argue that medical care and even health care as conventionally defined, make relatively little contribution to health compared to the contribution made by other social conditions. Nonetheless we feel that the health-care and medical-care system can, if appropriately structured and combined with other societal efforts, make a significant contribution to health.

Similarly, Ball (1978, 20–21) maintained,

> In spite of the current intellectual fashion of arguing to the contrary, national health insurance assumes that medical care is worth having.... Overall, genetic and environmental factors and personal habits may have more effect on health than medical care services, but that is not inconsistent with the conclusion that medical care frequently does make the difference between sickness and health and life and death. And it is this conclusion that makes ability to pay an unacceptable way to ration medical care in a democratic society and leads to the national health insurance objective of making good medical services available to all.

Davis's position (1975, 10) was similar:

> Many ... health problems cannot be totally eradicated by reducing the financial barrier to medical care; adequate incomes for all, sound nutrition, better sanitation, improved water supplies, and better housing will be required for that. However, making medical care more accessible to those with limited means is an important first step.

In summary, advocates of comprehensive NHI believed that, because some kinds of care were matters of life and death, the inequities resulting from deprivation of access to all care were unacceptable. Universal entitlement to comprehensive benefits would go far to reduce the glaring inequities by preserving the lives of those priced out of the market for lifesaving care; and it would generally enhance the social equity and solidarity of the country. The inefficacy of much medical care seemed irrelevant to these goals, and the expense of providing inefficacious care could be accepted subject to controls effected by regulation. Competitive theorists regarded the doubtful efficacy of health care as grounds for treating it as just another consumption good. Accordingly, there was little justification for limiting consumer sovereignty in health care, for dispensing with the market and the freedom it afforded the individual in registering preferences and meeting demands, or for supposing that social justice depended on equal access to health care services. What divided the two groups therefore was less their aspirations about the health of citizens than their differential views of equity, social solidarity, and individual autonomy.

NOTES

1. E.g., L. Brown 1981, Vladeck 1981, and Weiner 1981, all in a special issue of the *Milbank Memorial Fund Quarterly* on "Competition and Regulation in Health Care Markets"; Bovbjerg 1981 and Rosenblatt 1981 in the *Vanderbilt Law Review;* Dunham, Morone, and White 1982, Ginzberg 1982 and 1983, Luft 1982, American Public Health Association 1983.
2. In contrast to much of Starr's work, such as Starr 1979; Starr 1982a, especially book 2, chaps. 3–5; and Starr 1984 (though less so Starr 1982b, 133–38).

3. For example, Heclo 1974, Spek 1980, Ståhl 1980, Wilensky 1975 and 1981, Polsby 1984, Berkowitz 1984. Lowi (1969) emphasizes the point strongly for America since the New Deal; for a prospective view, see also Schultze 1977, p. 5. The forces making for policy change in the welfare state do not so much result from conventional politics as constitute the framework in which conventional politics takes place; cf. Fox 1985.

4. M. Feldstein 1971; Pauly 1971a, chap. 4; Pauly 1971b, pp. 33–44; Seidman 1980 and 1981; cf. also Marmor, Boyer, and Greenberg 1981, pp. 1006–7 (n. 13 and accompanying text), and McClure 1976, pp. 40–41, 44–47, 60–61.

5. Ellwood has published little, devoting himself instead to activism; see Ellwood et al. 1971a; Ellwood 1972b; Ellwood 1975; and Falkson 1980. McClure has long been connected with Ellwood's health policy research organization, InterStudy; see McClure 1976, 1978, and 1982. Enthoven is best known for his "Consumer-Choice Health Plan"; see Enthoven 1980. Many of Havighurst's papers are cited below; representative works are Havighurst 1977a and Havighurst 1981. For an overview of competition, both theoretical and empirical, see Langwell and Moore 1982.

6. There is some doubt, however, that the coalition that sponsored Medicare is properly regarded as a descendant of earlier campaigns for NHI; cf. Fox 1983, and Stevens and Stevens 1974, p. 53, with Polsby 1984, pp. 126–28, and Marmor 1970, pp. 14–30, 100–105.

7. For the politics of Medicare and Medicaid, see Marmor 1970, Stevens and Stevens 1974, and Sundquist 1968. These programs, by increasing demand for health services, intensified existing upward pressures on costs; see generally, P. Feldstein 1983, p. 228; Law 1974, chap. 4; Havighurst 1977b, p. 475; and Havighurst 1980, p. 335.

8. For overviews of the criticism and its persistence, see U.S. Congress 1970; Ginzberg and Ostow 1969; Kennedy 1972; McClure 1976, pp. 32–35; Sidel and Sidel 1977; and for a sobered view, Ginzberg 1977. For a radical perspective, which offers similar criticisms but concludes that there is a system—well organized in the pursuit of profit, research, and limited forms of pedagogy—see Ehrenreich and Ehrenreich 1970.

9. For the expanding conception of rights, see Starr 1982a, 388–93; Patterson 1981, chaps. 9–11; and Bell 1975. Cf. also Lubove 1982.

10. For an explicit rejection of incremental change, see Falk 1977, pp. 177–78.

11. For a similarly early expression of confidence in competitive HMOs, see Havighurst 1970c, pp. 720–22.

12. Schultze (1977, 19–20) makes the point for public policy generally.

13. For example, Harold S. Luft, having conducted a major review of the performance of health maintenance organizations, the most prominent and thoroughly investigated form of competitive delivery organization, remarks (Luft 1980, 283 and cf. 305–6) that "we still know far too little about HMOs to explain adequately their current performance, let alone predict accurately the outcome of HMO competition in a radically restructured market environment." Cf. also Bovbjerg 1981, especially p. 986, text and n. 70; Klein 1981, p. 198; and Ginzberg 1983, p. 1859.

14. In addition to the sources just cited, cf. McClure 1982 and Meyer 1985; but cf. also Luft 1985, pp. 394–98, for a sober view of the requirements posed for health services research by both competitive and regulatory policies.

15. The 27 studies published by the committee underlay its concluding report, *Health Care for the American People* (Committee on the Costs of Medical Care

1932). The work of the CCMC exercised a formative influence on much of American health economics and provided a base for the development of American health planning. For the CCMC, see Weeks and Berman 1985, chap. 2; Starr 1983; Pearson 1976, especially pp. 10–14, 43–48; May 1967, p. 17; and Walker 1979. For its persistent influence, see the papers in the *Milbank Memorial Fund Quarterly* 56 (1978), from a 1977 conference entitled "Medical Care for the American People: Unfinished Agenda."

16. In addition to the sources cited in the previous note, see Payton and Powsner 1980, p. 215; and Gottlieb 1974, especially p. 11.

17. Regionalization was therefore not, as Payton and Powsner 1980 (pp. 205–6) maintain, the invention of the voluntary hospital industry. Regionalization was tightly linked to planning, and, though these two topics are sometimes pursued independently in the professional literature, their conceptual linkage was close; cf. Klarman 1977, pp. 26, 34–35.

18. Payton and Powsner (1980) see the hospital elite and the public health establishment as sharing values and frequently exchanging personnel.

19. Law 1974; Payton and Powsner 1980; P. Feldstein 1983, pp. 219–23; Frech 1979 and 1980; cf. Arnould and Eisenstadt 1981. Entirely consistent with these analyses is the radical criticism of Ehrenreich and Ehrenreich 1970, chap. 10.

20. Law 1974; Ehrenreich and Ehrenreich 1970, p. 235; (but cf. also Anderson 1975, pp. 87–94, and Somers and Somers 1967, p. 189). For nonprofit institutions generally, cf. Lowi 1969, pp. 38–39, 84–85, 96; Weisbrod 1977; Hansmann 1980 and 1981.

21. Contrast Payton and Powsner 1980, pp. 223–24, 230, and Law 1974, chap. 4, with Anderson 1975, pp. 87–94. For developing methods of cost reimbursement, see Anderson 1975, pp. 34–35, 43–44; Somers and Somers 1967, chap. 8; Law 1974, chap. 4; and Weiner 1977.

22. M. Feldstein 1967, chap. 7; P. Feldstein 1966, especially pp. 136–38; Klarman 1977, pp. 25, 27, 29–32, 35; Fuchs 1968, p. 192; Fuchs 1974, pp. 60–63; Havighurst 1973, p. 1162; McClure 1976, p. 33; Langwell and Moore 1982, pp. 18–19. For a historical perspective on the "technological imperative," see Rosenberg 1979; and Vogel 1980, p. 66.

23. Somers and Somers 1961 (p. 196) quote one hospital administrator as saying in 1958, "If there is any valid complaint about our costs, it is that they are not high enough."

24. For planning under Hill-Burton, see May 1967, pp. 25–31; Klarman 1977; Payton and Powsner 1980, pp. 234–35; Yordy 1976, pp. 203–4; Gottlieb 1974, pp. 14–15; Weeks and Berman 1985, chap. 3.

25. For CHP, see May 1967, pp. 43–44; Dickey, Kestell, and Ross 1970, pp. 840–52; Payton and Powsner 1980, p. 262; Gottlieb 1974, pp. 17–19; Yordy 1976, p. 206; Rosenfeld and Rosenfeld 1975, pp. 447–48; cf. Somers and Somers 1971 pp. 208–9, 213–25. For the 1974 act, see Klarman 1977, pp. 33–34, 36; Rosenfeld and Rosenfeld 1975; Havighurst 1982, pp. 127–29; U.S. Congress 1974.

26. In this literature, the terms "franchising" and "licensing," though not synonymous, were often used interchangeably in the hospital industry; see Somers 1969a, p. 152n.

27. This discussion draws on Payton and Powsner 1980, a highly suggestive but scarcely definitive source. A comprehensive treatment of regulation in the hospital industry in relation to the structure and political economy of the market remains to be written. Cf. also Havighurst 1973, pp. 1148–51.

28. In the light of the literature on regulation described below, this interpretation does not seem farfetched. Richard Posner, a major analyst of regulation, does warn that newer theories of regulation demand "a confident rejection of the public-interest rationales" for regulation, but he also supposes that the economic theory of fraud may explain the routine invocation of public interest rhetoric; Posner 1974a, pp. 354–56. Payton and Powsner do point out that this misrepresentation was made possible, inter alia, by the then monopoly held by the voluntary hospital industry on discussion about hospitals; Payton and Powsner 1980, p. 211.

29. For overviews of the advance of planning and regulation in the 1970s, see Roemer 1975 and Somers and Somers 1977, pp. 239–44 (and cf. Luft 1985, pp. 383–88).

30. For the advisory role of planning, see Gottlieb 1974, pp. 9, 10; May 1974, pp. 67–68; Havighurst 1973, pp. 1197–98 and n. 186.

31. U.S. Congress 1974, p. 40. Students of planning and regulation were fully aware of the linkage between NHI and the advance of planning and regulation; e.g., Saward 1976, pp. ix–xi; Bice and Kerwin 1976, p. 63; Ginzberg 1976, p. 229; Newhouse and Acton 1974; D. Greenberg 1974; and Havighurst 1974.

32. Baumol 1952 (Baumol 1965 differs from Baumol 1952 by the addition of an informative introduction that "discusses the pertinent developments in welfare economics since the . . . first edition" [p. 1]); Mishan 1969; Schick 1966, pp. 254–55; Haveman 1969, p. 3; Krutilla 1969, pp. 277–80.

33. Schick 1966, pp. 249–51. For the subsequent decline of the PBB system, see Schick 1973.

34. For a brief overview, see Mishan 1968.

35. Anderson 1966 makes this point. With reference to Anderson's and related arguments, Fox 1979 maintains (pp. 325–27) that pluralism induces policy-oriented researchers to support the status quo.

36. Prest and Turvey 1965 is the best survey from the mid 1960s; see also Eckstein 1961.

37. For this point, Wolf 1979, pp. 110–11; for a general commentary on these three and related characteristics, see Weisbrod 1968.

38. Eckstein 1961, esp. pp. 441, 446–47, 464, 480, 483; Margolis 1968, pp. 540, 542, 548–56; Margolis 1977, pp. 210–11. Cf. Wildavsky 1966; Luft 1976; Wolf 1979, pp. 133–38.

    Though pluralism did emphasize social mechanisms for decision making, the policy niche that it seemed to offer economists (that of impartial analysts standing outside of interest-group conflicts) appears to have induced them to adopt the narrowest conception of the public interest.

    Pluralism is not alone to blame, however. The theoretical conundrums of welfare economics seemed to prevent its practitioners in principle from reaching their central goal, the clear identification of welfare-maximizing programs; see, for example, Baumol 1952, chap. 14; Eckstein 1961, pp. 439–49; Feldman 1969, p. 868; Weisbrod 1968, pp. 182–83; Blaug 1968, chap. 13.

39. Freeman 1967, Bonnen 1968, and Bonnen 1969 are similar in method and inspiration. For reactions of Weisbrod's colleagues, see Chase 1968b, pp. 20–29; Chase 1968a, pp. 209–22, 248–54.

40. The analyses were largely theoretical, though empirical experience with water resource projects, flood control measures, and utility pricing played a role.

41. Vickrey 1963, Krutilla 1969, Milliman 1969, Schultze 1969; cf. Noll 1971, p. 16.

    As Milliman points out, this deployment of user charges departed from the model provided by the literature on public utility pricing (the counterpart of user charges in other sectors) in which economic analysis was constrained by the legally required recovery of capital investments (historical or sunk costs). Pricing to recover sunk costs implied that user charges did not serve the goal of short-run efficiency, for they did not reflect current opportunity costs occasioned by use of the product; cf. Vickrey 1963; Prest and Turvey 1965, 692–93. Allocational inefficiencies resulting from preoccupation with sunk costs later marked criticism of governmental regulation generally (e.g., Noll 1971, p. 25) and were also aimed by competitive theorists at regulation of the hospital industry; for example, Havighurst 1973, pp. 1205–6 (following Noll); and Havighurst 1982, pp. 301–5.

42. Ibid., p. 309. In regard to certain kinds of program, Schultze 1977 adopted the same position (pp. 61–62).

43. Marglin 1963 provides an early precedent for this approach.

44. Cf. also Feldman 1969, pp. 880–81. Paul J. Feldstein subsequently endorsed Feldman's view, in analyzing national health insurance in his influential text, P. Feldstein 1979, p. 414, and, in the revised edition, P. Feldstein 1983, p. 515.

45. These perceptions may have resulted from Schultze's experiences as Budget Director in the late 1960s. Intimately involved with disseminating the PBB system from its source in the Department of Defense to the rest of the executive branch, Schultze may have come to share the conviction of some critics, such as Wildavsky 1969, that decision making under PBB could succeed only under a centralized regime that was inappropriate for the novel forms of governmental intervention in the private sphere.

46. Schultze 1977 actually discussed (pp. 46–64) four kinds of policy failures: regulation, capital grants (public investments in bricks and mortar), federal categorical grants (which often reveal a "failure to distinguish problems of supply and problems of demand" [p. 61]), and failures to identify and correct perverse incentives (previously labeled negative incentives). His discussion of the third topic, though strongly reminiscent of cost sharing, attracted little attention.

47. The theme was present in Schultze 1969, pp. 207–9, but more elaborately developed in Schultze 1977, pp. 8–15 and chap. 3.

48. Schultze argued (ibid., pp. 6–7, 17) that precisely because the opportunities for public intervention increase, coercive measures should be used sparingly. The market, by contrast, preserves and indeed increases the scope of choice. He also observed (pp. 17–18) that the incentives-based approach offers an alternative to the usual means of organizing society between the coercion that may result from democratic majoritarian rule and the "emotional forces" of compassion, patriotism, and brotherly love—that is, social solidarity.

49. Ibid., p. 5. Moreover, by providing his audience with two catch phrases— "command and control" and "perverse incentives"—for denigrating regulation, Schultze facilitated the marketing of his ideas.

50. Schultze 1977, pp. 28–46; but he did argue (pp. 46–47) that improper identification of market failure had typically resulted in faulty design of public programs.

51. Lowi 1969, chap. 2, provides a short introduction.

52. For the deleterious consequences of bargaining, see Lowi 1969, 85–93.
53. Though relying on certain precedents (described below) from political science, economists dominated the study of regulation from the late 1960s; see Noll 1985b and Noll 1985c.
54. Ibid., pp. 26–27, 27 n., 34–35. New targets included more than politics; as Stigler applied the methods of economics to political problems, Gary Becker applied them to sociological phenomena, and Richard Posner applied them to legal phenomena.
55. Though Peltzman (for whom see Reder 1982, p. 26, n. 52) preserves a role in policy making even for positive economics. Noll, who, as noted below, exploits Chicago even while preserving a normative view of regulation, finds social science research rather more important; for example, Joskow and Noll 1981, pp. 8–10; Noll 1985b, pp. 5–6; Noll 1985c, p. 43.
56. For a quick overview of developments in regulation from the Chicago perspective, see Stigler 1981.
57. Posner 1974a, p. 337; Noll 1985c, pp. 22–23. Lowi's view is one example of this kind of explanation.
58. Posner 1974a, pp. 339–40; Noll 1985c, p. 24. The intractability of regulatory tasks emphasized by Schultze falls under this heading; so does the "capture theory" discussed later in this section.
59. For example, Stigler and Friedland 1962 and Stigler 1971. For the skepticism of Chicago regarding supposedly irrational or inefficient behavior, see Reder 1982, p. 15.
60. For overviews of developments in the early 1970s, see Noll 1971, Posner 1974a, and Noll 1975.
61. Comanor and Mitchell 1972 call this procedure "planning by regulation."
62. Jordan 1972, pp. 152, 153–54; Posner 1974a, pp. 341–43. Cf. also Lowi 1969, pp. 153–54. The skepticism of capture Lowi exhibits here reflects his differences with the antecedent pluralist literature: instead of a decline in the commitments of regulators to their legal mandates, Lowi observes a decline in the willingness of Congress to stipulate these mandates clearly.
63. The quotation is from Peltzman 1976, p. 211. Peltzman's assessment of Stigler and Posner's 1974a inform this paragraph.
64. Noll 1975, a much-cited paper (for example by Enthoven 1980, pp. 111–12; and P. Feldstein 1983, pp. 265, 293). Noll there contrasted his theory with "capture," under which label he included Stigler 1971. More recently, (Noll 1985c) he presented his theory under the rubric of "external-signal" theory, while listing Stigler 1971 and Peltzman 1976 as an example of "capture-cartel theories." Noll's approach had taken form rather early; see Noll 1971, chap. 4.
65. As both Falkson 1980 (pp. 14–16) and Ellwood 1984 note, Ellwood's approach crystallized in part as a result of pondering Levine 1968, which possessed many similarities with Schultze's approach, and subsequently took on a patina of formality in the form of McClure's 1976 "structural incentives analysis."

    Havighurst 1984 reports that in the late 1960s, as a professor at the Duke University School of Law, he was teaching in the subjects of regulated industries and antitrust law and he was editing symposia for *Law and Contemporary Problems* on regulatory topics. These experiences created an interest in regulatory policy and law and economics, a skepticism about regulation, and a belief in the importance of incentives. A visit to HEW in 1970 incidentally brought him into contact with Rick Carlson, one of Ellwood's colleagues, whose presentation of Ellwood's ideas to the Nixon administration established the link between Havighurst's earlier interests and competitive plans. As shown in the final section of this chapter, this early interest in incentives is evident in Havighurst's writings of the early 1970s on the subject of competitive plans. In the late 1970s, he found that Schultze's book had encapsulated much of his own thinking, and he invoked Schultze as a general point of departure for reform of health care policy; for example, see Havighurst 1977a, pp. 310–11, and Havighurst 1982, pp. 21–22, 25, 109–11.

Enthoven 1986 reports that he had read Schultze's book shortly before devising his Consumer-Choice Health Plan and that he regards his book as the "working out" in the health care economy of an example of Schultze's general propositions; see also Enthoven 1978a, p. 655; Enthoven 1980, pp. 70–71, 112–13.

66. From Havighurst 1984, it is clear that his knowledge of the political economy of regulation issued from his early experiences as a teacher and editor at Duke University; and from Havighurst 1973, it is clear that he had a thorough knowledge of the antiregulatory literature.

Enthoven 1986 reports that he acquired his understanding of the political economy of regulation by direct involvement in the 1970s with health policy circles, to which he came after a career as an analyst of defense policy and an architect of the PBB system.

As shown in the final section of this chapter, Ellwood contented himself with merely asserting various theses about the political economy of the health sector; developing a case against them was largely the work of Havighurst and Enthoven.

67. This coarse generalization obscures the point that Enthoven demanded a significant body of procompetitive regulation. Another skeptic of regulation, Richard Posner, has similarly argued (but from a more nearly positive standpoint) that various social arrangements designed to maintain markets are better referred to a broad public interest than to narrow private interests; Posner 1973. However, as shown below, some of Enthoven's fellow advocates of competitive plans found his insistence on procompetitive regulation unsatisfactory.

68. Klarman 1965, p. 2 for the first quotation; p. 14, for the second (offered with a citation to M. Feldstein 1963).

69. Cf. Lowi 1969, p. 75 n. 18, with the account by Fox 1979, p. 325, of Odin Anderson's views; and see Anderson 1966; Anderson 1975, chap. 4; and Anderson 1985, chap. 1.

70. Ibid., p. 598, quoting Margolis 1977 in support.

71. Arrow 1965 replied that voluntary group insurance had arisen to reduce transaction costs by exploiting economies of scale and that the government, by encompassing the entire market, could do better.

72. Pauly 1978 follows a similar procedure.

73. Ibid., p. 7; he there concluded, in contradistinction to Feldstein, that "Government planners may want to maximize 'health,' but there is no basic reason why they should want to do so."

74. Cf. Pauly 1978, p. 17: "Consumers cannot evaluate quality. *But neither can anyone else*" (emphasis in the original). Weisbrod 1978 agreed but suggested that providers of services, possessing better information, can take advantage of consumers.

75. Seidman 1981 takes a similar position (p. 464).

76. "Attract" is used advisedly: Ellwood was aiming at voluntary change (for

example, Ellwood 1975, pp. 50–51); cf. Enthoven 1980, pp. 118, 141. For the virtues of HMOs just noticed, see Luft 1981, p. 1; Ellwood 1971, pp. 3–4; Ellwood 1972a, p. 31; Ellwood 1975, pp. 50–52, 65–66; Havighurst 1970c, p. 719.

77.   The most prominent empirical studies of regulation available to advocates of plans through the early 1980s resembled the state of the antiregulatory literature in the early 1960s: they aimed to determine the effects of regulation and typically showed that the announced effects had not been achieved, but that other, perhaps unintended effects did result from regulation. Leading examples of this genre include the investigations of certification of need by Salkever and Bice 1976 and Sloan and Steinwald 1980. Such studies are effective in undermining regulation only in juxtaposition with ideas about the structure of the market for health services and about the political economy of regulation; by themselves, they leave intact the argument that regulatory failure should be referred to the shortcomings of implementation (lack of experience or expertise, poor design of programs, insufficient breadth of regulatory powers, and the like) and not to the fundamental nature of regulation. This kind of empirical study can be regarded as justifying additional regulation just as easily as it justifies dismantling of existing regulation; cf. Havighurst 1982, pp. 69–72. Accordingly, this discussion concentrates on the ideas of competitive theorists about the political economy of regulation, not on their use of empirical evidence per se.

78.   Except where otherwise noted, this section is based on the following documents (which include some of the many unpublished items graciously provided the author by InterStudy): InterStudy 1970a; InterStudy 1970b; Ellwood et al. 1971a; Ellwood et al. 1971b; Ellwood 1972a; Ellwood 1972b; Schlenker and Ellwood 1973. The discussion also draws on Havighurst 1970c, especially pp. 718–24; McClure 1976; and Enthoven 1980, especially pp. 67–68. McClure 1978 and Havighurst 1981, pp. 1125–30, offer broader formulations of the ideas first articulated in the early 1970s. Additional citations to these sources are given only to locate a few ideas that, while common among advocates of plans, are either infrequently made explicit or not widely known.

79.   For medical care as a cottage industry, see, for example, Ellwood 1972b, pp. 74–75.

80.   For shifts in the locus of care out of the hospital and into the practitioner's office and out of specialties into primary care, see InterStudy 1972a, pp. I-5, I-7.

81.   For the entitlement issue, see InterStudy 1972a, section III; InterStudy 1972b, section II; Institute of Medicine 1974, p. 63.

82.   Competition for providers is a newer theme recently pressed by Havighurst (Havighurst 1982, pp. 116–17, 210, 256, 299) to stress the responsibility of providers to accept directly the burden of cost containment. The theme points to the link by which plans translate the competitive pressure applied by consumers into efficient modes of practice.

83.   For flexibility, Ellwood 1970, p. 1; InterStudy 1972a, p. I-2; InterStudy 1972b, pp. 2–3, 5; cf. also McClure 1978, pp. 304–7.

84.   For example, Havighurst 1973, p. 1226; Institute of Medicine 1974, pp. 13–14; Ellwood 1975, pp. 53–54; McClure 1976, p. 41; for a less sanguine view, see Enthoven 1980, pp. 90–91; and cf. Enthoven 1978b, pp. 262–73.

85.   For example, Havighurst 1970c, pp. 736, 743; Havighurst 1973, pp. 1223–24; Havighurst 1974, pp. 250, 251; Havighurst 1975, p. 577; Havighurst 1977a, p. 311; Ellwood 1975, pp. 64–65; McClure 1976, p. 44; P. Feldstein 1983, p.

283, and, for the same point with regard to hospital rate regulation, p. 310.

86. Havighurst 1970c, pp. 717, 739–42 (citing Kessel 1970, p. 268); Havighurst 1978b; cf. Frech 1981, pp. 56–60. Cf. also Ginzberg 1982, who agrees that "health care never conformed to the competitive market" (p. 392), but explains (p. 393) this departure from market arrangements as reflecting the will of the public, not of providers.

87. The conference proceedings are contained in Havighurst 1974; the analysis of cartelization is Havighurst 1973. For the role of the Health-PAC volume (Ehrenreich and Ehrenreich 1970) in suggesting cartelization, see Havighurst 1974, p. 44 and Havighurst 1973, p. 1149 and n. 22.

88. Havighurst 1973, pp. 1178–1224. For a similar but less detailed analysis, see Havighurst 1975 and Enthoven 1980, pp. 110–13.

89. For example, Havighurst and Blumstein 1975, pp. 34–35; the same point was made early by Ellwood et al. (1971b), p. I-9.

90. Enthoven 1980, p. 101. Ellwood and his colleagues doubted that an effective system of regulation was even technically possible; see, e.g., InterStudy 1970a, pp. 3–4, and Ellwood et al. 1971a, pp. 292–93.

91. For the amendments, see Havighurst 1980; Havighurst 1982, chap. 5.

92. Enthoven 1980, pp. xvi–xvii (emphasis in the original); the point is reiterated on p. 6. Cf. Enthoven's view with that of Karen Davis, a proponent of comprehensive NHI: "While medical care is only one factor contributing to health, it is often a matter of life and death"; Davis 1975, p. 9.

93. For the skepticism, see Starr 1982a, pp. 408–11; Fuchs 1972, p. 41; Fuchs 1974, p. 144; Cochrane 1972; Ginzberg 1977a, p. 153; Wildavsky 1977. The emphasis on consumer sovereignty may be understood as part of a more general shift toward renewed emphasis on individual as opposed to social responsibility for personal well-being; see Knowles 1977 and Rosenblatt 1981, pp. 1104–6.

94. Havighurst 1978a, p. 252, relying, for the "new class," on Kristol 1978, pp. 27–31, and Weaver 1978.

95. Havighurst 1982, p. 383; cf. also Meyer 1981, p. 448 and Enthoven 1981, p. 482. Critics of competitive theory have also noticed that its advocates seem to value it as much as an end as a means; see, e.g., Marmor, Boyer, and Greenberg 1981; Rosenblatt 1981.

96. As pointed out early by Ellwood and Havighurst; Ellwood et al. 1971b, p. I-5, and Havighurst 1970c, pp. 742–43, 754–55.

97. E.g., Enthoven 1981, p. 482; Havighurst 1981, p. 1132. Both agree that, in a market of competing health care plans, the number of options would be fewer than under the prevailing system.

98. Ibid., 407–8. Havighurst offered this recommendation despite his awareness that employee-management relations provide significant political obstacles to the assumption of a constructive role by unions and employers; removal of the tax subsidy was intended to diminish these obstacles.

99. Havighurst 1980, p. 335 for this and the next quotation; cf. also Havighurst 1981, pp. 1124–25. By "market advocates," Havighurst here means advocates of plans; proponents of cost sharing, who also value the market, proceeded from analysis of public programs.

100. The criticisms, as well as some of the justifications noted in the text, are summarized by Havighurst 1973, pp. 1164–65, 1188–92; Havighurst 1982, pp. 281–83; Posner 1974b; in turn, Havighurst and Posner rely heavily on Posner 1971, and Havighurst also exploits Noll 1971, and Comanor and Mitchell 1972.

101. Enthoven 1980, p. 139 for this and the next quotation. Here, Enthoven was mindful not of enforced charity, but of the incentives in third-party reimbursement for subsidizing costly care and the knowledge that Medicare pays more for the rich than the poor.

REFERENCES

American Public Health Association. 1983. "Growth of For-Profit Health Care Institutions." Policy Statement No. 8321. Washington, DC: The Association.

Anderson, Odin W. 1966. "Influence of Social and Economic Research on Public Policy in the Health Field: A Review." *Milbank Memorial Fund Quarterly/Health and Society* 44: 11–51.

———. 1975. *Blue Cross Since 1929: Accountability and the Public Trust.* Cambridge, MA: Ballinger.

———. 1985. *Health Services in the United States: A Growth Enterprise Since 1875.* Ann Arbor, MI: Health Administration Press.

Arnould, Richard, and David Eisenstadt. 1981. "The Effects of Provider-Controlled Blue Shield Plans: Regulatory Options." In *A New Approach to the Economics of Health Care,* ed. by Mancur Olson, 339–60. Washington, DC: American Enterprise Institute.

Arrow, Kenneth J. 1963. "Uncertainty and the Welfare Economics of Medical Care." *American Economic Review* 53: 941–73.

———. 1965. "Uncertainty and the Welfare Economics of Medical Care: Reply (The Implications of Transaction Costs and Adjustment Lags)." *American Economic Review* 55: 154–58.

Ball, Robert M. 1978. "National Health Insurance: Comments on Selected Issues." *Science* 200: 864–70. Reprinted in *Health Care: Regulation, Economics, Ethics, Practice,* ed. by Philip H. Abelson, 20–26. Washington, DC: American Association for the Advancement of Science, 1978.

Baroody, William J. 1980. "Foreword." In *National Health Insurance: What Now, What Later, What Never?* ed. by Mark V. Pauly. Washington, DC: American Enterprise Institute.

———. 1981. "Foreword." In *A New Approach to the Economics of Health Care,* ed. by Mancur Olson. Washington, DC: American Enterprise Institute.

———. 1983. "Foreword." In *Market Reforms in Health Care: Current Issues, New Directions, Strategic Decisions,* ed. by Jack A. Meyer. Washington, DC: American Enterprise Institute.

Baumol, William J. 1952. *Welfare Economics and the Theory of the State.* Cambridge, MA: Harvard University Press.

———. 1965. *Welfare Economics and the Theory of the State.* Rev. ed. Cambridge, MA: Harvard University Press.

Bell, Daniel. 1975. "The Revolution of Rising Entitlements." *Fortune* 91 (April): 98–103, 182, 185.

Berkowitz, Edward D. 1984. "Disability Insurance and the Limits of American History." Paper presented before the 99th annual meeting of the American Historical Association, Chicago, December 28.

Bice, Thomas W., and Cornelius Kerwin. 1976. "Governance of Regional Health Systems." In *The Regionalization of Personal Health Services,* ed. by Ernest W. Saward, 61–105. Rev. ed. New York: Prodist (for the Milbank Memorial Fund).

Blaug, Mark. 1968. *Economic Theory in Retrospect*. Rev. ed. Homewood, IL: Richard D. Irwin.

Bonnen, James T. 1968. "The Distribution of Benefits from Cotton Price Supports." In *Problems in Public Expenditure Analysis*, ed. by Samuel B. Chase, Jr., 223–48. Washington, DC: Brookings Institution.

———. 1969. "The Absence of Knowledge of Distributional Impacts: An Obstacle to Effective Public Program Analysis and Decisions." In *The Analysis and Evaluation of Public Expenditures: The PBB System, A Compendium of Papers . . . ,* U.S. Congress, I, 419–49. Joint Economic Committee, Subcommittee on Economy in Government, 91st Cong., 1st Sess., 3 vols. Joint Comm. Print.

Bovbjerg, Randall R. 1981. "Competition Versus Regulation in Medical Care: An Overdrawn Dichotomy." *Vanderbilt Law Review* 34: 965–1002.

Brown, Lawrence D. 1981. "Competition and Health Cost Containment: Cautions and Conjectures." *Milbank Memorial Fund Quarterly/Health and Society* 59: 145–89.

———. 1982. "The Political Structure of the Federal Health Planning Program." Staff Paper. Washington, DC: Brookings Institution.

———. 1983. *Politics and Health Care Organization: HMOs as Federal Policy*. Washington, DC: Brookings Institution.

Brown, Ray E. 1959. "Let the Public Control Utilization through Planning." *Hospitals* 33 (December 1): 108–10.

Chase, Samuel B., Jr., ed. 1968a. *Problems in Public Expenditure Analysis*. Washington, DC: Brookings Institution.

———. 1968b. "Introduction and Summary." In *Problems in Public Expenditure Analysis*, ed. by Samuel B. Chase, Jr., 1–32. Washington, DC: Brookings Institution.

Cochrane, Archibald Leman. 1972. *Effectiveness and Efficiency: Random Reflections on Health Services*. London: Nuffield Provincial Hospitals Trust.

Columbia University School of Public Health and Administrative Medicine. 1961. *Prepayment for Hospital Care in New York State: A Report on the Eight Blue Cross Plans Serving New York Residents*. (The Trussell Report.) New York: Columbia University Press.

Comanor, William S., and Bridger M. Mitchell. 1972. "The Costs of Planning: The FCC and Cable Television." *Journal of Law and Economics* 15: 177–231.

Committee on the Costs of Medical Care. 1932. *Health Care for the American People*. Committee on the Costs of Medical Care, Publication No. 28. Chicago: University of Chicago Press.

Curran, William J. 1974. "A National Survey and Analysis of State Certificate-of-Need Laws for Health Facilities." In *Regulating Health Facilities Construction*, ed. Clark C. Havighurst, 85–111. Proceedings of a Conference on Health Planning, Certificates of Need, and Market Entry. Washington, DC: American Enterprise Institution.

Davis, Karen. 1975. *National Health Insurance: Benefits, Costs, and Consequences*. Washington, DC: Brookings Institution.

Dickey, Walter J., James L. Kestell, and Carl W. Ross. 1970. "Comprehensive Health Planning—Federal, State, Local: Concepts and Realities." *Wisconsin Law Review* 3: 839–78.

Dunham, Andrew, James A. Morone, and William White. 1982. "Restoring Medical Markets: Implications for the Poor." *Journal of Health Politics, Policy and Law* 7: 488–501.

Eckstein, Otto. 1961. "A Survey of the Theory of Public Expenditure Criteria." In *Public Finances: Needs, Sources, and Utilization*, ed. by National Bureau of Economic Research, 439–94. Princeton, NJ: Princeton University Press.

Ehrenreich, Barbara, and John Ehrenreich. 1970. *The American Health Empire: Power, Profits, and Politics.* A Health-PAC Book. New York: Random House.

Ellwood, Paul M., Jr. 1970. "The Concept of the Health Maintenance Organization: Summary of Discussions between Executives of an Insurance Company and Paul M. Ellwood. . . ." Typescript. Minneapolis: InterStudy.

———. 1971. "Testimony Presented to the Subcommittee on Health of the Senate Committee on Labor and Public Welfare, 6 October 1971." Typescript. Minneapolis: InterStudy.

———. 1972a. "The Organizational Model Implications of Health Legislation and Current Proposals." Paper presented before the Sun Valley Forum on National Health, Inc., Sun Valley, Idaho, June 28, 1972. Typescript. Minneapolis: InterStudy.

———. 1972b. "Models for Organizing Health Services and Implications of Legislative Proposals." *Milbank Memorial Fund Quarterly/Health and Society* 50: 73–101.

———. 1975. "Alternatives to Regulation: Improving the Market." In *Controls on Health Care,* Papers of the Conference on Regulation of the Health Industry, January 7–9, 1974, 49–72. Washington, DC: National Academy of Sciences.

———. 1984. Telephone conversation with the author, May 25.

Ellwood, Paul M., Jr., Nancy N. Anderson, James E. Billings, Rick J. Carlson, Earl J. Hoagberg, and Walter McClure. 1971a. "Health Maintenance Strategy." *Medical Care* 9: 291–98.

Ellwood, Paul M., Jr., Patrick O'Donoghue, Earl J. Hoagberg, Robert Schneider, Walter McClure, and Rick J. Carlson. 1971b. "Comparative Analysis of a Competitive HMO System with Other Health Care Delivery Systems." Contract No. HSM 110-72-69. Typescript. Minneapolis: InterStudy.

Ellwood, Paul M., Jr., Patrick O'Donoghue, Walter McClure, Robert Holley, Rick J. Carlson, and Earl Hoagberg. 1973. *Assuring the Quality of Health Care.* Minneapolis: InterStudy.

Enthoven, Alain C. 1978a. "Consumer-Choice Health Plan." *New England Journal of Medicine* 298: 650–58, 709–20.

———. 1978b. "Competition of Alternative Delivery Systems." In *Competition in the Health Care Sector: Past, Present, and Future,* ed. by Warren Greenberg, 255–77. Proceedings of a Conference Sponsored by the Bureau of Economics, Federal Trade Commission, 1978. Germantown, MD: Aspen Systems.

———. 1980. *Health Plan: The Only Practical Solution to the Soaring Cost of Medical Care.* Reading, MA: Addison-Wesley.

———. 1981. "Supply-Side Economics of Health Care and Consumer-Choice Health Plan." In *A New Approach to the Economics of Health Care,* ed. by Mancur Olson, 467–89. Washington, DC: American Enterprise Institute.

———. 1986. Telephone conversation with the author, November 17.

Falk, I. S. 1970. "National Health Insurance: A Review of Policies and Proposals." *Law and Contemporary Problems* 35: 669–96.

———. 1977. "Proposals for National Health Insurance in the USA: Origins and Evolution, and Some Perceptions for the Future." *Milbank Memorial Fund Quarterly/Health and Society* 55: 161–91.

Falkson, Joseph L. 1980. *HMOs and the Politics of Health System Reform.* Chicago: American Hospital Association.

Feldman, Paul. 1969. "Prescription for an Effective Government: Ethics, Economics, and PBBS." In *The Analysis and Evaluation of Public Expenditures: The PBB System, A Compendium of Papers . . . ,* U.S. Congress, III, 865–85. 91st Cong., 1st

Sess., 3 vols., Joint Comm. Print.

——. 1971. "Efficiency, Distribution, and the Role of Government in a Market Economy." *Journal of Political Economy* 79: 508–26.

Feldstein, Martin. 1963. "Economic Analysis, Operational Research, and the National Health Service." *Oxford Economic Papers* 15(ns): 19–31.

——. 1967. *Economic Analysis for Health Service Efficiency: Econometric Studies of the British National Health Service.* Contributions to Economic Analysis, vol. 51. Amsterdam: North Holland.

——. 1971. "A New Approach to National Health Insurance." *Public Interest* 23: 93–105.

Feldstein, Paul J. 1966. "Research on the Demand for Health Services." In *Economic Aspects of Health Care: A Selection of Articles from the* Milbank Memorial Fund Quarterly, ed. by John B. McKinlay, 123–58. New York: Prodist (for the Milbank Memorial Fund), 1973.

——. 1979. *Health Care Economics.* New York: Wiley.

——. 1983. *Health Care Economics.* Rev. ed. New York: Wiley.

Fox, Daniel M. 1979. "From Reform to Relativism: A History of Economists and Health Care." *Milbank Memorial Fund Quarterly/Health and Society* 57: 297–336.

——. 1983. "The Decline of Historicism: The Case of Compulsory Health Insurance in the United States." *Bulletin of the History of Medicine* 57: 596–610.

——. 1985. "History and Health Policy: An Autobiographical Note on the Decline of Historicism." *Journal of Social History* 18: 349–64.

Frech, H. E., III. 1979. "Market Power in Health Insurance: Effects on Insurance and Medical Markets." *Journal of Industrial Economics* 28: 55–72.

——. 1980. "Blue Cross, Blue Shield, and Health Care Costs: A Review of Economic Evidence." In *National Health Insurance: What Now, What Later, What Never?* ed. by Mark V. Pauly, 250–63. Washington, DC: American Enterprise Institute.

——. 1981. "The Long-Lost Free Market in Health Care: Government and Professional Regulation of Medical Care." In *A New Approach to the Economics of Health Care,* ed. by Mancur Olson, 44–66. Washington, DC: American Enterprise Institute.

Freeman, A. Myrick, III. 1967. "Income Distribution and Planning for Public Investment." *American Economic Review* 57: 495–508.

Friedman, Bernard. 1980. "Rationales for Government Initiative in Catastrophic Health Insurance." In *National Health Insurance: What Now, What Later, What Never?* ed. by Mark V. Pauly, 85–103. Washington, DC: American Enterprise Institute.

Fuchs, Victor R. 1968. "The Growing Demand for Medical Care." *New England Journal of Medicine* 279: 190–95.

——. 1972. "The Basic Forces Influencing Costs of Medical Care." In *Essays in the Economics of Health Care and Medical Care,* ed. by Victor R. Fuchs, 39–50. New York: Columbia University Press for the National Bureau of Economic Research.

——. 1974. *Who Shall Live?: Health, Economics, and Social Choice.* New York: Basic Books.

Ginsburg, Paul B. 1981. "Medicare Vouchers and the Procompetition Strategy." *Health Affairs* 1: 39–52.

Ginzberg, Eli. 1976. "Summing Up." In *The Regionalization of Personal Health Services,* ed. by Ernest W. Saward 223–31. Rev. ed. New York: Prodist (for the Milbank Memorial Fund).

————. 1977. *The Limits of Health Reform: The Search for Reality.* New York: Basic Books.

————. 1982. "Procompetition in Health Care: Policy or Fantasy?" *Milbank Memorial Fund Quarterly/Health and Society* 60: 386–98.

————. 1983. "The Grand Illusion of Competition in Health Care." *Journal of the American Medical Association* 249: 1857–59.

Ginzberg, Eli, and Miriam Ostow. 1969. *Men, Money, and Medicine.* New York: Columbia University Press.

Gottlieb, Symond R. 1974. "A Brief History of Health Planning in the United States." In *Regulating Health Facilities Construction,* ed. by Clark C. Havighurst, 7–25. Proceedings of a Conference on Health Planning, Certificates of Need, and Market Entry. Washington, DC: American Enterprise Institute.

Grannemann, Thomas W. 1980. "Reforming National Health Programs for the Poor." In *National Health Insurance: What Now, What Later, What Never?* ed. by Mark V. Pauly, 104–36. Washington, DC: American Enterprise Institute.

Greenberg, Daniel S. 1974. "Preparing for National Health Insurance, and Other Matters." *New England Journal of Medicine* 291: 1205–6.

Greenhouse, Samuel M. 1966. "The Planning-Programming-Budgeting System: Rationale, Language, and Idea-Relationships." *Public Administration Review* 26: 271–77.

Grosse, Robert N. 1974. "The Need for Health Planning." In *Regulating Health Facilities Construction,* ed. by Clark C. Havighurst, 27–31. Proceedings of a Conference on Health Planning, Certificates of Need, and Market Entry. Washington, DC: American Enterprise Institute.

Hansmann, Henry. 1980. "The Role of Nonprofit Enterprise." *Yale Law Journal* 89: 835–901.

————. 1981. "Reforming Nonprofit Corporation Law." *University of Pennsylvania Law Review* 129: 497–623.

Harris, Seymour E. 1964. *The Economics of American Medicine.* New York: Macmillan.

Haveman, Robert. 1969. "The Analysis and Evaluation of Public Expenditures: An Overview." In *The Analysis and Evaluation of Public Expenditures: The PBB System, A Compendium of Papers . . . ,* U.S. Congress, I, 1–10. Joint Economic Committee, Subcommittee on Economy in Government, 91st Cong., 1st Sess., 3 vols., Joint Comm. Print.

Haveman, Robert H., and Julius Margolis, eds. 1970. *Public Expenditures and Policy Analysis.* Chicago: Markham.

————, eds. 1977. *Public Expenditure and Policy Analysis.* 2d ed. Chicago: Rand McNally.

Havighurst, Clark C. 1970a. "Foreword." *Law and Contemporary Problems* 35: 229–32.

————. 1970b. "Foreword." *Law and Contemporary Problems* 35: 667–68.

————. 1970c. "Health Maintenance Organizations and the Market for Health Services." *Law and Contemporary Problems* 35: 716–95.

————. 1973. "Regulation of Health Facilities and Services by 'Certificate of Need.'" *Virginia Law Review* 59: 1143–1232.

————. 1974. "Speculations on the Market's Future in Health Care." In *Regulating Health Facilities Construction,* ed. by Clark C. Havighurst, 249–69. Proceedings of a Conference on Health Planning, Certificates of Need, and Market Entry. Washington, DC: American Enterprise Institute.

————. 1975. "Federal Regulation of the Health Care Delivery System: A Foreword in the Nature of a 'Package Insert.'" *University of Toledo Law Review* 6: 577–90.

————. 1977a. "Health Care Cost Containment Regulation: Prospects and an Alternative." *American Journal of Law and Medicine* 3: 309–22.

————. 1977b. "Controlling Health Care Costs: Strengthening the Private Sector's Hand." *Journal of Health Politics, Policy and Law* 1: 471–98. Also available, with the same pagination, as Offprint No. 68, Washington, DC: American Enterprise Institute, 1977.

——. 1978a. "More on Regulation: A Reply to Stephen Weiner." *American Journal of Law and Medicine* 4: 243–53.

——. 1978b. "Professional Restraints on Innovation in Health Care Financing." *Duke Law Journal* 1978: 303–87.

——. 1980. "Prospects for Competition under Health Planning-cum-Regulation." In *National Health Insurance: What Now, What Later, What Never?* ed. by Mark V. Pauly, 329–59. Washington, DC: American Enterprise Institute.

——. 1981. "Competition in Health Services: Overview, Issues, and Answers." *Vanderbilt Law Review* 34: 1117–58.

——. 1982. *Deregulating the Health Care Industry: Planning for Competition.* Cambridge, MA: Ballinger.

——. 1984. Letter to the author, November 6.

Havighurst, Clark C., and James Blumstein. 1975. "Coping with Quality/Cost Trade-Offs in Medical Care: The Role of PSROs." *Northwestern University Law Review* 70: 6–68.

Heclo, Hugh. 1974. *Modern Social Politics in Britain and Sweden: From Relief to Income Maintenance.* New Haven: Yale University Press.

Hodgson, Godfrey. 1973. "The Politics of American Health Care: What Is It Costing You?" *Atlantic Monthly* 282: 1973, 45–61.

Institute of Medicine. 1974. "Health Maintenance Organizations: Toward a Fair Market Test." A Policy Statement by a Committee of the Institute of Medicine, IOM Publication 74-03. Washington, DC: National Academy of Sciences.

InterStudy. 1970a. "A Resource Paper for Decision-Makers: Health Care Issues of Importance to Minnesota." Minneapolis: InterStudy.

——. 1970b. "Health Maintenance Organization Option under Medicare." Consultation Summary, Department of Health, Education, and Welfare. Typescript. Minneapolis: InterStudy.

——. 1972a. "Testimony Presented on April 13, 1972, to the Subcommittee on Public Health and Environment of the House Committee on Interstate and Foreign Commerce." Typescript. Minneapolis: InterStudy.

——. 1972b. "Testimony Presented on May 25, 1972, to the Subcommittee on Health of the Senate Committee on Labor and Public Welfare." Typescript. Minneapolis: InterStudy.

Jewkes, John, and Sylvia Jewkes. 1961. *The Genesis of the British National Health Service.* Oxford: Basil Blackwell.

Joint Committee of the American Hospital Association and U.S. Public Health Service. 1961. *Areawide Planning for Hospitals and Related Health Facilities.* U.S. Public Health Service Publication No. 855.

Jordan, William A. 1972. "Producer Protection, Prior Market Structure, and the Effects of Government Regulation." *Journal of Law and Economics* 15: 151–76.

Joskow, Paul L., and Roger G. Noll. 1981. "Regulation in Theory and Practice: An Overview." In *Studies in Public Regulation,* ed. by Gary Fromm, 1–65. Cambridge, MA: MIT Press.

Kennedy, Edward M. 1972. *In Critical Condition: The Crisis in America's Health Care.* New York: Simon & Schuster.

Kessel, Reuben A. 1958. "Price Discrimination in Medicine." *Journal of Law and Economics* 1: 20–53.

——. 1970. "The A.M.A. and the Supply of Physicians." *Law and Contemporary Problems* 35: 267–83.

Klarman, Herbert E. 1965. *The Economics of Health.* New York: Columbia University Press.

———. 1977. "Planning for Facilities." In *Regionalization and Health Policy,* ed. by Eli Ginzberg, 25–35. DHEW Publication No. (HRA) 77-623. Washington, DC: U.S. Department of Health, Education, and Welfare, Public Health Service, Health Resources Administration.

———. 1982. "The Road to Cost-Effectiveness Analysis." *Milbank Memorial Fund Quarterly/Health and Society* 60: 585–603.

Klein, Rudolf. 1981. "Reflections on the American Health Care Condition." *Journal of Health Politics, Policy and Law* 6: 188–204.

Kneese, Allen V., and Ralph d'Arge. 1969. "Pervasive External Costs and the Response of Society." In *The Analysis and Evaluation of Public Expenditures: The PBB System, A Compendium of Papers . . . ,* U.S. Congress, I, 87–115. Joint Economic Committee, Subcommittee on Economy in Government, 91st Cong., 1st Sess., 3 vols., Joint Comm. Print.

Kneese, Allen V., and Charles L. Schultze. 1975. *Pollution, Prices, and Public Policy.* Washington, DC: Brookings Institution.

Knowles, John H., ed. 1977. *Doing Better and Feeling Worse: Health in the United States.* New York: Norton.

Kristol, Irving. 1978. *Two Cheers for Capitalism.* New York: Basic Books.

Krutilla, John V. 1969. "Efficiency Goals, Market Failure, and the Substitution of Public for Private Action." In *The Analysis and Evaluation of Public Expenditure: The PBB System, A Compendium of Papers . . . ,* U.S. Congress, I, 277–89. Joint Economic Committee, Subcommittee on Economy in Government, 91st Cong., 1st Sess., 3 vols., Joint Comm. Print.

Langwell, Kathryn M., and Sylvia F. Moore. 1982. *A Synthesis of Research on Competition in the Financing and Delivery of Health Services.* DHHS Publication No. (PHS) 83-3327. Washington, DC: U.S. Department of Health and Human Services, National Center for Health Services Research.

Law, Sylvia. 1974. *Blue Cross: What Went Wrong?* New Haven: Yale University Press. 2d ed. 1976.

Lee, Roger I., and Lewis Webster Jones. 1932. *The Fundamentals of Good Medical Care: An Outline of the Fundamentals of Good Medical Care and an Estimate of the Service Required to Supply the Medical Needs of the United States.* Committee on the Costs of Medical Care, Publication No. 22. Chicago: University of Chicago Press.

Lees, Dennis S. 1960. "The Economics of Health Services." *Lloyds Bank Review* 56(ns) (April): 26–40.

———. 1961. *Health Through Choice: An Economic Study of the British National Health Service.* Hobart Paper No. 14. London: Institute of Economic Affairs.

———. 1962. "The Logic of the British National Health Service." *Journal of Law and Economics* 5 (October): 111–18.

Lees, Dennis S., and Robert G. Rice. 1965. "Uncertainty and the Welfare Economics of Medical Care: Comment." *American Economic Review* 55: 141–54.

Levine, Robert A. 1968. "Rethinking our Social Strategies." *Public Interest* 10: 86–96.

Lowi, Theodore J. 1969. *The End of Liberalism: Ideology, Policy, and the Crisis of Public Authority.* New York: Norton.

Lubove, Roy. 1968. *The Struggle for Social Security, 1900–1935.* Cambridge, MA: Harvard University Press.

———. 1982. "The Right to Health Care: Ethical Imperatives vs. Enforceable Claims." In *Compulsory Health Insurance: The Continuing Debate,* ed. by Ronald

L. Numbers, 145–54. Contributions in Medical History, No. 11. Westport, CN: Greenwood Press.

Luft, Harold S. 1976. "Benefit-Cost Analysis and Public Policy Implementation: From Normative to Positive Analysis." *Public Policy* 24: 437–62.

———. 1980. "Health Maintenance Organizations, Competition, Cost Containment, and National Health Insurance." In *National Health Insurance: What Now, What Later, What Never?* ed. by Mark V. Pauly, 283–306. Washington, DC: American Enterprise Institute.

———. 1981. *Health Maintenance Organizations: Dimensions of Performance.* New York: Wiley.

———. 1985. "Competition and Regulation." *Medical Care* 23: 383–400.

Lyons, Gene M. 1969. *The Uneasy Partnership: Social Science and the Federal Government in the Twentieth Century.* New York: Russell Sage Foundation.

Marglin, Stephen A. 1963. "The Social Rate of Discount and the Optimal Rate of Investment." *Quarterly Journal of Economics* 77: 95–112.

Margolis, Julius. 1968. "The Demand for Urban Public Services." In *Issues in Urban Economics,* ed. by Harvey S. Perloff and Lowdon Wingo, 527–64. Baltimore: Johns Hopkins University Press for Resources for the Future, Inc.

———. 1977. "Shadow Prices for Incorrect or Nonexistent Market Values." In *Public Expenditure and Policy Analysis,* ed. by Robert H. Haveman and Julius Margolis, 204–20. Chicago: Rand McNally.

Marmor, Theodore R. 1970. *The Politics of Medicare.* London: Routledge and Kegan Paul.

Marmor, Theodore R., Richard Boyer, and Julie Greenberg. 1981. "Medical Care and Procompetitive Reform." *Vanderbilt Law Review* 34: 1003–28.

May, J. Joel. 1967. *Health Planning: Its Past and Potential.* Health Administration Perspectives, No. A5. Chicago: Center for Health Administration Studies, University of Chicago.

———. 1974. "The Planning and Licensing Agencies." In *Regulating Health Facilities Construction,* ed. by Clark C. Havighurst, 47–68. Proceedings of a Conference on Health Planning, Certificates of Need, and Market Entry. Washington, DC: American Enterprise Institute.

McClure, Walter. 1976. "The Medical Care System under National Health Insurance: Four Models." *Journal of Health Politics, Policy and Law* 1: 22–68.

———. 1978. "On Broadening the Definition of and Removing Regulatory Barriers to a Competitive Health Care System." *Journal of Health Politics, Policy and Law* 3: 303–27.

———. 1982. "Implementing a Competitive Medical Care System through Public Policy." *Journal of Health Politics, Policy and Law* 7: 2–44.

Mechanic, David. 1970. "Problems in the Future Organization of Medical Practice." *Law and Contemporary Problems* 35: 233–51.

———. 1978. *Medical Sociology.* 2d ed. New York: Free Press.

Meyer, Jack A. 1981. "Health Care Competition: Are Tax Incentives Enough?" In *A New Approach to the Economics of Health Care,* ed. by Mancur Olson, 424–49. Washington, DC: American Enterprise Institute.

———, ed. 1983. *Market Reforms in Health Care: Current Issues, New Directions, Strategic Decisions.* Washington, DC: American Enterprise Institute.

———, ed. 1985. *Incentives vs. Controls in Health Policy: Broadening the Debate.* Washington, DC: American Enterprise Institute.

Meyer, Jack A., and Rudolph G. Penner. 1980. "Impact of National Health Insurance Proposals on the Budget." In *National Health Insurance: What Now, What*

   Later, What Never? ed. by Mark V. Pauly, 11–30. Washington, DC: American
      Enterprise Institute.
Milliman, Jerome W. 1969. "Beneficiary Charges and Efficient Public Expenditure
      Decisions." In *The Analysis and Evaluation of Public Expenditures: The PBB System, A Compendium of Papers . . . ,* U.S. Congress, I, 291–318. Joint Economic
      Committee, Subcommittee on Economy in Government, 91st Cong., 1st Sess.,
      3 vols., Joint Comm. Print.
Ministry of Health, Consultative Council on Medical and Allied Services. 1920. *Interim Report on the Future Provision of Medical and Allied Services.* London: H.M.
      Stationery Office.
Mishan, E. J. 1968. "Welfare Economics." *International Encyclopedia of the Social Sciences*
      XVI: 504–12. New York: Macmillan.
———. 1969. *Welfare Economics: Ten Introductory Essays.* 2d ed. New York: Random
      House.
Mushkin, Selma J. 1962. "Health as an Investment." *Journal of Political Economy* 70
      (October suppl.): 129–57.
Newhouse, Joseph P., and Jan P. Acton. 1974. "Compulsory Health Planning Laws
      and National Health Insurance." In *Regulating Health Facilities Construction,*
      ed. by Clark C. Havighurst, 249–69. Proceedings of a Conference on Health
      Planning, Certificates of Need, and Market Entry. Washington, DC: American Enterprise Institute.
Noll, Roger G. 1971. *Reforming Regulation: An Evaluation of the Ash Council Proposals.*
      Washington, DC: Brookings Institution.
———. 1975. "The Consequences of Public Utility Regulation of Hospitals." In *Controls on Health Care,* Papers of the Conference on Regulation of the Health Industry, January 7–9, 1974, 25–48. Washington, DC: National Academy of
      Sciences.
———, ed. 1985a. *Regulatory Policy and the Social Sciences.* Berkeley: University of
      California Press.
———. 1985b. "Introduction." In *Regulatory Policy and the Social Sciences,* ed. by
      Roger G. Noll, pp. 3–8. Berkeley: University of California Press.
———. 1985c. "Government Regulatory Behavior: A Multidisciplinary Survey and
      Synthesis." In *Regulatory Policy and the Social Sciences,* ed. by Roger G. Noll,
      9–63. Berkeley: University of California Press.
Olson, Mancur, ed. 1981. *A New Approach to the Economics of Health Care.* Washington,
      DC: American Enterprise Institute.
Ostow, Miriam, and Karen Brudney. 1977. "Regional Medical Programs." In *Regionalization and Health Policy,* ed. by Eli Ginzberg, 60–70. DHEW Publication No.
      (HRA) 77-623. Washington, DC: U.S. Department of Health, Education, and
      Welfare, Public Health Service, Health Resources Administration.
Patterson, James T. 1981. *America's Struggle against Poverty, 1900–1980.* Cambridge,
      MA: Harvard University Press.
Pauly, Mark V. 1968. "The Economics of Moral Hazard: Comment." *American Economic Review* 58: 531–37.
———. 1971a. *Medical Care at Public Expense: A Study in Applied Welfare Economics.* New
      York: Praeger.
———. 1971b. *National Health Insurance: An Analysis.* Washington, DC: American Enterprise Institute.
———. 1978. "Is Medical Care Different?" In *Competition in the Health Care Sector: Past,
      Present, and Future,* ed. by Warren Greenberg, 11–35. Proceedings of a Conference Sponsored by the Bureau of Economics, Federal Trade Commission,
      1978. Germantown, MD: Aspen Systems.

————, ed. 1980a. *National Health Insurance: What Now, What Later, What Never?* Washington, DC: American Enterprise Institute.

————. 1980b. "Introduction." In *National Health Insurance: What Now, What Later, What Never?* ed. by Mark V. Pauly, 1–7. Washington, DC: American Enterprise Institute.

Payton, Sallyanne, and Rhoda Powsner. 1980. "Regulation Through the Looking Glass: Hospitals, Blue Cross, and Certificate-of-Need." *Michigan Law Review* 77: 203–77.

Pearson, David A. 1976. "The Concept of Regionalized Personal Health Services in the United State, 1920–1955." In *The Regionalization of Personal Health Services,* ed. by Ernest W. Saward, 3–51. Rev. ed. New York: Prodist (for the Milbank Memorial Fund).

Peltzman, Sam. 1976. "Toward a More General Theory of Regulation." *Journal of Law and Economics* 19: 211–40.

Polsby, Nelson W. 1984. *Political Innovation in America: The Politics of Policy Initiation.* New Haven: Yale University Press.

Posner, Richard A. 1971. "Taxation by Regulation." *Bell Journal of Economics and Management Science* 2: 22–50.

————. 1973. *Economic Analysis of Law.* New York: Little, Brown.

————. 1974a. "Theories of Economic Regulation." *Bell Journal of Economics and Management Science* 5: 335–58.

————. 1974b. "Certificates of Need for Health Care Facilities: A Dissenting View." In *Regulating Health Facilities Construction,* ed. by Clark C. Havighurst, 113–17. Proceedings of a Conference on Health Planning, Certificates of Need, and Market Entry. Washington, DC: American Enterprise Institute.

Prest, A. R., and R. Turvey. 1965. "Cost-Benefit Analysis: A Survey." *Economic Journal* 75: 683–735.

Priest, A. J. G. 1970. "Possible Adoption of Public Utility Concepts in the Health Care Field." *Law and Contemporary Problems* 35: 839–48.

Reder, Melvin W. 1982. "Chicago Economics: Permanence and Change." *Journal of Economic Literature* 20: 1–38.

Roemer, Milton I. 1961. "Bed Supply and Hospital Utilization: A Natural Experiment." *Hospitals* 35 (November 1): 36–42.

————. 1970. "Controlling and Promoting Quality in Medical Care." *Law and Contemporary Problems* 35: 284–304.

————. 1975. "The Expanding Scope of Governmental Regulation of Health Care Delivery." *University of Toeldo Law Review* 6: 591–616.

Rosen, George. 1976. "Social Science and Health in the United States in the Twentieth Century." *Clio Medica* 11: 245–68.

Rosenberg, Charles E. 1979. "Inward Vision and Outward Glance: The Shaping of the American Hospital, 1880–1914." *Bulletin of the History of Medicine* 53: 346–91.

Rosenblatt, Rand E. 1981. "Health Care, Markets, and Democratic Values." *Vanderbilt Law Review* 34: 1067–1115.

Rosenfeld, Leonard S., and Irene Rosenfeld. 1975. "National Health Planning in the United States: Prospects and Portents." *International Journal of Health Services* 5: 441–53.

Russell, Louise B. 1980. "Commentary." In *National Health Insurance: What Now, What Later, What Never?* ed. by Mark V. Pauly, 275–79. Washington, DC: American Enterprise Institute.

Salkever, David S., and Thomas W. Bice. 1976. "The Impact of Certificate-of-Need Controls on Hospital Investment." *Milbank Memorial Fund Quarterly/Health and*

Society 54: 185–214. In slightly revised form, these results are also available as idem, *Hospital Certificate-of-Need Controls: Impact on Investment, Cost, and Use.* Washington, DC: American Enterprise Institute, 1979.

Saward, Ernest W. 1976. "Preface." In *The Regionalization of Personal Health Services,* ed. by Ernest W. Saward, ix–xiii. Rev. ed. New York: Prodist (for the Milbank Memorial Fund).

Schick, Allen. 1966. "The Road to PBB: The Stages of Budget Reform." *Public Administration Review* 26: 243–58.

―――. 1973. "A Death in the Bureaucracy: The Demise of Federal PBB." *Public Administration Review* 33: 146–56. Reprinted in *Public Expenditure and Policy Analysis,* ed. by Robert H. Haveman and Julius Margolis, 556–76. Chicago: Rand McNally.

Schlenker, Robert E., and Paul M. Ellwood, Jr. 1973. "Medical Inflation: Causes and Policy Options for Control." Typescript. Minneapolis: InterStudy.

Schultze, Charles L. 1969. "The Role of Incentives, Penalties, and Rewards in Attaining Effective Policy." In *The Analysis and Evaluation of Public Expenditures: The PBB System, A Compendium of Papers . . . ,* U.S. Congress, I, 201–25. Joint Economic Committee, Subcommittee on Economy in Government, 91st Cong., 1st Sess., 3 vols., Joint Comm. Print. Rev. version available in *Public Expenditures and Policy Analysis,* ed. by Robert H. Haveman and Julius Margolis, 145–72. Chicago: Markham, 1970.

―――. 1977. *The Public Use of Private Interest.* Washington, DC: Brookings Institution.

Seidman, Laurence S. 1980. "Income-Related Cost Sharing: A Strategy for the Health Sector." In *National Health Insurance: What Now, What Later, What Never?* ed. by Mark V. Pauly, 307–28. Washington, DC: American Enterprise Institute.

―――. 1981. "Consumer-Choice Health Plan and the Patient Cost-Sharing Strategy: Can They Be Reconciled?" In *A New Approach to the Economics of Health Care,* ed. by Mancur Olson, 448–66. Washington, DC: American Enterprise Institute.

Shain, Max, and Milton I. Roemer. 1959. "Hospital Costs Relate to the Supply of Beds." *Modern Hospital* 92 (April): 71–73, 168.

Sidel, Victor, and Ruth Sidel. 1977. *A Healthy State: An International Perspective on the Crisis in United States Medical Care.* New York: Pantheon. 1983.

―――, eds. 1984. *Reforming Medicine: Lessons of the Last Quarter Century.* New York: Pantheon.

Sloan, Frank A., and Bruce Steinwald. 1980. "Effects of Regulation on Hospital Costs and Use." *Journal of Law and Economics* 23: 81–109.

Somers, Anne R. 1969a. *Hospital Regulation: The Dilemma of Public Policy.* Princeton, NJ: Industrial Relations Section, Princeton University.

―――. 1969b. "These Are the Questions about Regulation: What Kind? How Much? By Whom? Why?" *Modern Hospital* 113 (September): 137–41.

―――. 1971. *Health Care in Transition.* Chicago: The Hospital Research and Educational Trust.

Somers, Anne R., and Herman M. Somers. 1977. *Health and Health Care: Policies in Perspective.* Germantown, MD: Aspen Systems.

Somers, Herman M., and Anne R. Somers. 1961. *Doctors, Patients, and Health Insurance: The Organization and Financing of Medical Care.* Washington, DC: Brookings Institution.

―――. 1967. *Medicare and the Hospitals: Issues and Prospects.* Washington, DC: Brookings Institution.

Spek, Jan-Erik. 1980. "Why is the System So Costly? Problems of Policy and Management at National and Regional Levels." In *The Shaping of the Swedish Health*

System, ed. by Arnold J. Heidenheimer and Nils Elvander, 181–207. New York: St. Martin's.

Ståhl, Ingemar. 1980. "The Growth of Health Care: Two Model Solutions." In *The Shaping of the Swedish Health System,* ed. by Arnold J. Heidenheimer and Nils Elvander, 208–19. New York: St. Martin's.

Starr, Paul. 1979. "Kennedy's Conservative Health Plan." *New Republic* 180 (June 9): 18–21.

———. 1982a. *The Social Transformation of American Medicine: The Rise of a Sovereign Profession and the Making of a Vast Industry.* New York: Basic Books.

———. 1982b. "Transformation in Defeat: The Changing Objectives of National Health Insurance, 1915–1980." In *Compulsory Health Insurance: The Continuing Debate,* ed. by Ronald L. Numbers, 115–43. Contributions in Medical History, No. 11. Westport, CN: Greenwood Press.

———. 1983. "Medical Care and the Pursuit of Equality in America." In *Securing Access to Health Care: The Ethical Implications of Differences in the Availability of Health Services,* President's Commission for the Study of Ethical Problems in Medicine and Biomedical Research, II, 3–22. Washington, DC: U.S. Government Printing Office.

———. 1984. "Review [of Sidel and Sidel 1984]." *New York Times Book Review* 89: 25.

Steiner, Peter O. 1969. "The Public Sector and the Public Interest." In *The Analysis and Evaluation of Public Expenditures: The PBB System, A Compendium of Papers . . . ,* U.S. Congress, I, 13–45. Joint Economic Committee, Subcommittee on Economy in Government, 91st Cong., 1st Sess., 3 vols., Joint Comm. Print.

Stevens, Robert, and Rosemary Stevens. 1974. *Welfare Medicine in America: A Case Study of Medicaid.* New York: Free Press.

Stevens, Rosemary, and Robert Stevens. 1970. "Medicaid: Anatomy of a Dilemma." *Law and Contemporary Problems* 35: 328–435.

Stigler, George J. 1971. "The Theory of Economic Regulation." *Bell Journal of Economics and Management Science* 2: 3–21.

———. 1981. "Comment on Joskow and Noll." In *Studies in Public Regulation,* ed. by Gary Fromm, 73–77. Cambridge, MA: MIT Press.

Stigler, George J., and Claire Friedland. 1962. "What Can Regulators Regulate?" *Journal of Law and Economics* 5: 1–16.

Sundquist, James L. 1968. *Politics and Policy: The Eisenhower, Kennedy, and Johnson Years.* Washington, DC: Brookings Institution.

U.S. Congress. 1969. *The Analysis and Evaluation of Public Expenditures: The PBB System, A Compendium of Papers. . . .* Joint Economic Committee, Subcommittee on Economy in Government, 91st Cong., 1st Sess., 3 vols., Joint Comm. Print.

———. 1970. *Medicare and Medicaid: Problems, Issues, and Alternatives.* Senate, Staff of Committee on Finance, 91st Cong., 2d Sess., Comm. Print.

———. 1974. *National Health Planning and Resources Development Act of 1974: Report to Accompany S. 2994.* Senate, Staff of Committee on Finance, 93rd Cong., 2d Sess., S. Rept. 93-1285.

Vickrey, William S. 1963. "General and Specific Financing of Urban Services." In *Public Expenditure Decision in the Urban Community,* ed. by H. G. Schaller. Washington, DC: Resources for the Future. Corrected and abridged version in *Readings in Welfare Economics,* ed. by Kenneth J. Arrow and Tibor Scitovsky, 561–87. Republished Articles on Economics, Vol. 12. Homewood, IL: Richard D. Irwin for the American Economic Association, 1969.

Vladeck, Bruce R. 1981. "The Market *vs.* Regulation: The Case for Regulation." *Milbank Memorial Fund Quarterly/Health and Society* 59: 209–23.

Vogel, Morris J. 1980. *The Invention of the Modern Hospital: Boston, 1870–1930.* Chicago:

University of Chicago Press.

Walker, Forrest, A. 1979. "Americanism vs. Sovietism: A Study of the Reaction to the Committee on the Costs of Medical Care." *Bulletin of the History of Medicine* 53: 498–504.

Weaver, Paul H. 1978. "Regulation, Social Policy, and Class Conflict." *Public Interest* 50: 45–63.

Weeks, Lewis E., and Howard J. Berman. 1985. *Shapers of American Health Care Policy: An Oral History.* Ann Arbor, MI: Health Administration Press.

Weiner, Stephen M. 1977. "'Reasonable Cost' Reimbursement for Inpatient Hospital Services under Medicare and Medicaid: The Emergence of Public Control." *American Journal of Law and Medicine* 3: 1–47.

———. 1978. "Governmental Regulation of Health Care: A Response to Some Criticisms Voiced by Proponents of a 'Free Market.'" *American Journal of Law and Medicine* 4: 15–33.

———. 1981. "Reflections on Cost Containment Strategies." *Milbank Memorial Fund Quarterly/Health and Society* 59: 269–96.

Weisbrod, Burton A. 1968. "Income Redistribution Effects and Benefit-Cost Analysis." In *Problems in Public Expenditure Analysis,* ed. by Samuel B. Chase, Jr., 177–209. Washington, DC: Brookings Institution.

———. 1969. "Collective Action and the Distribution of Income: A Conceptual Approach." In *The Analysis and Evaluation of Public Expenditures: The PBB System, A Compendium of Papers . . . ,* U.S. Congress, I, 177–97. Joint Economic Committee, Subcommittee on Economy in Government, 91st Cong., 1st Sess., 3 vols., Joint Comm. Print.

———. 1977. *The Voluntary Nonprofit Sector: An Economic Analysis.* Lexington, MA: Lexington Books.

———. 1978. "Comment [on Pauly 1978]." In *Competition in the Health Care Sector: Past, Present, and Future,* ed. by Warren Greenberg, 37–42. Proceedings of a Conference Sponsored by the Bureau of Economics, Federal Trade Commission, 1978. Germantown, MD: Aspen Systems.

Wildavsky, Aaron. 1966. "The Political Economy of Efficiency: Cost-Benefit Analysis, Systems Analysis, and Program Budgeting." *Public Administration Review* 26: 292–310.

———. 1969. "Rescuing Policy Analysis from PPBS." In *The Analysis and Evaluation of Public Expenditures: The PBB System, A Compendium of Papers . . . ,* U.S. Congress, III, 835–64. Joint Economic Committee, Subcommittee on Economy in Government, 91st Cong., 1st Sess., 3 vols., Joint Comm. Print.

———. 1977. "Doing Better and Feeling Worse: The Political Pathology of Health Policy." In *Doing Better and Feeling Worse: Health in the United States,* ed. by John H. Knowles, 105–23. New York: Norton.

Wilensky, Harold L. 1975. *The Welfare State and Equality: Structural and Ideological Roots of Public Expenditures.* Berkeley: University of California Press.

———. 1981. "Leftism, Catholicism, and Democratic Corporatism: The Role of Political Parties in Recent Welfare State Development." In *The Development of Welfare States in Europe and America,* ed. by Peter Flora and Arnold J. Heidenheimer, 345–82. New Brunswick, NJ: Transaction Books.

Wolf, Charles, Jr. 1979. "A Theory of Nonmarket Failure: Framework for Implementation Analysis." *Journal of Law and Economics* 22: 107–39.

Yordy, Karl D. 1976. "Regionalization of Health Services: Current Legislative Directions in the United States." In *The Regionalization of Personal Health Services,* ed. by Ernest W. Saward, 201–15. Rev. ed. New York: Prodist (for the Milbank Memorial Fund).

3

The New Competition in Health Care: Implications for the Future

Walter W. McMahon

Powerful economic forces are transforming health care delivery. This transformation, which is becoming the second major revolution affecting health care in modern times, is a reaction to the first, an extraordinarily rapid diffusion since 1945 of health insurance and third-party reimbursement, unfortunately accompanied by escalating health care costs. The rapid expansion of private health insurance was followed in 1965 by public health insurance, through Medicare and Medicaid, which piggybacked on the private Blue Cross/Blue Shield cost-based reimbursement methods. This first health care revolution and its reimbursement methods encouraged high use and even permitted padding to creep into health care costs and billing.

The escalation of health care costs has fueled the second revolution— a radical change in the way in which hospitals and physicians are reimbursed, coupled with deregulation of the health sector and the emergence of competition. This "new competition" is the result of efforts by the major buyers of health care (the large employers, the federal government, and the state governments) to contain health care costs. These buyers are the ones that must bear most of the health care bills. They now negotiate in advance to contract for the price of a package of health care services under conditions of increasing competition among providers. The use of these more competitive contracts is extremely likely to continue so long as health care costs continue to rise. It is a new kind of competition that has profound implications for the way in which health care services will be provided and for the structure of the health care system of the future.

This chapter explores the implications for the future of the health care system of the emergence of the new competition, which combines deregulation with advance negotiation for "bundles" of health care services. It is to the advantage of providers to consider, as they plan ahead, the nature of the change and its implications. The development of health policies—at the state level and by employers—also will proceed better if influenced by an awareness of the economic forces at work and of the economic implications of current trends.

To enhance this awareness, the chapter first characterizes the escalation in health care costs that has motivated the continuing interest by government and business in attaining greater efficiency. It explains how cost-based retrospective reimbursement by insurers contributes to the escalation of health care costs, including those resulting from expensive novelties in medical technology and from inappropriate hospital utilization. It then describes the forms of the new competition emerging in health care and considers the rationale (the way in which competition is *supposed* to work to bring down costs). As the implications for the structure of the industry are developed, the chapter suggests some of the forms that a sound competitive health care policy should take to meet the needs of marginal groups, such as the working poor and the elderly, and to keep them from falling through the gaps in the system. Finally, the discussion turns to some of the implications for the activities and training of health care professionals as they become more involved with management decisions and grow more concerned with efficient use of resources.

UPHEAVAL, CHANGE, AND CHALLENGE

Deregulation, moves toward more competition, and shifts away from retrospective reimbursement are all producing dramatic change. A description of the economic forces causing this change will set the stage for a description of its nature.

Health Care Costs—A Few Facts

To appraise the scope of the forces producing change, it is necessary to look briefly at the current level and trend of health care costs. Health care costs reached 11.0 percent of gross national product (GNP) in 1987, as compared with 4.4 percent of the nation's output in 1950. In recent years, health expenditures in real terms have been growing at four times the nation's growth rate (Fuchs 1986). In absolute dollars, health care costs come to $6,936 each year for an average family of four, and more than this for those whose family income is above average. Also in absolute dollars, the total health care bill in the United States has increased 11-fold since 1960.

The chief administrator of the federal Health Care Financing Administration, Carolyne Davis, estimated that 58 percent of the increase is due to the rising price per unit of physician and hospital services (Davis

1983, 13). The hospital room rate, for example, rose 457 percent from 1967 to 1983, and physician fees rose by 227 percent, but during the same time the overall Consumer Price Index rose 189 percent (Bureau of Labor Statistics 1985, 1987). Various regulatory approaches, such as the application of price "guidelines" during the Carter administration and, more recently, the freeze on physicians' Medicare reimbursement rates have not succeeded very well, in that the rate of increase has remained overall at about double the nation's inflation rate. However, there is some recent evidence that increased competition, together with other factors, has begun to slow the increase in physicians' incomes. Following the enactment of the Health Professionals Education Assistance Act in 1963, federal subsidies to expand the number and size of the nation's medical schools significantly increased the number of physicians; Korock (1984) estimates that, by 1990, 43 percent of the nation's doctors will have been graduated since 1978. There has been an increase in the number of physicians serving rural areas, small towns, and other physician shortage areas, and in the number of physicians accepting Medicare assignment (American Medical Association 1985; Korock 1984; Feldstein 1986). Increased supply, together with the freeze in rates of reimbursement, contributed to a .3 percent-per-year decline in the average real income of physicians between 1973 and 1983 (American Medical Association 1985, 61). The withdrawal of most federal assistance and a resultant decline in medical school admissions presage reductions in the supply of physicians and potential reversal of many of currently observable effects of the supply increase since 1963.

At the individual level, Senator Metzenbaum from Ohio, who investigated hospital prices, cites routine hospital charges of $275 a day for a double room; additional charges can easily raise the average price to over $1,000 a day for a short hospital stay. Physician charges are normally additional to hospital bills. As more states collect and publicize rates paid by third-party payers for each city and each hospital, the public is becoming increasingly aware of local prices. This is not to suggest that the public is likely to do much about this (since the insurance company, Medicare, or Medicaid normally pays the bills), but it does suggest that the public is likely to be more permissive as governmental units and employer groups begin to act.

The Forces Propelling Change

The moves toward the new competition, consisting of both deregulation and negotiation in advance on the prices of bundles of services (prospective reimbursement), continue to be motivated by these sharp increases in health care costs. Various political coalitions have emerged to propel continuing change. These include employers, who are concerned about the large and rising costs that they must bear for their employee health benefit plans; state governments, which are deeply concerned about the rising cost of Medicaid; and the federal government (and the retirees it serves through Medicare), who are concerned that the Social Security trust fund remain solvent. Though the moves toward competition began at the federal level, employers and state governments increasingly recognize their joint interests in containing costs, and state-level restructuring of the health care delivery system is therefore becoming common. As long as the price increases continue, federal, state, and employer motivations to act are strengthened.

The Basic Problem with Incentives—Leading to More Change

Cost-based reimbursement without prior agreement on the total price for the necessary bundle of treatments provides perverse incentives, inducing providers to increase costs. Retrospective reimbursement rewards with more revenue those who pad the costs and penalizes those who seek to be efficient and not to waste resources. This disincentive to be efficient is now widely recognized as a primary cause of escalating health care costs among those researching the economics of the operation of our health care system (see, for example, Feldstein 1985; Fuchs 1986; and Davis 1983).

When retrospective reimbursement is coupled with third-party payment—95 percent of those who require health care services do not pay their own bill—health care users lack incentive to police costs. After all, "the insurance company pays," or "Medicare pays," so why bother? Third-party payers include the federal government, which reimburses for Medicare patients; the state governments, which still reimburse for most Medicaid services on the old retrospective basis (and often in costly emergency room and Medicaid-mill settings); and private insurers, such as Blue Cross/Blue Shield. In virtually all other spheres of economic activity, the final buyer agrees on the price beforehand.

Cost-based retrospective reimbursement, furthermore, offers incentives to prescribe unnecessary services.[1] Studies have found that 50 percent of second opinions about the need for surgery, for example, are that the surgery is unnecessary. This result may overstate the percentage of the contemplated operations that are unnecessary, since it undoubtedly also reflects the absence in some situations of a consensus concerning appropriate medical practice. Nevertheless, it does provide an opportunity for a more balanced opinion, and many insurers are now requiring a second opinion before they will agree to reimburse.[2] Extra days in the hospital for a Blue Cross/Blue Shield patient help to keep the beds filled at a time when prospective reimbursement has limited this practice for Medicare and Medicaid patients, leaving hospitals with excess capacity. With some unnecessary utilization and cost shifting to privately insured patients, the cost to employer health benefit plans of the traditional Blue Cross/Blue Shield cost-based reimbursement insurance continues to rise.[3]

Getting away from cost-plus as a method of reimbursement is not the only way to contain costs, of course. In Canada, as Evans points out, the rise in health care costs was contained in 1980, with Canada spending then about what it spent in 1970, and by 1985, spending 20 to 30 percent less per capita than is spent in the United States (Evans 1983, 1984, 1985). However, the situation in Canada is quite different from that in the United States: There is a single public payer in each Canadian province, instead of our multiplicity of third-party payers. (Britain's National Health Service also has the equivalent of this 100 percent monopsony budget control, which is effective but seems unlikely to appear in the United States, at least in the current political environment.) In spite of this Canadian containment, the unbundled cost-based reimbursement method there permits Evans to marshal extensive evidence that a rise in the supply of hospital beds may lead not only to greater overall utilization, but also to constant or rising prices as the cost of these additional facilities is built into total health care costs and passed along, perhaps resulting in some loss in economic efficiency. It is also true that health care expenditures as a percent of GNP began to rise again in Canada in 1982 (Evans 1985, 451). Evans stresses that these problems are not generated by external forces such as an aging population, the extension of technology, or the demands of ethical standards, but are rooted in the current incentives within the health care system itself.

Another important trend causing cost-based reimbursement to contribute to rising costs in the United States (as well as in Canada) is the acquisition of expensive, high-technology equipment. In most industries the producer has an incentive to purchase new equipment that will do the job as well as or better than existing equipment and will save on labor and other costs. In health care, however, the full cost of the new equipment can be passed on to the third-party payer as part of the patient's bill. The kind of equipment purchased can therefore be indifferently cost-increasing or cost-reducing. Furthermore, the hospital's image with physicians, and therefore its ability to fill beds, may be enhanced by having the most recent, most expensive machines readily available. The result under cost-based reimbursement is the incentive to purchase too many new machines (because their costs are passed through to third-party payers) and to select machines that are not necessarily technologically appropriate (since they unnecessarily increase rather than reduce costs).[4]

A final illustration of how overutilization under third-party retrospective reimbursement provides weak incentives to manage costs is the example of standing orders for laboratory tests.[5] Several tests will always be more revealing than a few, of course, but tests have diminishing returns. At some point there must be a balance between the additional information yielded and the additional cost, not just to the third-party payer, but also in the form of the cost of the patient's time and the risks to his or her health.

Deregulation

To turn to the changes now taking place, it is important to recognize that health care is an industry in which entry is heavily regulated. There are cash investment requirements for health care plans; extensive state licensure requirements for physicians, nurses, and other providers; quality requirements; and state laws requiring certificates of need for new hospitals and high-technology equipment (McMahon and Blumberg 1985).

But things are changing very fast. The current federal administration is heavily committed to fostering competition as a means of containing escalating health care costs and encouraging greater efficiency in the use of health resources (Davis 1983, for example). Disillusioned with regulation as a means to these ends, as was the preceding administration, the Reagan administration is rapidly dismantling certificate-of-need requirements and is cutting back on the funding for health systems planning agencies. The courts have joined the trend by holding, in a recent Kansas City case, that state certificate-of-need laws bar entry and foster monopoly in violation of the antitrust laws. Similarly, the Supreme Court, in *Goldfarb v. Virginia State Bar,* has held that self-regulation by the "learned professions" is not exempt from antitrust scrutiny (Goldfarb 1975). These moves toward deregulation and competition have a significant effect in shifting the locus of economic power in health care from the self-regulation by the health care industry (especially by the American Medical Association and by county medical societies) to the demand side and to the discipline of the market.

Other aspects of deregulation and the moves toward more competition include the recent information that the administration will no longer enforce the regulations that require hospitals that have received Hill-Burton funds for expansion to care for their share of the poor.[6] One result is the widely publicized "dumping" of patients whose funds have run out by many not-for-profit hospitals as the hospitals face competitive pressures. Dumping is the transfer of patients who are often ill, elderly, and in the (very costly) last few days of their lives to underfunded public hospitals like Cook County Hospital in Chicago. Also, at the federal level, the Federal Trade Commission has insisted that the American Medical Association remove from its code of ethics the statement that advertising is unethical and notify its members of this change.[7] Hospitals and health maintenance organizations (HMOs) are already advertising widely.

States are also moving gingerly toward efforts to use competition to contain costs. Iowa and Illinois have established cost containment councils, for example, to increase consumer information on health care prices, which is necessary if competition is to be able to work.[8] Similarly, Massachusetts has released data relevant to the quality of care and to fees for comparable procedures. Following California, Illinois and Arizona are also trying new competitive bidding procedures to serve Medicaid recipients.[9]

However, most state licensure and certificate-of-need legislation is still in place. It is possible that with the greater influence of trade associations at the state level, health care will follow the earlier pattern established in the deregulation of trucking, with some states preserving islands of state-sponsored monopoly under the guise of (ineffective) economic regulation. However, there is increasing awareness that excessive requirements for cash investment and overly costly standards for facilities and licensure increase costs, as well as growing reconsideration of the economic impact of certificate-of-need requirements and other barriers to entry. As the federal government moves to dismantle the barriers to entry for which it has been responsible, and as states move to expand the information about prices available to consumers and to reexamine the barriers to entry that remain at the state level, genuine competition is likely to grow rather than diminish.

The New Competition

The new competition involves a combination of these two major changes—the shift toward negotiating the price beforehand, and the reduction of barriers to entry.

Since the federal government is a major purchaser of health services, its shift to prospective reimbursement for Medicare patients sets one significant part of the tone. Its steps to declare in advance the price it will pay by diagnosis for each of the original 470 diagnosis-related groups (which have come to be known by the acronym DRGs) is by now well known, but some of the underlying implications are less well understood. A key element is that prospective reimbursement forces hospitals to establish an accounting "cost center" for each of the 470 DRGs (the number will undoubtedly change somewhat over time), and then to allocate all hospital costs to one or another of these bundles of final treatment regimens that they sell. Because data of this kind were never available before, within the hospital none of these "product lines" has ever had a cost manager, and management to achieve economic efficiency was impossible. The main task of containing costs previously had been centralized in Blue Cross/Blue Shield data banks and state and federal Medicaid-Medicare offices, for use with the separate cost-based reimbursement rates that they establish for the many services now included within each DRG. The commercial insurers, as well as Medicaid and Medicare, have had the impossible task of monitoring the level and volume of procedures for which they would reimburse providers for patients they never saw. With indemnity (fixed-price) reimbursement for unbundled separate charges for separate procedures, the physician, who orders almost all of the services on behalf of the patient, has had no incentive to combine these services in the most economically efficient proportions and has lacked the cost data with which to do so. Without the information about the total cost and cost effectiveness of the bundle of treatments prescribed for each diagnosis, and without the capacity to compare those total product costs to the cost effectiveness of the bundle of treatments performed in response to the same diagnosis by others, even if the physician did have the incentive, it would be next to impossible to become a truly efficient cost manager.

The new steps by hospitals to collect data on the basis of the 470 cost centers is perhaps the most fundamental and revolutionary change involved in the newly emerging health care system. It permits the delegation of more power of a different kind to physicians—power to become managers, power that had been centralized (and still is for private and Medicaid patients) in those who enforce the reimbursement regulations in private health insurance companies and in state government offices. This decentralization of managerial decision-making responsibility is a very new and different kind of power that many physicians have not been trained to exercise. On whether or not it is exercised wisely rests the fate of many clinics and hospitals.

The excess capacity in hospital beds now resulting from the advent of DRGs is causing many hospitals to seek to eliminate local competition by arranging for mergers. Except for the advantage in raising funds nationally, mergers offer no major cost advantages after hospitals reach a medium size (see Berry 1967). Although mergers may still be economically advantageous to the hospital as local monopolies are created, there are always the problems of violation of the antitrust laws and the even higher hospital prices that can result from the elimination of local competition. Although some mergers of extremely small hospitals can be justified on cost grounds and can be induced by competition, many mergers that result in local near-monopolies probably should be viewed as anticompetitive moves.

Many new forms of health care delivery have emerged in the wave of the new competition: health maintenance organizations, independent practice associations, preferred provider organizations, primary care networks, management groups, and even some traditional fee-for-service clinics with surgicenter feeder networks.

Health maintenance organizations (HMOs), which agree beforehand to provide comprehensive services for a single annual capitation fee, are now growing in number very rapidly (see Punch and Johnson 1984). Research by Luft, Liebowitz, and others suggests that HMOs lower rates of hospital admission and shorten lengths of stay (Luft 1980; Manning et al. 1985). The result, according to some administrators, is a cost advantage of about 40 percent, allowing them consistently to offer lower out-of-pocket payments and larger benefits to those individuals choosing HMOs. Large private insurance companies such as Prudential have become involved in developing HMOs in Dallas, Austin (Texas), Nashville, Oklahoma City, Atlanta, Chicago, and elsewhere. There are Maxicare statewide networks, and most of the larger hospitals and clinics in most cities have become involved in setting up and advertising their own Personal Care, Heartland Care, Carle Care, or Other Care HMOs.

Independent practice associations (IPAs) are more loosely knit groups of physicians from the fee-for-service sector who bid together as providers of medical services for employer or state health plans. Many IPAs do not have the internal management structures to manage costs and therefore are less likely to be able to win bids and to survive in localities in which competition is severe.

Preferred provider organizations (PPOs) are a new form of competitive health plan negotiated with employers that offer financial incentives to employees to go to designated "preferred providers," that is, physicians and hospitals that have agreed to combine more cost-effective practice styles with lower fees. Employees are free to go to whatever physician they choose, but they pay no out-of-pocket fee if they choose a preferred provider.

Primary care networks (PCNs) are groups of primary care physicians, usually general practitioners, who act as gatekeepers to health care, providing primary care themselves and overseeing the use of specialist and hospital services. PCNs contract with hospitals, and after selling their services for a prospective reimbursement rate, set aside a fund, called a risk pool, to cover both specialists and hospitalization.

Management groups combine employers into groups to purchase health insurance. Because employer benefit plans are very costly, large employers such as IBM, Polaroid, John Deere, General Mills, Honeywell, and Caterpillar have begun to circumvent Blue Cross/Blue Shield and contract directly with more cost-effective providers. This has caused Blue Cross/Blue Shield to offer additional options in coverage and has given a boost to those health care plans that have abandoned fee-for-service in favor of a prepaid capitation rate.

State governments, as mentioned earlier, are also beginning to solicit competitive bids for serving Medicaid recipients on a capitation basis (see McMahon and Blumberg 1985). Following Medi-Cal in California, Arizona, which formerly had no state Medicaid program, has now written Medicaid-

Figure 3.1—Short Term HI Trust Fund Ratios. Adapted and Reproduced with Permission of Anthony J. Jannetti, Inc., Publisher, *Nursing Economic$,* Vol. 1, No. 1, pp. 10–17. Figure 5.

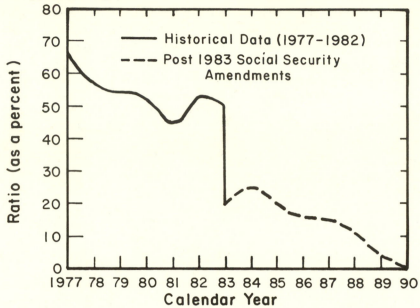

HMO contracts in all communities in which there were two or more competitive bids. Illinois has funded six large Medicaid-HMO contracts in Chicago. Experiments with Medicaid HMOs are underway in several other states, including the demonstration experiments funded by the Health Care Financing Administration in Florida, Missouri, and Minnesota.

A large portion of both Medicare and Medicaid payments goes for long-term care of the elderly in nursing homes. These services include medical appliances, which can cost as much as $195 per month to rent (and must often be rented for years) or as much as $2,000 to purchase (in the case of a padded wheelchair). Despite the recent increases in Social Security taxes, the continuing rise in health care costs for the elderly means that the Social Security trust fund will be bankrupt by 1990 (as shown in fig. 3:1), even after the effect of the 1983 increase in Social Security taxes is taken into account. Under these conditions it would appear virtually certain that the decision to proceed with DRGs will not be reversed. There are inevitable adjustment strains, and problems with "diagnosis creep"; but DRGs are beginning to reduce hospital utilization rates and hence slow down the escalation of Medicare hospital costs.

The Health Care Financing Administration, furthermore, is now experimenting with the extension of the prepayment approach to Medicare and Medicaid HMOs for long-term nursing home care, which is important because long-term care accounts for such a large percentage of public health care costs. Some research problems remain to be solved, especially with respect to how to share the risks and the total fee among those admitted when their health conditions differ widely (see Thomas et al. 1983).[10] If these problems are solved, the HMO concept is likely to be extended soon to long-term nursing home care for Medicaid recipients.

THE RATIONALE: HOW ARE COMPETITION AND PREPAYMENT SUPPOSED TO WORK?

It must first be emphasized more strongly that the most important kind of competition, the kind for which accurate information on the price and quality of health care needs to be available, is the competition among health plans. Competition after a person is sick is far less meaningful—at that point he or she is not in a good position to shop around. It is during an annual enrollment period (when employers are reconsidering their health insurance contracts with alternative providers and employees are selecting from among health insurance plans) that competition among providers is most effective. It is in this situation that the most cost-effective plans, which are likely to be those based on prospective reimbursement, are gradually winning out.

The Rationale

But how is this combined effect of prepayment and competition, together with the retention of some necessary minimum quality regulations, supposed to work?

The combined effect is illustrated in figure 3:2, in which the curve CC illustrates the minimum cost of production at each level of health care quality. Quality must be measured in terms of an ordinal index, with higher quality reflecting greater health effectiveness further to the right, and lower quality to the left. (There is no cardinal measure of exactly how much the levels of quality differ.) Higher quality, of course, means higher costs, so the cost curve slopes upward to the right. Eventually, however, more dollars do less and less to increase the health effectiveness of the care, and the curve becomes vertical. That is, diminishing returns set in as expenditures for treating a given diagnosis increase. Eventually additional outlays of cost simply do not further increase the true quality of care, and with the complications that arise with medical procedures, additional outlays and procedures could even eventually reduce the health effectiveness of the care.

In principle, health services may be provided at any combination of quality and cost located on or above the curve CC. However, in practice, certain combinations must be ruled out. Minimum quality regulations rule

Figure 3:2—Abandonment of Cost-Based Reimbursement

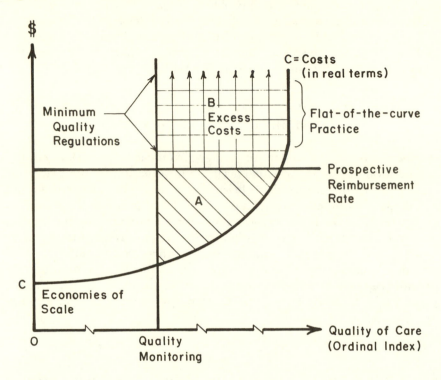

out the entire area to the left of the vertical line in figure 3:2—inadequate nursing homes, untrained health care professionals, unsanitary hospital conditions. Regulations of this type will always be needed; hence, a blend between regulation and competition can reasonably be expected to be a permanent feature of the new competition. The kinds of regulation being eliminated at the federal level, such as certificates of need and extraordinary initial requirements for HMO plans, are those that set up excessive barriers to entry and thereby serve to foster monopoly. At the state level, few regulations of this type have been dismantled and, as mentioned, trade association influence remains very strong. Anticompetitive economic regulation and islands of monopoly may therefore persist in some states for many years to come.

The most severe current problems are illustrated in figure 3:2 in the area to the right of the minimum quality regulations and above the cost curve CC. Here, as discussed above, cost-plus reimbursement, much like the cost-plus contracts in nuclear plant construction, provides incentives to all providers to increase costs. The area of excess costs (area B in fig. 3:2) is without an upper bound for most episodes of medical treatment, since additional costs can be incurred and passed on to the insurance company or

Figure 3:3—Rationalization of Health Care Delivery

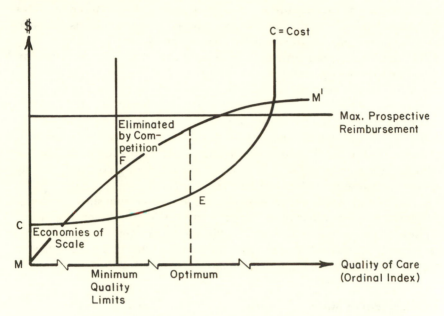

the government. Furthermore, not only is the red tape unpleasant to providers, regulators, and patients, but the large amount of paper work required is also costly and wasteful.

Prospective reimbursement via DRGs is not a form of regulation that involves the use of laws and the police power of the state; it involves instead a use of market power on the demand side by the government to reach a price agreement between buyer and seller before services are rendered. Health maintenance organizations are also reimbursed prospectively rather than retrospectively, but in their case the stipulated price covers preventive care, ambulatory care, and full-service hospital care. As Medicare DRGs are bundled to produce a single price for full-service coverage, they will approach a prospective-reimbursement HMO basis. With negotiation beforehand to fix a price for bundles of services, there is a stronger incentive to bring costs under control. The result of combining minimum quality regulations with the abandonment of cost-based reimbursement is to place an upper bound on the feasible region in figure 3:2, limiting it to area A—that is, to care of good quality, but at prenegotiated cost.

However, reasonable prospective reimbursement rates require that there be competitive bidding among health care insurance plans. So, as shown in figure 3:3, the new competition is designed to limit the feasible region further, providing a curved upper bound symbolizing the discipline of the market. Curve MM′ is a total revenue curve based on the final effective demand from both public and private insurance plans (assuming that now all patients, rather than just Medicare patients, are included in the analysis). This new competition among health care plans offered by HMOs and other health insurance providers is intended to provide disincentives to those providing the lowest quality care at the highest cost (area F in fig. 3:3). The largest opportunities to grow, and the largest net revenues, are available to those operating at the most cost-effective point, point E. The net revenues are much smaller or negative for those providing the lower-quality care at high cost (in area F) although a few may be able to survive, especially in those states that retain protective anticompetitive legislation. The net revenue will also be smaller for those who provide costly increments to health care that do not contribute significantly to health effectiveness (near point M'). Their high costs are not being covered, and the survival of these providers will be in jeopardy.

Increasing the intensity of competition beyond that shown in figure 3:3 would have the effect of shifting the curve MM' (representing the discipline of the market) downward. This would further limit the feasible region and squeeze more of the providers toward the area around the single most cost-effective range (near E).

Requirement of Multiple Choice

Requiring employers to offer their employees a choice of several health insurance plans, at least one of which uses prospective reimbursement, encourages competition among plans and the creation of prospective-reimbursement plans in localities now lacking them. It enables employees to compare and to choose the most cost-effective plan, that is, the plan that offers the greatest benefits, or the one that has the lowest out-of-pocket costs, or one that balances these features. The requirement that employers go a step further and rebate some fraction of the cost savings to those choosing the more cost-effective health plans would drastically increase the amount of competition because it would alert employees and give them a strong incentive to compare plans. This is a step that the federal government has not as yet been willing to take.

To make competition more effective, it is now necessary to reduce sharply the state-level economic regulations that bar entry and foster monopoly. State certificate-of-need legislation and state licensing requirements must be reduced. If state cost-based Medicaid reimbursement methods were replaced with prospective reimbursement, empty hospital beds that now can be used to raise cost-based rates would instead become a strong deterrent to increasing hospital room rates. Instead of raising rates to pass on the costs, the empty beds would be an incentive to hospital managers to lower rates to attract additional business from employers. Underused technology also would be avoided in favor of technology that could either reduce costs, be fully utilized, or both, and therefore be more cost-effective. Increased admission to medical schools, rather than the decreasing enrollments that are now occurring, would continue to restrict the rise in physicians' incomes, while also continuing to increase the supply of physicians to underserved areas. Reduction of the barriers encountered by nurse practitioners, who can perform a range of the more standard and simpler medical treatments and refer other cases to specialists, would also help to lower costs. In these ways the states could greatly help to reduce cost escalation and, instead of being part of the cost-escalation problem, become part of the solution.

INEQUITY: THE BIGGEST CRACK IN
THE EMERGING SYSTEM

As competition increases, the discretion available to nonprofit institutions to serve those whose insurance is inadequate and who are unable to pay is squeezed. The working poor, who are ineligible for Medicaid and yet are underinsured, are increasingly denied access or are forced onto the already overcrowded public hospitals.

Uncompensated Hospital Care

About 90 percent of all short-term hospital beds are in not-for-profit institutions of the type that dominate the health care industry. As these institutions meet competition, their traditional roles—of serving the poor and of providing care in an environment where patients have little information—come under increasing pressure. Largely as a result of this pressure, cracks in the newly emerging system are beginning to appear.

It is a serious and vexing problem to continue to provide health care throughout the nation to those who lack health insurance. Hospitals have borne these costs in the past largely through cost shifting, that is, recouping the costs for charity care by charging more to those patients who have full private insurance coverage. This route is increasingly barred, however, as a safety valve. As competition increases, Blue Cross/Blue Shield and other private insurers are becoming increasingly chary about reimbursement for services that they know are being charged at a rate above their true full cost. This attitude puts the squeeze on not-for-profit and for-profit hospitals alike. Consistent with this point, Hadley and Feder present data that show that hospitals are no longer increasing their markups from privately insured patients when revenues are squeezed. Instead they reduce personnel, postpone pay increases, and *limit charity care*. In fact, as early as 1980 to 1982, the period covered by Hadley and Feder's study, 24.4 percent of hospitals that had increased need for cost shifting (due to the costs of caring for noncommercially insured patients that exceeded their sources of funds from all other activities) responded by adopting explicit limits on charity care (Hadley and Feder 1985).

Health Care for the Working Poor, the Unemployed, and the Uninsured

Complex new issues are raised, therefore, about how to finance health care for the working poor, those who are temporarily unemployed, and others who are not totally destitute and thereby eligible for Medicaid but who are uninsured for long run catastrophic illness. Gail Wilensky estimates the scope of the problem, based on the American Hospital Association's Annual Survey of Hospitals in 1982, at $4.5 billion in bad debt and $1.7 billion in charity care for patients who were not expected to pay—a total of $6.2 billion in uncompensated care. She cites also National Medical Care Utilization and Expenditures Survey data that suggest that 18 million people were uninsured and an additional 16 million people were underinsured—almost one-fifth of the U.S. population (Wilensky 1984).

A tax-supported health care plan is obviously needed to deal with this problem. One would think that at least some of the savings achieved in the health care system through the shift to prepayment, capitation, and greater competition could and should be devoted to this problem. However, in the current fiscal environment of large deficits, resistance to restoring revenue lost as the result of tax cuts, and efforts to pare government expenditure further, a clear demonstration may be needed of savings in Medicare and Medicaid before any new program can be passed. Problems in public financing notwithstanding, if the system is to remain humane, grants are needed for the working poor, the unemployed, the underemployed, and the low-income underinsured to help them cover at least a fraction of the annual premium—not, one hopes, in a cost-plus reimbursement but in a prospective-reimbursement health plan (see National Center for Health Services Research 1985).

Opportunities and Problems in Implementation

In addressing this problem, there is a real danger of continuing a low, flat threshold for Medicaid eligibility. A prospective-reimbursement plan with a scaled copayment has the potential of increasing both the efficiency and the equity of the whole health care system. A new "Healthcare Plan" of this type would use capitation-type prepayment rather than a cost-plus reimbursement, while also scaling public contributions inversely and more precisely to recipients' ability to pay. Such a plan would have the potential for increasing the economic efficiency of private physicians by the incentives inherent in prepaid, longer-term, capitation reimbursement. It also has the potential for increasing social efficiency by serving a segment of the population that is currently less healthy and underserved. This segment now contributes to the fact that U.S. health statistics compare poorly with those of Britain, Canada, Japan, and several other developed nations. Finally, equity also would be served by the greater sensitivity of this Healthcare Plan to ability to pay, a feature that would also serve to minimize the tax cost of such a plan.

Approaches that involve targeting providers, targeting individuals, and targeting grants to local governments have been discussed in the literature, and different states are trying a number of them (Wilensky 1984; Jones and Kilpatrick 1986). Each approach has situations in which it is particularly advantageous; hence examples of each are likely to persist. For example, a publicly owned and operated hospital (such as Cook County Hospital in Chicago) that serves a unique set of purposes is common in most localities, and could be viewed as a part of a broader attempt to target providers. However, expanding this approach to systems of subsidization or private for-profit and not-for-profit hospitals (such as exist in Maryland and New Jersey), to reimburse providers for uncompensated care, has major disadvantages. It does not direct users to the most efficient providers, and it requires heavy regulation—probably more than most states would find acceptable. New York, which is also an all-payer reimbursement state, grants funds to providers who need not be tied to the system from a common pool of revenues. Nevertheless, the practice remains in these systems of reimbursing hospitals according to current utilization patterns, thereby rewarding inefficient delivery and penalizing innovations that increase efficiency.

The approach of targeting grants to local governments also has both virtues and drawbacks as the basis for a greatly expanded system. It would probably incur higher costs than a program more precisely targeted to individuals in need (witness the problems with some of the housing and urban development programs, which must have a local government's involvement, or the federal subsidization of local urban transit). There is the further problem of the on-off nature of federal revenue-sharing programs, which are currently undergoing dramatic cuts. This instability can be wasteful, but may be more sustainable in physical capital investment in housing or buses than in health programs, where ongoing hospital staff changes and an immediate impact on the health and lives of many people are involved.

The most attractive approach is that of targeting individuals so that those without the ability to maintain adequate insurance coverage can pay their bills. There are various groups and types of coverage involved: catastrophic coverage, insurance for the unemployed, insurance for the indigent, and so forth. Several states are making piecemeal efforts. Alaska,

Maine, and Rhode Island have catastrophic insurance programs for individuals, for example. To enable high-risk individuals to secure coverage, Connecticut and five other states have risk-sharing pools. Several states have considered expanding Medicaid to larger numbers of unemployed and others who are underinsured. However, this approach has the severe disadvantages of the "all-or-nothing" feature inherent in Medicaid, and it entails higher average tax cost per person served because it recovers no resources from those who do have some ability to pay.

A more advantageous approach, similar to the Pell Grants used relatively successfully in higher education, may be merely to target all individuals who are underinsured due to insufficient ability to pay. A voucher, scaled inversely to income, would be provided to each person whose adjusted gross income (on his or her 1040 income tax form) is below a predetermined level. When supplemented with the family's expected contribution, it could be used to purchase annual coverage in a comprehensive health maintenance organization or other prospective reimbursement health plan of the individual's choice, so long as the plan met certain minimal standards of coverage. The reduction in paper work and in filing and processing public and private insurance claims would be enormous.

The situation in health care is much more comparable to that in higher education than it is to the case of primary and secondary education, in which vouchers are so seriously burdened with problems that, in this author's opinion, they are quite inappropriate. Primary and secondary schools are overwhelmingly publicly owned and operated, in sharp contrast to hospitals and clinics in the health care system. Racial segregation in the schooling of young children and the undercutting of support for a comprehensive citywide public school system are major implications of using vouchers for public schooling, problems that do not arise with equal force in health care.

A major attraction of health care vouchers is that they provide consumers with strong incentives to be cost-conscious in their choice of health care plans. Safeguards would have to be provided to prevent adverse and preferred risk selection—requiring a physical examination as each individual joins an HMO, for example—and then some quota system to ensure that each plan accepts an equal balance of the poorest and most preferred patients. This is a familiar problem with employer-based insured groups as well, and not unsolvable.

Another major advantage of targeting individuals is that the cost of the health care voucher plan to the taxpayers can be reduced by relating the size of the voucher to the recipient's ability to pay, as measured by income. This approach is far less costly, since it allows for considerable resource recovery. It simultaneously increases the equity of the system, since it reduces the large arbitrary distinctions between private patients who pay their own way and Medicaid patients who pay nothing but must first prove that they are totally destitute. Sophisticated methods of financial need analysis are widely used in awarding college tuition waivers and grants. In the case of health care, a one-page form, requiring the applicant to copy a few lines from his or her last income tax return, would be sent to a central processing center to produce a timely report of the patient's unmet need. This report then would be used directly to determine both the size of the grant that is provided and the patient's expected contribution to his or her own health care costs.[11]

Targeting individuals with partially structured Healthcare Plan vouchers would not be without problems. On the contrary, the likely problems would include those of new financing and risk selection (alluded to above), of consumer education, and of avoiding too much specialization among providers. These problems are not unique to the approach of targeting individuals, however, and no approach is free of all difficulties. Targeting individuals does seem realistic in the current context. It could be phased in and its funding increased to the extent that resources become available from the costs saved through the new competition. When combined with prospective reimbursement and capitation, it also shows promise of contributing positively to the social efficiency of the health care system. A financial need analysis system to determine the family's expected contribution (and the size of the voucher) would certainly involve a significant improvement in the crude state of equity in the system of health care financing.

The simple procedure of a scaled family contribution is far less costly than providing free care to all who are eligible, and makes sense for those above the Medicaid threshold. If Medicare also were to be means-tested in this way, additional problems would be raised, since those eligible for Medicare have paid into the Social Security trust funds. However, the huge savings that would be realized from Medicare alone could be more than enough to fund at no additional cost to the taxpayers a new health care system for the working poor, unemployed, uninsured, and underinsured who are eligible neither for Medicare nor Medicaid. It is this in-between group that is currently being dumped out of the for-profit *and* not-for-profit hospitals.

IMPLICATIONS FOR HEALTH CARE PROFESSIONALS

Prospective reimbursement that involves a capitation rate covering the entire health care for the patient is requiring greater attention to cost management by physicians and greater attention to the cost effectiveness of alternative treatments (for example, hospitalization versus outpatient care). This change in incentives, in turn, implies the need for greater attention to the cost-effectiveness training of new physicians in the medical schools, as well as training that increases their awareness of the nature of the new competition. Training in cost effectiveness is therefore likely to put the health professional who possesses it at a premium. Those physicians who have not learned how to combine medical services in cost-effective (and health-effective) ways are likely to be under increasing discomfort in the hospitals in which they practice.

Professionals on boards of hospitals and clinics need to alert their institutions to the need to meet the new competition by offering prepaid health plans, if they are not already doing so. Physicians are also likely to continue to combine in groups to bid for contracts with employers. Those remaining in solo practice or continuing to work on a fee-for-service basis are likely to come under increasing economic pressure as they serve a declining share of the market and are not positioned to bid for new business.

CONCLUSIONS

The newly emerging health care system shows promise of reducing cost escalation. There is acute need, however, to use part of the savings to help maintain access to health care by the working poor, the unemployed, the underemployed, and the uninsured.

Achieving these combined goals requires a continuing shift away from cost-based reimbursement and toward prospective reimbursement. When combined with the emergence of competition, this shift is likely to encourage physicians to practice in larger groups, as well as lead to hospital and hospital-clinic mergers.

A shift of power is occurring that enhances the role of physicians as economic managers. In a sense, it increases their responsibility and gives them a new kind of power by shifting from state and insurance-company administrators to physicians the basic decisions about the number of hospital days and other health care services used. This is a more appropriate locus for this power, since physicians have the patients' needs in view. It means, however, that physicians are at risk for wasting resources under prospective reimbursement. Physicians therefore need to be more adequately trained, as are engineers, architects, and other professionals, to make managerial decisions of this kind.

State-level economic regulations that continue to bar entry and foster monopoly power need to be reexamined and reduced, and cost-based reimbursement gradually abandoned, if states wish to join in using the new competitive approach to curtail rising health care costs. Medicaid especially needs to shift over to prospective reimbursement as the results of the experiments in process come in.

The result, after an adjustment period, should be a health care system with incentives to operate both more health-effectively and much more cost-effectively. Prepayment implies stronger incentives to provide preventive care and not just crisis care. Such a system also should be more satisfactory to providers, who will encounter less waste, less red tape, and more independent responsibility. It will be possible, if new legislation is passed, to be more equitable and humane in using the savings realized by the new competition to provide health care for those members of the working poor and other underinsured groups who are increasingly being denied adequate access.

NOTES

1. Feldstein 1985, 92, surveys a number of studies that conclude that the rate of surgical procedures is higher when the physician is reimbursed on a fee-for-service basis.
2. In a study of over 11,000 consultations, it was consistently shown that "33% of those voluntarily seeking a second opinion and roughly 18% of those required to seek a second opinion consultation were not confirmed for surgery by a board-certified panel consultant." The highest rate of nonconfirmation was for hysterectomies, prostatectomies, bunionectomies, and knee surgery; see McCarthy, Finkle, and Ruchlin 1981.
3. Medical care prices and insurance rates continued to rise at a 7.54 percent annual rate in 1986–87 as shown by the Medical Care Price Index; Bureau of Labor Statistics 1987, 73.
4. Garrison and Wilensky 1986, 49–51. These authors also develop (pp. 50–53) many of the specific changes that can be expected with the reversal of economic incentives that has accompanied Medicare's prospective payment system, including a greater emphasis on cost-saving technologies.
5. This and the preceding illustration are implications of Feldstein 1985, 130–34.
6. The information is based on inquiries made by the physicians in charge of the admissions department at Cook County Hospital in Chicago, who feel under pressure as other Chicago hospitals dump patients onto Cook County Hospital.
7. Regarding the American Medical Association: 94 FTC 701 (1979) modified and enforced by 638 F.2d 443 (2d Cir. 1980) affirmed by the Court 452 US 960 (1982) (per curiam).
8. See the Illinois Health Reform Act enacted by the state of Illinois in 1984, and patterned to some extent on the Iowa law, that sets up a cost containment council with this charge.
9. See McMahon and Blumberg 1985 for further description of these developments.
10. Steven Wallach in Boston has been actively working on this problem.
11. See, for example, the description of the American College Testing Program's 1986 financial need analysis criteria and methods.

REFERENCES

American College Testing Program. 1986. "Revisions of the ACT Student Financial Need Analysis Services for 1987–8." Iowa City, IA: The Program.

American Medical Association. 1985. "Reports of the Council on Long Range Planning and Development." Chicago: The Association.

Berry, Ralph. 1967. "Returns to Scale in the Production of Hospital Services." *Health
Services Research* 2: 123–39.

Bureau of Labor Statistics. 1985. *Monthly Labor Review.* Washington, DC: U.S. Department of Labor, September and later issues.

———. 1987. *Handbook of Labor Statistics: CPI Detailed Report.* Washington, DC: U.S.
Department of Labor, various issues.

Davis, Carolyne. 1983. "The Federal Role in Changing Health Care Financing."
Nursing Economics 1: 10–17.

Evans, Robert G. 1983. "Health Care in Canada: Patterns of Funding and Regulations." *Journal of Health Politics, Policy and Law* 8: 1–43.

———. 1984. *Strained Mercy: The Economics of Canadian Health Care.* Toronto: Butter-
worths.

———. 1985. "Illusions of Necessity: Eroding Responsibility for Choice in Health
Care." *Journal of Health Politics, Policy and Law* 10: 439–66.

Feldstein, Paul J. 1985. *Health Care Economics.* 2d ed. New York: Wiley.

———. 1986. "The Emergence of Market Competition in the U.S. Health Care System: Its Causes, Likely Structure, and Implications." *Health Policy* 6: 1–20.

Fuchs, Victor R. 1986. "Paying the Piper, Calling the Tune: Implications of Changes
in Reimbursement." N.B.E.R. Working Paper No. 1605. New York: National Bureau of Economic Research.

Garrison, Louis P., and Gail Wilensky. 1986. "Cost Containment and Technology."
Health Affairs 5: 46–58.

Goldfarb v. Virginia State Bar. 1975. 421 U.S. 773.

Hadley, Jack, and Judith Feder. 1985. "Hospital Cost Shifting and Care for the Uninsured." *Health Affairs* 4: 67–80.

Jones, Katherine, and K. Kilpatrick. 1984. "State Strategies for Financing Indigent
Care." *Nursing Economics* 4: 61–65.

Korock, Milan. 1984. "Marketplace Medicine in the United States." *Canadian Medical Association Journal* 130: 785–88.

Luft, Harold S. 1980. "Assessing the Evidence on HMO Performance." *Milbank
Memorial Fund Quarterly/Health and Society* 58: 501–36.

Manning, W., A. Leibowitz, G. A. Goldberg, W. H. Rogers, and J. P. Newhouse. 1984.
"A Controlled Trial of the Effect of a Prepaid Group Practice on Use of Services." *New England Journal of Medicine* 310: 1505–10.

McCarthy, Eugene, Madelon Finkle, and Hirsch Ruchlin. 1981. *Second Opinion Elective Surgery.* Boston: Auburn House.

McMahon, Walter W., and Linda J. Blumberg. 1985. "The Road to Competitive
Health Care through State Initiatives." Working Paper, University of Illinois
College of Medicine at Urbana-Champaign.

National Center for Health Services Research. 1985. "Who Are the Uninsured: Data
Preview 1." National Health Care Expenditures Study (PHS) 80-3276, PB
82-257064. Washington, DC: U.S. Department of Health and Human
Services.

Punch, Linda, and Donald E. L. Johnson. 1984. "HMOs Predict Rapid Enrollee
Growth as Consumers' Cost Concerns Mount." *Modern Healthcare* (January):
54–58.

Thomas, J. William, R. Lichtenstein, L. Wyszewianski, and S. Berki. 1983. "Increasing Medicare Enrollment in HMO's: The Need for Capitation Rates Adjusted for Health Status." *Inquiry* 20: 227–37.

Weisbrod, Burton A. 1985. "America's Health-Care Dilemma." *Challenge* 28: 30–34.

Wilensky, Gail R. 1984. "Solving Uncompensated Hospital Care: Targeting the Indigent and the Uninsured." *Health Affairs* 3: 50–62.

4

Integration as a Provider Response to Shrinking Health Care Dollars

Richard J. Arnould, John W. Pollard, and Charles B. Van Vorst

The health care sector in the United States and in many other countries consists of various independent provider groups. Each group plays a highly specific role in supplying health care services to consumers. Close functional relationships exist between many providers, such as physicians and hospitals. Many of these relationships are complementary in nature and are essential to providing certain types of health care. However, formal economic relationships between these provider groups, from limited contractual relationships to full integration through common ownership, have been almost nonexistent.

Various structural inefficiencies in providing health care services have resulted from this lack of coordination and integration. Structural inefficiencies exist when disharmony arises between means (efficient utilization inputs) and goals (health status). These inefficiencies take many forms, including overlapping responsibility, unnecessary duplication of facilities, unnecessary tests and services, misplacement of needed care, use of inefficient facilities, excess capacity, and limited quality control.

In the United States the most impelling cause of inefficiencies in production and consumption has been the availability of public (Medicare and Medicaid) and private (Blue Cross/Blue Shield) insurance systems that transfer the financial risk associated with providing health care services to third-party payers. The third-party reimbursement system institutionalized the independent roles of provider groups. Providers of individual services were not linked in any economic manner when rendering services to the same patient. No financial incentive to coordinate or include services existed. Communication among providers on basic patient-care data was not formally established as an operating norm.

Thus, our health care system was built on a model with limited incentives for efficient resource use. The cumulative result was a rapid escalation of total expenditures for health care services in the United States. In 1965, $41.7 billion, or 6 percent of gross national product (GNP) was spent on health care in the United States. These costs had risen to $321.4 billion, or 10.2 percent of GNP, in 1982. Total health care costs are expected to increase to over $462 billion by 1985 (U.S. Department of Health and Human Services, various years). Clearly, some of this increase is the result of improved technology and changing demographic characteristics of the U.S. population. However, a significant portion of the increase in these expenditures can be attributed to inefficiencies in the demand for and the supply of health care services.

This rapid increase in health care costs, coupled with major changes in the nation's economy, has caused a reevaluation of the basic philosophical goals of health care and significant changes in the insurance systems in the private and public sectors. Both sectors have adopted more market-oriented approaches that shift part of the financial risk to providers and consumers. Clearly, the changes represent only a partial move toward reliance on the "free market." Since they concentrate on reimbursement programs, health service providers continue to be heavily regulated.

By shifting some of the insurance risk back to the provider and consumer, these changes to prospective pricing systems (discussed in more detail later) provide incentives for more efficient production and consumption of health care services. (However, often prospective prices are set by purchasers with some monopsonistic power, leaving room for elements of market failure.) These changes will result in a substantial reevaluation of the traditional roles, structures, and responsibilities of providers. Various forms of provider integration that will bring more economic incentives to various provider groups are rapidly emerging. The form of this integration will be determined by the efficiencies realized through the various "linking" arrangements among providers. This discussion will provide a theoretical basis for health care provider integration, a documentation of certain types of integration, and an assessment of certain gains in efficiency.

Because these gains are difficult to measure, long-run experimentation with different market forms will be necessary, and firms in the industry will go through forms of integration and disintegration. Hospitals, for example, will find that the costs of some services can be reduced by integration, and that other services can be produced more efficiently by specialized vendors.

The next section of this chapter describes the nature of production and consumption of health care services and identifies six groups of participants in these activities. The third section describes existing contractual relations between these participant groups and explains how changes in these relationships are changing the agency roles of providers. The fourth section describes types and sources of efficiency from integration.

NATURE OF PRODUCTION AND
CONSUMPTION OF HEALTH CARE SERVICES

An understanding of the nature of production and consumption of health care services in the United States is essential to an analysis of past structural inefficiencies and the emerging role of provider integration. There are six broad groups of participants that interact to provide health care services: government, consumers, insurers, first-level providers, second-level providers, and third-level providers.

Government

Government exerts authority over the health care system at all levels in society. The federal government greatly expanded its activities as a purchaser of health care services through the enactment of Medicare and Medicaid. Cooperative planning efforts during the 1960s were strengthened in the 1970s through the passage of PL 93-641 and the subsequent development of state certificate-of-need (CON) activities.

Tax treatment of health insurance premiums in the United States has eliminated the normal effect of higher insurance prices on consumers' incomes and, thus, the incentive for the insurer to function as the efficiency control mechanism (Feldstein 1972). Other governmental actions have resulted in a similar lack of efficiency incentives. Selective cost controls engendered the transfer of costs from regulated inputs to unregulated inputs, and from publicly reimbursed patients to privately insured patients (Sloan and Steinwald 1980). Subsidies to expand the number of physicians and hospital beds without controls on demand resulted in supply-created demand (Arnould and Van Vorst 1985).

The professions have used self-regulation to restrict infringement in their production areas by different types of cost-effective supplier (Havighurst and King 1983). Other forms of regulation have promoted the divergent interests of various input providers (Sloan and Steinwald 1980; Arnould and Van Vorst 1985).

As long as purchasers' budgets expanded, health care service providers had no incentive to become more efficient by integrating. In the past decade, attention has focused on the rapidly increasing resources being devoted to health care. Employee health care costs were a factor in causing U.S. firms to lose their competitive edge in world markets (Arnould and Van Vorst 1985). Rapidly escalating costs of governmental programs placed great strains on the federal budget. The aging U.S. population is increasing the number of people in the high medical cost category. The rapid increase in high-cost, life-improving, technological developments further increased costs. Without changes in governmental policies, costs in this sector will continue to place strains on the economy.

The government established methods to control resource expenditures in health care. Professional standards review organizations (PSROs), created in 1972 to provide external review of procedures prescribed by physicians, have failed to control the elements under their jurisdiction (Sloan and Steinwald 1980). This failure is due in part to PSROs' having no authority over costs per unit of service. Certificate-of-need laws, established to reduce excess capacity by limiting the availability of services, have not effectively controlled costs. Finally, selective controls on certain inputs have controlled those inputs, but have caused costs to be shifted to other inputs, resulting in higher overall costs (ibid.). Thus, governmental actions have failed to negate the perverse effects of incentives generated by third-party payment mechanisms.

Consumers

Consumers are individuals who use health care services. Their role includes a unique function: the consumer provides substantial input into the production process in the form of the information he or she relates before the other inputs are prescribed (Arnould 1982). This interaction gives the physician knowledge about the consumer's health status and psychological state. Using this knowledge, the physician acts as an agent and prescribes the other inputs necessary to provide the desired health outcome (Arrow 1963; Evans 1983). Consumer knowledge of health care production is generally limited. The consumer may be able to identify symptoms but is usually unable to diagnose the cause or draw together appropriate inputs to produce a desired result. The physician-agent determines what tests are needed, whether the problem can be treated with drugs or surgery, whether hospitalization is necessary and, if so, for how long, and whether specialists are required.

Typically, agency relationships occur in single economic units when owners and managers have different objectives (Jensen and Meckling 1976). Also, these relationships occur in markets in which competition places some, if not ultimate, control over deviations of firm behavior from cost minimization and profit maximization. The agency relationship in health care encompasses two economic units: the consumer and one of the provider units. Evans (1983) argues that this arrangement amounts to incomplete vertical integration because it does not encompass economic or contractual relationships between the physician-agent and the consumer or other input providers. Therefore, the physician-agent bears no financial risk[1] for other inputs prescribed and has no financial responsibility to the consumer. Finally, the behavior of governments and insurers has removed competitive market forces that would control the extent to which the agency behavior deviates from cost-minimization behavior.

Third-Party Payers

Third-party payers finance and insure health care services for consumer groups. Third-party payers consist of various governmental units, private insurers, and self-insured employers. More than 40 percent of all U.S. health care expenditures are made by federal and state governments, largely for Medicare and Medicaid recipients. Similarly, Blue Cross/Blue Shield plans, which vary across states, accounted for about half of the private health insurance in force in the United States in the late 1970s. Thus, there has been a substantial amount of concentration in the insurance and third-party markets.

Various forms of cost-plus pricing have been common in private and government health insurance contracts. Prices have been determined retrospectively. This pricing policy has led to a significant amount of cost-plus pricing. To be efficient, cost-plus pricing requires the third-party payer to control the cost of a unit of service and the number of units of each service provided. Health insurance contracts failed in both demands, resulting in a significant degree of moral hazard.[2] Output limits were not clearly delineated in insurance contracts. External cost monitoring, as provided, for example, by PSROs, has been costly and, often, based on incomplete information. The external monitors were not provided with tools to influence the incentives of providers. Though private and government third-party payers have had the authority to audit the costs of providers, auditors have usually had no independent method to determine true minimum cost levels. They therefore resorted to comparing the costs of individual cases to industry wide norms. Since no providers had incentives to minimize costs, the industry cost norms were inflated.

Prices paid for some services may have been set at artificially high levels for an additional reason. The reimbursement policies of many major private insurers have been controlled or significantly influenced by providers who bear no risk for default of the plans. Providers have used their control of plans to establish input prices and coverage levels that ultimately resulted in excessive insurance coverage (Feldstein 1973; French and Ginsberg 1978), provision of excessive and inefficient services (Goldberg and Greenberg 1977), and higher input costs, particularly physician fees (Arnould and DeBrock, forthcoming). A market in which providers bear some risk of financial default will force insurers to control use and price services competitively, increasing efficiency in the production and consumption of health care services. Insurers and providers unwilling to do so will find that their prices to consumers, and their market shares, decline.

First-Level Providers

First-level providers typically have the initial agency relationship with the consumer.[3] These providers are physicians, usually in the primary care specialties of family practice, general internal medicine, pediatrics, and obstetrics. There are approximately 202,117 licensed primary care physicians in the United States, more than 148,655 of whom are solo practitioners. First-level providers have traditionally been the point of entry of the patient into the health care system and in earlier times represented the bulk of services available to the populace. The growth of specialization and advancements in technology have changed the historical role of the primary-care provider. Competition in health care markets and the development of prepaid and prospectively determined reimbursement methods are increasing the importance of primary care providers in controlling use and are conferring on them a more formalized gatekeeper role.

Second-Level Providers

Second-level providers provide services that are used by the consumer under the direction of first-level providers or as intermediate products to first-level or other second-level providers. Second-level providers include the physician-specialists, who, like first-level physicians, are organized primarily as solo practitioners. Numbering 299,841, they play an important role in bringing advancements in information and technology to medicine.

The largest expenditure of health care dollars for second-level providers is for hospital services, though the relationship between the hospital and the physician (whether first- or second-level) normally lacks an economic link or output control mechanism. Traditionally, the contractual relationships between the hospital and the physician take the form of practice privileges. This relationship limits the types of practice and procedures of physicians but places no limit on the output of either the hospital or physician. Direct agency relationships do exist in hospitals that are owned or controlled by physicians. Pauly and Redisch (1973) argue that physician control turns the hospital into a physician cooperative, and that the agency role of the physicians induces the hospital to operate according to policies that maximize the physicians' incomes.

Other second-level providers supply services for patient care as the hospital does, generally in an indirect role; these services are consumed upon prescription by the physician-agent, not purchased directly by the consumer.

Third-Level Providers

Third-level provider services typically are used directly by the consumer with minimal input from the first and second levels. Third-level providers supply a broad range of services designed to treat general health problems with a social focus on the individual as a member of society. Third-level providers include, but are not limited to:

— Housing services, including senior citizen apartments, and assisted living, foster care, and life care communities

— Home health services, including Medicare-certified and private in-home services, hospice, homemaker services, and home infusion therapies

— Durable medical equipment, including beds, walkers, oxygen equipment, and related supplies

The six broad groups outlined above provide a conceptual model of the various health care production entities. These definitions are not precise, and many participants play multiple roles. The pluralism of the current health care system and the lack of economic integration and coordination among its various components are evident.

Input-output relationships in the health care system are not totally analogous to those in many areas of manufacturing. For example, in petroleum markets the input-output relationships start with exploration for crude oil and extend through refining, distribution, and retailing. In health care the closest analog is the continuum from wellness to illness. To motivate the discussion of mutual integration that follows in a later section of this chapter, we might think of the patient as the ultimate consumer of health care. The production of wellness occurs over a continuum with the consumer entering the system through the many inputs from first-level providers. The consumer then moves on to purchase inputs provided by second-level providers, as prescribed by the first-level provider and as necessary to produce wellness. These inputs could include physician specialists, hospital care, drugs, and so on. The third-party payment system provides an umbrella over producers and consumers. It may be viewed as a combination payment-insurance mechanism. As such, it can be integrated into the consumer function, in which case the consumer is self-insuring, or into the producer function.

The traditional unintegrated system lacks a central unifying authority responsible for the efficient coordination of the various inputs. The physician-agent, though responsible for the patient's health, has no contractual obligation to see that the patient's needs are met efficiently. The lack of provider integration suggests that either integration will not cause increased efficiency or certain characteristics of health care markets have eliminated incentives for more efficient production. Evidence suggests that the latter is the appropriate conclusion.

CONTRACTUAL RELATIONSHIPS IN THE HEALTH CARE SECTOR

Contractual relations among consumers, third-party payers, and providers have been poorly defined and often open-ended. A complete contract must specify the prices, quantities, and quality of the services to be provided. Contractual relations between third-party payers and providers have been deficient in all three respects. Providers have been reimbursed on the basis of retrospectively determined cost-plus prices for each individual unit of service provided. The costs were not necessarily minimum costs, and the prices may have been administered by provider influence over the third parties. Also, difficulties in specifying, in the contract, the number of units of each service necessary to treat a specific ailment (such as blood transfusions, days in hospital, and level of nursing care) have left the quantity dimension of the contract virtually open-ended. Finally, quality has been specified only loosely in terms of very general standards. These relationships are summarized in figure 4:1.

The incompleteness of the third-party contracts and the reimbursement systems adopted in those contracts has permitted the physician-agent to pass all financial risks on to the third party, thereby generating the potential for a significant amount of moral hazard.

Purchasers of health care services in search of more efficient market-oriented health care systems are changing these contracts, especially those between third-party payers and providers, to close some of the open-endedness and shift financial risk to providers. The three most prominent types of contractual relationship developing in the United States are health maintenance organizations (HMOs), which are complete, prepaid health plans; prospective payment systems (PPSs), in which prices are based on an episode of a specific health problem rather than each unit of service provided; and preferred provider arrangements (PPAs), featuring direct purchase negotiations between payers and providers. Each plan closes various loopholes in the previous contractual arrangements.

HMOs provide the most complete shift of risk from third-party payers to providers. Purchasers of health care services (governments or private entities) contract with one source to meet all of the health care needs of a consumer group for a predetermined premium. This inclusive premium will be competitively determined if the HMOs must compete with other plans for the contract. Further, most moral hazard will be eliminated be-

Figure 4:1—Market Relationship

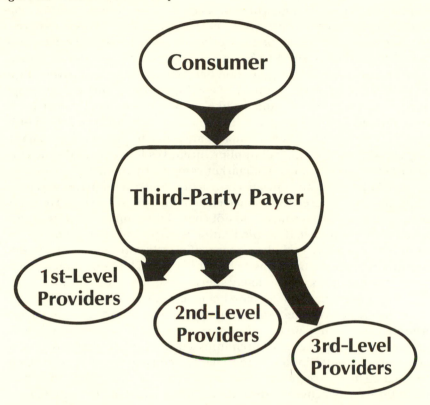

cause providers' revenues are fixed for the duration of the coverage period, usually one year. Thus, their incomes are maximized only if their costs are minimized.

PPSs and PPAs are contractual arrangements between third-party payers and providers in which prices for services are determined prospectively, though the two systems use different definitions of the units of services provided.

The most prominent PPS in the United States is the system of diagnosis-related groups used to reimburse hospitals for service provided to Medicare beneficiaries. Currently that system delineates units of health care services in terms of 468 DRGs, each of which represents an illness or health problem. Hospital reimbursement for each DRG is based not only on the primary diagnosis, but also on secondary diagnosis and the patient's age and sex. Physician, ancillary, and outpatient services, and hospital capital costs currently are not included in the system. If the hospital's cost of providing the services is less than the predetermined prices, the hospital keeps the surplus; if the cost is greater, the hospital suffers the loss. This system encourages hospitals to treat patients efficiently and to minimize ancillary services and lengths of stay. It closes the price and quantity loopholes in fee-for-service contracts for each DRG treated. However, there is no incentive to reduce admissions, and there may be an incentive to use more highly reimbursed DRGs when secondary diagnoses offer an option.

PPAs involve direct negotiation between providers and payers. Typically, a third-party payer, insurer, or employer will negotiate daily hospital rates, physician charges, and the like with each provider (Trauner 1983). The PPA usually provides price discounts in return for guaranteed business. This arrangement is particularly attractive to providers in markets plagued with excess supply. Supplier incentives for increased efficiency result as various suppliers in a market compete by reducing prices.

PPAs provide appropriate contractual controls on prices and units of specific services used to produce each of the priced services. However, these contractual arrangements do not control the number of units of each priced service supplied. If hospitalization is priced on a per diem rate, the hospital will produce each day of care efficiently, but the hospital has no incentive to reduce admissions or lengths of stay. Thus, one dimension of the contract remains incompletely specified, as in the case of PPSs.

Less substantial changes have been made in the contractual arrangements between consumers and third-party payers. The reduction in the real insurance premium paid by consumers, resulting from the favorable tax treatment of health insurance premiums and the low marginal cost of services, provides only limited incentives for consumers to seek efficient providers. The tax treatment of premiums has not changed. Studies have found that co-payments and deductibles, which increase the marginal cost of medical services to the consumer, also reduce the units of health services consumed (Phelps 1982; Phelps and Newhouse 1972).

The Rand group found that 25 percent and 50 percent co-insurance rates reduced average total ambulatory and hospital expenditures by 19 percent and 30 percent, respectively (Newhouse 1978; Phelps 1982; Phelps and Newhouse 1972). Similarly, an income-related deductible and a flat $150 deductible that applied only to ambulatory care reduced average total expenditures by 31 percent and 23 percent, respectively. In all cases, the reductions in expenditures for ambulatory care were greater than those for hospital care. Contrary to earlier beliefs, reductions in expenditures for hospital care were significant and related mainly to reductions in admissions. The study reported no differences in cost per hospital admission.

Phelps (1982) argues that additional forms of cost sharing could reduce health care expenditures. These devices include limiting the tax deductibility of employer health insurance contributions and including those premiums as taxable income to the employee. Phelps estimates that taxing the private insurance premiums would reduce health care expenditures by $12 or $13 billion. Of this reduction, expenditures for services provided by hospitals and physicians would decline by $7.6 and $3.8 billion, respectively.

Those cost-sharing devices have a direct influence on providers. As consumers reduce their expenditures for health care, competition increases among providers for health care dollars. Consumers seek the most efficient health care providers.

There has been concern about the influence of competition on quality. Much of this concern has been misplaced. First, both price and quality are important dimensions of competition. Competition is expected to enforce minimum prices and costs for a predetermined quality level. However, providers may decide to compete on quality dimensions as well as price dimensions. Therefore, some providers will offer services of high quality and some services of low quality. The former cost more to produce than the latter. Importantly, if the markets are competitive, producers will be forced to produce and price services of every quality efficiently.

Second, increased competition need not reduce the quality of health care for the indigent. Effective competition could increase the efficiency of producing health services of the desired quality, thereby permitting the purchase of more units of service for the same cost. A reduction in quality will be forced on the indigent only if the government fails to reimburse providers sufficiently to cover their costs of producing services of the desired quality. However, exactly the same conclusion is drawn from systems of providing health care to the indigent population that are not market-oriented.

CHANGES IN CONTRACTUAL CONDITIONS RESULT IN CHANGES IN AGENT ROLES

The major effect of the changes in contractual relationships among consumers, third-party payers, and providers, discussed in the previous section, is the coupling of the traditional agency role of the physician with a new agent-coordination role that assumes responsibility for the economic efficiency of the production process of the physician and of the providers of other medical services prescribed. The new role responds to the increased risk imposed on providers. The physician may maintain the agency role of prescribing medical services purchased from the various provider levels to consumers, but may concede the agent-coordinator role of minimizing costs to other units. Shifts in financial risk and their effect on the agency role may be explored with several models of contractual relations between third-party payers and providers. These models are summarized in figure 4:2.

Figure 4:2—Market Relationships and Agency Roles

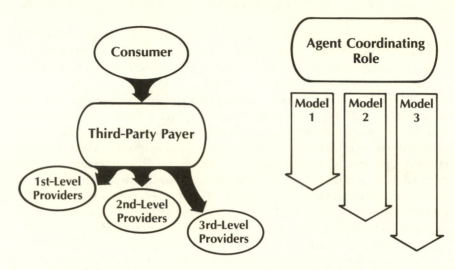

   In the first model, an independent third-party payer contracts with
each provider type, such as physicians, hospitals, and skilled nursing facilities (SNFs). In this model we assume that these contracts pay each provider
a capitation rate based on the number of consumers entitled to services.
If the capitation rates are competitively determined, each provider must
maximize production efficiency to maximize economic surplus. In this
model, the third-party payer assumes the overall agent-coordinator role.
The physician-agent may continue to prescribe units of his or her own
medical services and those provided by providers at other levels, but is constrained by the agent-coordinator to prescribe them from specified
providers.

   In the second model, the third-party provider is integrated with first-
level physicians. (In the United States, for example, physician group practices often form HMOs.) This model combines the agent-coordinator role
with the physician-agent role. The physician-agents continue to prescribe
medical services supplied by providers at other levels. However, unlike the
previous model, in which an independent third-party payer selected the
other-level providers, the physician-agent does so under economic cost constraints.

   In the third model, the third-party payer is fully integrated downstream with all provider levels. All contracting with external provider levels
is eliminated because these providers are under common ownership. The
physician-agent role continues to be held by first-level physicians, but the
agent-coordinator role is fulfilled by the system or unit as a whole. Each
provider level has some influence over the decisions of the overall agent-

coordinator but is not responsible for its own provider function or for the efficiency of the unit as a whole. Unlike the second model, in which the physician-agents controlled the choice of other providers, in this model all providers have some authority over the choice of all other providers.

These three models provide a limited sample of various relationships that are emerging from the changes in contractual arrangements among consumers, third-party payers, and providers. Many other levels of integration between the first and third models are possible. Providers at any level could increase efficiency by integrating upstream, downstream, or horizontally with other providers. For example, hospitals that have signed a capitation agreement to provide services to a group of consumers could increase efficiency by integrating downstream with SNFs and home health care providers or integrating upstream with physicians.

In the next section, we will define various types of integration and discuss sources of gains in efficiency from some of these. It is the shift of risk to the providers that will incorporate economic constraints in the agent role and induce incentives for efficiency among providers.

TYPES AND SOURCES OF EFFICIENCY FROM INTEGRATION

In this section, we assume that changes in the economic system responsible for providing health care (whether that system is characterized by highly centralized planning or decentralized decision making) have been instituted to place economic constraints on consumers and health care service producers. These constraints require consumers to seek efficient producers. Various types and levels of producer integration may increase production efficiency. This section defines these types of integration and sources of gains in efficiency and describes specific examples of integration taking place in the United States.

Types of Integration

Integration of provider units is occurring horizontally (within existing local markets or by geographical market extension or product extension) and vertically (between providers at different stages of the production process, one of which acquires ownership of the other). It exhibits various levels of completeness, from short-term contracting between providers to complete ownership. Although we describe all types of integration in this section, we concentrate on vertical integration.

Long-standing structural changes have generally involved horizontal growth of existing firms, i.e., expansion within generally homogeneous lines of business in the same geographic service area. These organizations achieve increased production efficiencies through economies of scale.

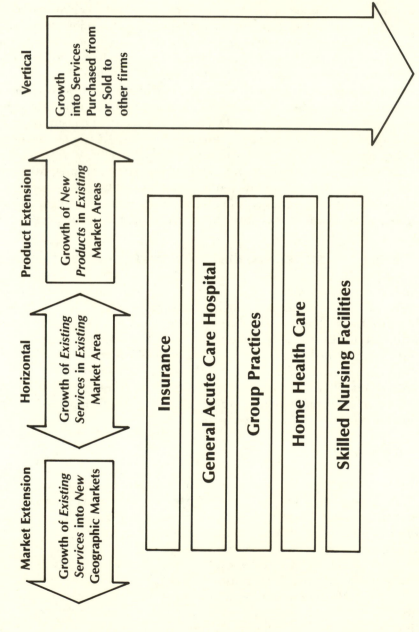

Figure 4:3—Forms of Growth

Figure 4:3 depicts the historical growth of hospitals. Until recently this growth resulted from the expansion of bed capacity and services offered within existing general, acute care hospitals. In the past decade, there has been substantial growth in proprietary and nonproprietary multi-hospital systems (Ermann and Gabel 1984). Some of this expansion has been through mergers of hospitals located within the same geographic area (horizontal groups), while some has involved mergers of hospitals located in different market areas (geographic market extension).

Similarly, independent physicians have formed group practices, generally within the same geographic market (horizontal). Often these groups have comprised physicians with differing specialties. Generally, if these physicians are exclusively first- or second-level providers, the group is horizontal; if they combine first and second levels, the growth is vertical.

Provider organizations are responding to the current health care environment by vertically integrating with other provider types. Vertical integration occurs when a provider either expands or acquires other health care input suppliers who produce products or services that were purchased from or sold to others prior to integration. Examples of vertical integration include group practices or hospitals offering HMOs, hospitals merging with skilled nursing facilities, and providers insuring themselves against malpractice claims. Other examples are shown in figure 4:3.

The various types of integration are summarized in figure 4:3. The number of cases of each type is not known, though Ermann and Gabel (1984) compiled the extensive summary of integration by multihospital systems shown in table 4:1. The activities listed do not always fit neatly into the traditional growth categories. For example, the expansion of hospitals into SNFs represents vertical integration to the extent that patients are transferred from one unit to the other. This growth might be considered a form of product extension because some hospital patients do not use SNFs or vice versa. However, the activities listed do show evidence of hospital system growth into virtually every aspect of health care and into many unrelated activities.

Sources of Gains in Efficiency

Types of integration are depicted in figure 4:3. Each type of integration provides potential gains in efficiency. The source of these gains in efficiency varies by the type of integration and the nature of exogenous conditions in the health care provider's market. Gains in efficiency from horizontal integration result when the firm achieves greater economies of scale. Therefore, the cost per unit of service produced declines as the firm expands output. The economies of scale result from factors such as increased specialization of functions within the provider unit and increased efficien-

Table 4:1—Percentage of Multihospital Systems Operating Health and Nonhealth Lines of Business, 1982

LINE OF BUSINESS	PERCENTAGE
Health Care Services	
1. Health promotion programs	55.7
2. Ambulatory care facilities	55.1
3. Nursing homes	50.6
4. Hospices	34.8
5. Alcoholism or drug treatment centers	33.8
6. Surgery centers	22.2
7. Ambulance companies	20.3
8. Convenience medical centers	18.4
9. HMO/IPA	12.6
10. Preferred provider organizations	11.4
Administrative Health Care Services	
1. Physician office buildings	71.8
2. Group purchasing plans	57.5
3. Health care management consulting	43.0
4. Department management	26.6
Nonhealth Care Businesses	
1. Office building management	23.4
2. Real estate development	21.6
3. Retirement settlements	14.6
4. Warehousing	13.3
5. Insurance company management	12.6
6. Hotel/restaurant/resort management	4.5

Source: *American Hospital Association Survey of Multi-Hospital Systems: Executive Summary 1983.* Adapted from Ermann and Gabel (1984).

cy of technologies at larger scales of operation. Larger hospitals and group practices may be able to subdivide various managerial functions efficiently, allowing them to hire more qualified administrators than is efficient for small hospitals and independent practitioners. Similarly, larger hospitals and group practices may be able to utilize accounting and data management technologies that operate efficiently at large scales but are not feasible on smaller scales.

Integration by geographic and product market extension provides potential gains in efficiency due to economies of scope. Whereas economies of scale result from expansion within a horizontally related line of business, economies of scope result from successfully taking advantage of joint cost opportunities. The capital input is a common example of a source of economies of scope. A hospital may have access to capital at an efficient rate, but may not wish to use that capital for local horizontal expansion, because, for example, the market may be adequately supplied with hospital beds. That capital may be more efficiently used to build or acquire hospitals in other markets or purchase providers at other levels of production, such as SNFs or home health care providers. In addition to being an outlet for excess capital funds, diversification and market expansion may reduce the financial risk associated with owning the hospital's capital instruments (stocks, bonds, or both), thereby reducing the cost of capital to the integrated firm. Risk often is measured by the degree of profit variability over time. Diversification and integration may reduce this variability if the profit streams are uncorrelated or negatively correlated. Excess capacity in the marketing or any other function within the firm may be more efficiently used by expansion into other activities that use these functions. There may be other inputs in the production of services that can be efficiently shared by provider types within and between the various provider levels.

Vertical integration has three potential sources of gains in efficiency.[5] First, gains in technical efficiency result from characteristics of the physical production process. The processing of iron ore into fabricated steel products provides an example of technical economies. Vertically integrating processing and fabricating levels eliminates the costs of reheating and cooling the product at each fabrication stage. In the health care sector, information describing a patient's health status provides a similar example. Each provider level may need the patient's medical record. A contract between providers could specify the transfer of that record between providers. However, that contract must specify that the information be transferred according to a common information system. Further, the contract must specify the quality of the information and provide for patient approval of the transfer of information. The difficulties of establishing these contractual conditions may make vertical integration a more efficient alternative. Technical economies may also result from cases in which, while a patient is having a procedure such as surgery, another health-related problem is discovered that requires use of other provider specialists. Having direct access to those other providers may permit multiple procedures to be conducted, with anesthesia or some other input administered only once.

Second, contractual costs provide a source of incentives for firms to integrate vertically and to increase efficiency. Contractual costs are incurred in the process of haggling over price, quantity, and quality dimensions of the contract. Further costs are incurred if, once negotiated, the conditions of the contract permit moral hazard.

Third, vertical integration may result in information economies if redevelopment of the information at various procedure levels is eliminated. This elimination permits the high fixed costs associated with information gathering to be spread over more units of output. Information economies also may result if parties negotiating a contract disagree on the interpretation of the information.[6] Examples of vertical integration induced by each of these sources of efficiency will be provided in the next section.

Third-party payer/first-level provider integration. Probably the most extensive and visible integration has occurred between third-party payers and various levels of provider. In most cases, these integrated systems offer complete coverage of the enrollees' medical needs. By bringing the insurance function and the medical provider function under common control, risk is shifted to providers, thereby generating incentives for provider efficiency. The extent of integration ranges from including only third-party payers and first-level providers (in which case contractual relations are established for services required from providers at other levels), to including almost all provider levels under common ownership, as shown in models 2 and 3 in figure 4:3. The major gains in efficiency from this form of integration result from eliminating various contractual costs. The cost reductions from these sources will vary with the structural relations between third-party payment mechanism and the first-level providers.

Integration between prepaid plans and first-level providers has taken three general structural forms, two of which encompass forms of group practice. The staff plan employs physicians who provide services exclusively to HMO-plan enrollees. Staff physicians may be salaried, as in the Kaiser-Permanente Plan, or compensated in whole or in part on a capitation rate, as in Group Health Cooperative of Puget Sound. In the closed-panel structure, group practice physicians enter into a contractual agreement to provide services to HMO enrollees while continuing to serve fee-for-service patients. As in the staff plan, physicians may be salaried or paid a capitation rate. However, in some closed panels in which HMO enrollees make up a small percentage of total patients served, the individual physicians are paid on a fee-for-service basis, although the panel is paid by a capitation method.

The third structure, independent practice associations, contract with independent physicians to provide services to enrollees. The IPA, if integrated, is owned by the independent physicians. Physicians may bill the IPA on a fee-for-service basis or share the IPA revenues on a capitation basis.

In any of these structures, the method of reimbursing physicians has an important effect on the extent to which incentives are changed by shifting risk to the HMO. The HMO will have minimal effect on physician behavior if physician salaries are based on production, that is, number of services provided. Alternatively, if physicians receive salaries based on a capitation rate, costs from providing unnecessary services are minimized.

Integration between staff or group practice physicians and prepaid plans may have additional advantages over IPAs. IPAs require that internal contracting be established between the "insurance" function and the independent physicians, each of whom may have different operating costs. These internal agreements are likely to be more difficult to establish than in group practices, in which each provider's operating costs are shared by all group members. Also, because the IPA involves physicians who operate independent businesses in various locations, it will be much more difficult to police free-rider problems in the IPA model than in the group practice model.[7]

Cost reduction from integration may also result from increased incentives to keep patients well. Recall that prepaid plans avoid the problems of specifying the coverage limits by covering almost all of the health care needs of enrollees. Therefore, physicians should practice more preventive medicine, assuming preventive services are less costly to provide than treatments for contracted health problems. Many groups have developed wellness programs. Examples are educational programs to lose weight, to stop smoking, and to exercise sensibly.

HMOs, common forms of prepaid health plans, are having a substantial effect on U.S. health care. In 1970, there were 33 HMOs in the United States serving approximately 3 million enrollees (National Industry Council for HMO Development 1984). In 1983, there were 280 HMOs serving 12 million enrollees. HMOs have a market penetration of 33.7 percent in San Francisco, 26.4 percent in Minneapolis, 25.1 percent in Los Angeles, and 23.4 percent in Portland, Oregon. Only one metropolitan area with a population of over 1 million is not served by an HMO. Numerous studies confirm the lower cost of HMOs.[8]

Most cost savings in HMOs are the result of reductions in total health care expenditures, hospital admissions, and lengths of hospital stay (Luft and Trauner 1981). Luft (1980) found total hospital days per 1,000 enrollees to be 35 percent lower for HMO patients than for fee-for-service patients. Most of these reductions are due to reduced hospital admission rates. Hospital admission rates were found to be 20 percent to 40 percent lower for HMO enrollees, but length of stay was not found to be perceptively lower (Luft 1980; Arnould, DeBrock, and Pollard 1984). Some evidence indicates that HMOs devote more attention to preventive care. However, this incentive may be explained because HMOs cover preventive care, whereas most fee-for-service plans do not, resulting in a real change for HMO enrollees (Berki et al. 1977). Arnould, DeBrock, and Pollard (1984) found that HMOs produce certain specific health services more efficiently; Richardson, Martin, and Diehr (1984), in a comparative analysis of a staff-plan HMO and an IPA, found total costs, hospital admissions, and average lengths of stay adjusted per number of enrollees to be significantly lower for staff plans than for IPAs.

Clearly integration of the insurance and provider functions changes provider behavior, reduces transaction costs, and results in significant gains in efficiency. One caveat is necessary. The HMOs included in the empirical evidence vary in degrees of integration. In some, integration is limited to third-party payers and first-level physicians; in others, integration encompasses all levels of providers. Thus, some cost reductions may be the result of integration among first-, second-, and third-level providers. Empirical evidence of gains in efficiency from integration among providers in these levels is not available.

Horizontal and vertical integration among first- and second-level physicians. The proportion and number of physicians organized into group practices in the United States have grown. In 1980, 26.2 percent of the physicians were in 10,762 group practices. The average group practice consisted of eight physicians. By 1984, 29.3 percent of the physicians were in 15,485 groups.[9] The average group practice consisted of nine physicians. Some groups consist of first-level physicians; others combine the first and second levels. Gains in efficiency may result from economies of scale, reduced contractual costs, and information economies. Economies of scale may result from the horizontal growth at various levels of the system. For example, if providers own a prepaid plan, economies of scale in the insurance function may dictate the size of the patient base and, therefore, the group practice necessary for the insurance function to operate efficiently. Economies of scale in the provision of insurance are well documented (Arrow 1963).

Forming group practices reduces the number of contracts negotiated between providers; it also provides access to internal mechanisms to control quality and costs. Group practices may need to expand into other geographic markets to attract an adequate patient base that will support an efficient insurance function. Contracting with independent providers in various locations presents problems in quality and utilization control similar to those attributed to IPAs and nonintegrated plans. To overcome these problems, providers are diversifying into new geographic markets. Kaiser-Permanente has physician staffs in 12 states and hospitals in 22 cities. Second-level physician centers are establishing satellite first-level provider facilities to guarantee an adequate patient base and to support the second-level care center efficiently. Mayo Clinic, a second-level physician group practice, has announced plans to develop satellite facilities in southern states. Carle Clinic, also a second-level physician group practice, has provider satellites in a 50-mile radius of its tertiary care center and plans further geographic expansion.

Finally, information economies may be gained through group practices if the practice provides a common level and quality of information to first- and second-level physicians.

Integration among second-level providers. This integration permits input factors to be rearranged functionally and to respond more readily to the extent of care required and to the most cost-effective means for its provision. If these facilities are vertically integrated, the flow of patients from hospitals, nursing homes, and home care services is not impeded in the short run by economic constraints or by the need of each input provider to maximize profits. For example, hospitals reimbursed on capitation or payment per DRG can lower costs by reducing the lengths of patients' stays. Those patients continuing to need care can be transferred to SNFs, where costs per diem average $46 in the United States compared with $368 for acute care hospitals. Patients needing lower levels of care than that provided by SNFs may be transferred to their homes and treated by home care agencies at even lower per diem costs.

All three levels of provider group discussed in the preceding paragraph stand in a variety of relations with each other as well as exist as freestanding units. More than 50 percent of the multihospital systems own nursing homes, more than 40 percent have home care agencies. In some cases, SNFs own home care agencies (Ermann and Gabel 1984). In fact, 84 percent of the nation's home care agencies are owned by organizations other than freestanding visiting nurse associations, usually hospitals or SNFs (Lundberg 1984). Clearly, these services could remain freestanding, attracting patients by referral from physician-agents. This relationship may not provide necessary economic ties among the provider groups to promote efficiency.

Management service contracts are being used to establish contractual relationships among these providers in many cases. Other providers are finding a number of advantages from full integration. SNFs require long-term investments in capital facilities. It is difficult for health care providers to develop satisfactory long-term contracts because they operate in an environment of rapid technological change in which quality standards are difficult to establish and coordination is essential for cost efficiency. Profits or surpluses will be captured by the integrated system regardless of where the service is provided within the system. Thus, there are more incentives to provide the most appropriate care to meet patient needs in the integrated system than in a nonintegrated system.

The contractual completeness in an integrated approach allows short-range efficiencies to accrue while the larger health delivery system attends to the longitudinal need for overall economic efficiency.[10] In addition, greater flexibility exists in meeting external competitive pricing. The internal system has the ability to alter payment structures on a dynamic basis to meet market demand and to deter market entry (Schmalensee 1973). The integrated system may be able to price certain services at levels that discourage entry into the market. If the threat of entry is short-lived, short-run reduction in earned surplus may be more than compensated by long-term gains in surplus. Although this discouragement of market entry does not increase economic efficiency as do the other factors, it remains a potential reason for integration. Thus, temporal market and price fluctuations can be effectively addressed without harm to the overall system. This ability is important to second- and third-level providers, which tend to be more capital-intensive and wish to protect the long-term viability of their capital investment.

The creation of information-sharing and information-processing systems is an essential element in the continued viability of integrated relationships. Data processing systems with high fixed costs can be expanded to encompass the information needs of each provider level at a relatively low marginal cost and with internal quality controls. More complete information on operating costs allows the most prudent use and arrangement of inputs. These systems also facilitate demand forecasting and modeling over a greater number of production units and inputs, thus improving the overall predictability of services needed and resources required. Savings also can occur through inventory control and variable staffing patterns.

The common data base applied directly to patient care provides the physician-agent with more integrated input information, which may have a positive effect on reducing duplicated services. The data base serves as a source of quality control and peer evaluation, and as a research base to track the efficiency of various input configurations and the quality of the results. Perhaps most important, an integrated system of financial and clinical data can be used to effect change. Objective data can be used by providers at all levels to evaluate the causes and effects of various resource-consumption decisions. The data can assist providers in making decisions and balancing the interests of the individual patient and the economic interests of the system of integrated providers.

Standardization also may reduce input costs by increasing purchasing power. The ability of the patient to "transfer" information and procedures from one input provider to another could be a significant factor in increasing patient compliance with prescribed interventions. Greater compliance may lead to greater clinical efficacy, thereby reducing overall resource consumption.

Integrated providers may be able to hire and retain more capable functional specialists once they are able to spread the specialists' knowledge and costs over a larger number of units. The improved forecasting capability of the integrated system will enable it to plan the human resources it needs and to develop methods for the recruitment and training of these providers. The health care industry's needs for human capital are growing, both in the number of people wanted and the skills required of them. An integrated system has the added potential to stimulate individual and system growth through the interaction of managers and providers at various levels. The structure of the interaction within an integrated system tends to promote more focused problem solving and a need to understand the points of view of providers at different levels. The integrated system provides a built-in mechanism for individuals to change their "perceptual set" on how things can be done, and begins to expand understanding on a system level.

Technical efficiencies may be gained through the availability of complementary technologies. Integration can ensure referrals within the various divisions of the integrated system and allow priorities to be established. The assured access to regulated production inputs (nursing home ownership under certificate of need) is essential in priority setting and may avoid monopoly input distortions if the integrated firm sells inputs to other units within the system at marginal cost (Vernon and Graham 1971). The aggregation of similar inputs throughout the system may allow CON volume thresholds to be reached to gain access to or expand regulated activities. Specific exceptions such as HMO volume may also accrue to other system inputs. Last, the ability of an integrated system to move inputs from regulated to nonregulated provider levels (hospital services to physician offices) represents potential market and financial advantages.

Providers, mainly physician groups and hospitals, have integrated into various types of self-insurance. Typically, these include self-insurance of malpractice claims and employees' health care needs. Self-insurance against workers' compensation has been practiced by many firms for several years. There are four ways in which self-insurance may result in lower costs. First, the cost of a malpractice liability will detract from the ability of the group practice or hospital to pay employees or engage in other necessary activities. This cost increases the incentives for the organization to develop stringent quality controls. Peer pressure from those affected financially by the actions of individuals also will affect quality control. Second, insurance fees are determined by group rating organizations. Organizations with better than average risk experiences subsidize those with worse than average experiences. Therefore, the former can reduce insurance costs by self-insurance. Third, certain organizations may believe that their exposure to risk is less than the insurance market perceives it to be. This divergence of expectations may be due to straightforward differences in interpretation, to quality controls, or to other limits on exposure the benefits of which cannot easily be conveyed to the private insurer. Again, if the hospital or group practice correctly interprets the information, insurance costs will be reduced by vertical integration. Fourth, truly integrated insurance coverage may provide economies in combined legal representation. United insurance eliminates the ability of the plaintiff's attorney to increase the total settlement by seeking individual settlements. The economic savings are difficult to project but may be significant for cases involving large and complex litigation.

Finally, all of these forms of integration have in common their inclusion of those provider services prescribed by a prescribing agent. In the traditional nonintegrated system in the United States, the primary care physician served this agency role. The agency role has been constrained by utilization review procedures enacted by other provider groups and by integrated systems in which an agent coordinator for the system looks over the shoulder of all provider types. Diversification and integration also abolish the freedom of the physician to prescribe outside the system of the providers, capturing clients of one provider for all elements of the system.

SUMMARY

Vertical integration has the potential to increase significantly the efficiency of health care provision. We have discussed types of integration that could increase technical efficiency, reduce contractual, informational, and transactional costs, and provide appropriate provider incentives.

Vertical integration to provide more efficient production of health care services and coordination of patient needs is a relatively recent phenomenon in the United States. Therefore, only limited empirical evidence of its effects on health care costs can be provided. Yet those cost savings are substantial in some areas. The integration of the patient insurance function into the provider functions is a case in point. The integration of hospitals, SNFs, and home care agencies also provides a strong potential for large cost reductions due to the differences in daily costs among these units. However, no estimates are available of the potential reductions in lengths of stay at the higher cost facilities. Also, it remains unclear whether integration of these services is more efficient than a more limited contractual agreement.

Although the forms of vertical integration discussed in this chapter are appearing at a rapid pace, and some evidence was provided of benefits from some forms of integration, there is contrary evidence within the same decentralized economic markets of the United States. For example, freestanding outpatient surgery centers and facilities that treat only obstetric and gynecologic cases are being constructed in many cities. Generally, this countermovement is occurring in localities where facilities exist that are insufficient, inefficient, or both. However, even though more empirical evidence is necessary before final judgment can be made on relative efficiencies, most existing evidence suggests that some types of integration promote efficient patient care. The sources of other types of integration are dependent upon individual market conditions and characteristics of the vertical linkages yet to be discovered.

NOTES

1. Throughout this chapter the term *financial risk* is used to identify situations in which health care services might be sold below cost, resulting in inadequate profits or producing surplus to cover debt requirements. This terminology is not, as in the standard corporate finance literature, used to indicate a change in the leverage of the provider.
2. Moral hazard exists when the introduction of the insurance mechanisms changes the probability of occurrence of the insured event.
3. The terminology used to define first-, second-, and third-level providers should not be confused with the common use of primary, secondary, and tertiary provider designations.
4. These providers include, but are not limited to, specialty inpatient hospitals, including psychiatric, rehabilitation, and alcohol/substance abuse; extended inpatient care, including skilled nursing, intermediate care, and swing bed programs; outpatient clinics; emergency response systems; psychosocial counseling; adult day care; day hospital; cardiac rehabilitation programs; and outreach services, including screening clinics, emergency centers, and mobile diagnostic facilities.
5. This section draws heavily from Williamson 1971.
6. Williamson 1971 calls this problem "information impactedness."
7. Free-rider problems exist when someone gains from the resource commitment of others without contributing proportional resources to the effort.
8. For a detailed summary, see Luft 1981.
9. Information provided to the authors by Medical Group Management Association.
10. In effect, complete integration provides for contractual completeness by eliminating the contractual arrangement between the integrated parties.

REFERENCES

American Hospital Association. 1983. *Survey of Multi-Hospital Systems: Executive Summary, 1983*. Chicago: The Association.

Arnould, R. J. 1972. "Pricing Professional Services." *Southern Economic Journal* 31 (April): 495–507.

Arnould, R. J., and L. W. DeBrock. 1985. "The Effects of Provider Control of Blue Shield Plans on Health Care Markets." *Economic Inquiry* 23: 449–74.

Arnould, R. J., L. W. DeBrock, and J. W. Pollard. 1984. "Do HMO's Produce Services More Efficiently?" *Inquiry* 21 (Fall): 243–53.

Arnould, R. J., and C. B. Van Vorst. 1985. "Supply Responses to Market and Regulatory Forces in Health Care." In *Health Care Cost Management*, ed. by J. Meyer, 107–31. Washington, DC: American Enterprise Institute.

Arrow, K. J. 1963. "Uncertainty and the Welfare Economics of Medical Care." *American Economic Review* 53: 941–73.

Berki, S. E., M. L. Ashcraft, R. Penchansky, and R. S. Fortus. 1977. "Enrollment Choice in a Multi-HMO Setting: The Roles of Health Risk, Financial Vulnerability, and Access to Care." *Medical Care* 15: 95–104.

Ermann, D., and J. Gabel. 1984. "Multi-hospital Systems: Issues and Empirical Findings." *Health Affairs* 3: 50–64.

Evans, R. G. 1983. "Incomplete Vertical Integration in the Health Care Industry: Pseudomarkets and Pseudopolicies." *Annals of the American Academy of Political and Social Sciences* 468 (July): 60–87.

Feldstein, M. S. 1973. "The Welfare Loss from Excess Health Insurance." *Journal of Political Economy* 81: 251–80.

Frech, H. E., III, and P. Ginsburg. 1978. "Competition among Health Insurers." In *Competition in the Health Care Sector: Past, Present, and Future,* ed. by W. Greenberg, 168–87. Germantown, MD: Aspen Systems.

Gibson, R. M., and D. R. Waldo. 1981. "National Health Expenditures, 1980." *Health Care Financing Review* 3: 1–54.

Goldberg, L. G., and W. Greenberg. 1977. "The Effect of Physician Controlled Health Insurance." *Journal of Health Politics, Policy and Law* 2 (Spring): 48–78.

Havighurst, C. C., and N. M. King. 1983. "Private Credentialing of Health Care Personnel: An Antitrust Perspective." *American Journal of Law and Medicine* 9: 131–201, 263–334.

Jensen, M., and W. Meckling. 1976. "Theory of the Firm: Managerial Behavior, Agency Costs and Ownership Structure." *Journal of Financial Economics* 3: 305–60.

Khogali, M. 1978. "Vertical Integration for Providing Health Services in Developing Countries." *Tropical Doctor* 8 (July): 157–59.

Luft, H. S. 1980. "Trends in Medical Care Costs: Do HMO's Lower the Rate of Growth?" *Medical Care* 18: 1–16.

———. 1981. *Health Maintenance Organizations: Dimensions of Performance.* New York: Wiley.

Luft, H. S., and B. Trauner. 1981. *The Operation and Performance of Health Maintenance Organizations.* Washington, DC: National Center for Health Services Research.

Lundberg, C. J. 1984. "Home Health Care: A Logical Extension of Hospital Services." *Topics in Health Care Financing* 10 (Spring): 22–33.

National Industry Council for HMO Development. 1984. *The Health Maintenance Organization Ten Year Report: 1973–83.* Washington, DC: The Council.

Newhouse, J. P. 1978. "Insurance Benefits, Out-of-Pocket Payments and the Demand for Medical Care: A Review of the Literature." *Health and Medical Care Services Review* 1 (4): 3–5.

Palley, H. A., Y. Yishai, and P. Ever-Hadani. 1983. "Pluralist Social Constraints on the Development of a Health Care System: The Case of Israel." *Inquiry* 20 (Spring): 65–75.

Pauly, M. V., and M. Redisch. 1973. "The Not-for-Profit Hospital as a Physicians' Cooperative." *American Economic Review* 63: 87–100.

Phelps, C. E. 1982. *Health Care Costs: The Consequences of Increased Cost Sharing.* R-2970-RC. Santa Monica, CA: RAND Corporation.

Phelps, C. E., and J. P. Newhouse. 1972. *The Effects of Co-insurance on the Demand for Physicians' Services.* R-976-OEO. Santa Monica, CA: RAND Corporation.

Radner, R. 1970. "Problems in the Theory of Markets under Uncertainty." *American Economic Review* 60: 454–60.

Richardson, W., D. Martin, and P. Diehr. 1984. "Consumer Choice and Cost Containment: Safeco United Healthcare Plan." *Health Care Financing Grants and Contracts Report.* 017-00164-0. Washington, DC: U.S. Government Printing Office.

Schmalense, R. 1973. "A Note on the Theory of Vertical Integration." *Journal of Political Economy* 81: 442–49.

Scitovsky, A. A., and N. McCall. 1977. "Co-insurance and the Demand for Physician Services." *Social Security Bulletin* 40 (5): 19–27.

Sloan, F., and B. Steinwald. 1980. *Insurance Regulation and Hospital Costs.* Lexington, MA: Heath.

Trauner, J. B. 1983. *Preferred Provider Organizations: The California Experiment.* Berkeley: University of California Press.

U.S. Department of Health and Human Services. 1982. *Health, United States.* Hyattsville, MD: The Department.

Vernon, J., and D. Graham. 1971. "Profitability of Monopolization by Vertical Integration." *Journal of Political Economy* 79 (July/August): 924–25.

Williamson, O. E. 1971. "The Vertical Integration of Production: Market Failure Considerations." *American Economic Review* 61: 112–23.

5

Consumer Sovereignty in a Competitive Market: Fact or Fiction?

Thomas W. O'Rourke

One element underlying the competitive approach to medical care is the expanded role of the consumer. The term *consumer* will be defined here in a functional sense, as any purchaser of medical goods or services. Consumers may be individuals who pay for medical services "out-of-pocket" or "third-party" payers, such as businesses, industries, labor groups, and the government, who purchase medical services on behalf of individual recipients. Proponents of competitive models envision enlightened consumers shopping for health services while providers compete vigorously for their business. In their view, sovereign consumers, by expressing demand in the market, will determine the behavior of those supplying health services. Proponents argue that, under a competitive approach, health care services will more closely follow the patterns of production and distribution of other goods and services within our society. Ultimately, health care services, along with toothpaste, soap, widgets, and bubble gum, will be guided by the laws of supply and demand.

This chapter considers whether the emergence of a competitive approach genuinely fosters consumer sovereignty in the health care market. It first argues that the present health care "system" is more myth than reality, it provides a rationale for consumer involvement in the medical area, it questions whether consumer sovereignty exists, and it identifies a number of significant obstacles to the realization of such sovereignty.

The chapter also argues that competition beneficial to the patient-consumer is not, and has never been, an element of our health care services. It suggests that proposals that seek to foster a truly competitive market are unlikely to satisfy the best interests of consumers. Tinkering with organizational structures and reimbursement methods will not significantly affect health. Only when we seek to maximize the quality of life, rather than to bandage an irrational sick care system, will we be on the way to developing a true health care system.

THE HEALTH CARE SYSTEM: MYTH OR REALITY?

The term *health care system* requires some clarification. The concept as it exists now is a myth; the term is a popular euphemism that will not be used in this chapter without qualification. Hamilton (1982, 10–11) maintains that each word in the phrase is misleading. The term *health* seems inappropriate when the criterion for entry is a diagnosis of illness. *Care* seems likewise inappropriate, since the present system focuses on treatment, not on caring (listening, touching, and reassuring). The word *system* is simply inaccurate; it implies that services by professionals, institutions, suppliers, and third-party payers are organized and coordinated on a large scale to serve those in need. In fact, services in most areas are unequally distributed, devoted to a narrow range of the health spectrum (usually emphasizing acute care and minimizing prevention, rehabilitation, and long-term services), and varied in quality. More accurate than health care system might be *medical treatment chaos* or *nonsystem*. Critics also charge that ours is not a health care system but a disease care system whose structure, function, and financing are dominated by medical providers to the detriment of the consumer (Ehrenreich and Ehrenreich 1971; Gleen 1980; Duhl and Blum 1981, 271–87).

Medical care in America is a collage of programs and acronyms. It is HSAs, HMOs, PSROs, PPOs, and CATs. It is Medicare, Medicaid, and private health insurance. It is hospitalization and monopolization. It is nursing home care and home care nursing. It is medicalization and demedicalization. The system is complex, fragmented, and, many say, in need of reform.

Some maintain that bold new initiatives are needed:

> The delivery of health services is faltering so badly that we will have to shake the present system literally to its foundation. . . . Revolutionary changes are needed. . . . The nation must have new careers, new professions, new kinds of manpower; and we do not have thousands of years, perhaps not even thousands of days, to lose. . . . We will have to question every cherished belief about how health care ought to be provided. (*Washington Post* 1969).

Corry (1983, 14) contends that it "sometimes borders on being a three-ring circus. It is complicated, cumbersome, sometimes dishonest and hurtful but also occasionally the very best in the world." For the sake of familiarity, the term *medical care system* will be used in this chapter.

WHAT IS A CONSUMER?

In the health care arena, the term consumer presents some confusion. Until recently, *patient* was satisfactory, particularly among providers; for others *client* was preferred. Consumer was the term least likely to be used in the jargon of health providers.

Under the National Health Resources and Planning Development Act of 1974 (PL 93-641), consumers were defined by default and in negative terms. This historic act created a nationwide network of some 200 health systems agencies (HSAs) to address access, quality, cost, and other major health care issues of the day. Each HSA board comprised health "providers" and "consumers." Providers were defined as those who earned an income from the medical system; consumers were defined as those who did not.

In most sectors a consumer is thought of as a person who purchases and uses certain goods and services. In medical care, however, defining a consumer is more complex. From the standpoint of our mortality, everyone may be viewed as a potential consumer. Beyond this, Hamilton (1982, 6–9) provides an excellent argument for the theory that virtually everyone is a consumer of medical care regardless of the extent to which he or she receives it. While only patients use health care services, virtually everyone bears the costs of these services. Through taxes we all subsidize the education of providers, medical research, provider evaluation through PSROs, and direct care for others through programs such as Medicare and Medicaid. Thus, practically everyone is a consumer.

In addition, the consumer is not only the individual. For example, Blue Cross and Blue Shield plans, commercial insurance companies, and prepaid and self-insured plans paid an estimated $107 billion in medical benefits in 1984. This amount represented 31 percent of personal health care expenditures (Levit et al. 1985, 15). The private health insurance plans often originate in the workplace, where the employer frequently pays a major share of the premium. These costs are then transferred to consumers through the price of the employer's product. Similarly, government— especially at the federal level—is another major consumer of medical care. For example, the federal government, which contracts for care through Medicare and Medicaid, acts as a consumer of care for millions of citizens. In 1984, the $99 billion spent through these programs translated into 29 percent of all personal health care in the nation. By 1990, governmental expenditures for medical care for all programs are projected to be $267.2 billion, with the federal government paying 72 percent of that total (Arnett et al. 1986, 6).

Because health care consumers or purchasers are not only individual patients but also businesses and industries, labor unions, and the govern-

ment, they should not be viewed simply as patients or individuals who compare drug prices or seek out a specific provider to meet their needs. To
avoid confusion, the term consumer in this chapter is used quite generally to encompass any individual or organization that pays for health care,
regardless of the use of medical care services.

The distinction between patient and consumer is important to many
providers. The image of the doctor-patient relationship often conflicts with
that of physicians or institutions that market themselves to consumers. The
term patient has many appeals to providers—patients, by their very nature,
are more passive and dependent than consumers. Some people find the
term consumer rather mercenary. While useful, the term is often inappropriate to medical care, which often deals with issues of life and death.
Whether the term patient or client is used is a moot point. Both are inadequate, failing to acknowledge the complexity of an individual, institutional,
or organizational relationship to the medical care system. Both terms merely describe an individual's relationship to the medical care system at a
specific time, usually in relation to a perceived illness. Consumer is more
appropriate since it describes an ongoing relationship of an individual or
a larger entity to the medical care system over an indefinite period of time
(Hamilton 1982, 8).

Medical care is also a business—a very big business. With a total price
tag in 1984 of $387 billion, a per capita expenditure of approximately
$1,580, and a 10.6 percent share of the GNP (Levit et al. 1985, 1), medical
care is the second largest industry in the United States. Recent projections
indicate that by 1990 national health expenditures will grow to $640 bil-
lion, have a per capita cost of $2,476, and consume 11.3 percent of GNP
(Arnett et al. 1986, 6). Access to medical care in our free-market economy
is largely dependent upon economic factors. Money fuels the system. For
this reason, too, the term consumer seems appropriate.

THE EMERGENCE OF THE CONSUMER

The past two decades in particular have witnessed the emergence of consumer activism in many areas. Underlying the consumer movement was the
notion that the status quo was not always equitable, ethical, or legal. Dissatisfaction led various groups such as blacks, women, and environmen-
talists to voice their concerns, educate the public, and sometimes
demonstrate and organize for social, political, and economic change
(Boston Women's Health Book Collective 1973). Concomitant with these
movements was the extension of the concept of rights to areas where they
may have been lacking or considered privileges. Pleas were heard for civil
rights for members of racial minority groups, women, and gay people;
others insisted on the public's right to a safe environment and to health
care.

During this period, there was a growing skepticism of business and industry, as exemplified by Senator Edward Kennedy's statement about the medical industry: "It is an industry in which there is very little incentive to offer services responsive to the people's needs and demands. It is an industry which strongly protects the profit and rights of the provider, but only weakly protects the healing and the rights of the people" (Kennedy 1972, 16). Existing institutions designed to address solutions to problems began to be viewed by many in the consumer movement as the sources of those problems and protectors of the status quo.

Evidence of an emerging political recognition of the consumer led President John F. Kennedy in 1962 to develop a consumer Bill of Rights that included the rights to safety, information, choice, and a voice (Consumers Advisory Council 1963). Others have reinforced the importance of an informed and involved consumer. For example, Virginia H. Knauer, former special assistant to the president for consumer affairs, stated that

> Our greatest challenge is to heighten the consumer's awareness of his rights and to educate him about the marketplace and his role in it. . . . We need a consuming public that shops for value, demands more information about products, is discriminating about advertisements, suspects offers of something-for-nothing and is vocal about the abuses of the marketplace. (Coniff 1971, 18)

Ralph Nader supported and amplified Knauer's comment when he remarked, "There can be no daily democracy without daily citizenship. If we do not exercise our civic rights, who will? If we do not perform our civic duties, who can? The fiber of a just society in the pursuit of happiness is a thinking, active citizenry" (McGarrah 1974). The growing consumer movement has been further refined and integrated into mainstream society. Materials to assist consumers in the purchase of virtually every good and service are now commonplace. Thousands of consumer organizations exist and continue to grow. Today, because of these past events and a more educated public, a more discriminating consumer has emerged.

RATIONALE FOR CONSUMER INVOLVEMENT IN MEDICAL CARE

As one might expect, health care providers, particularly physicians, are not overly enthusiastic about greater consumer involvement in the medical system. A classic statement is "I wouldn't tell an airline pilot how to fly a plane, and I don't want a patient telling me how to practice medicine." To the providers, medicine is too esoteric for the consumer to understand, much less control. Others maintain that consumer involvement only "slows things down," "confuses the issues," or is a short-lived phenomenon that, if ignored, will go away. These arguments are bogus; they distort the real issues.

Hamilton (1982, 2–3) rejects the airline analogy, maintaining that consumers do not want to tell pilots how to fly. The rationale for consumer involvement has never been based on the idea of technical expertise. However, consumers do want to have access to transportation, to be able to afford a ticket, to pick their destination, and to be free to take the bus if they prefer. In the health sector, consumers increasingly want less emphasis on treating acute illness and more emphasis on promoting wellness; they want the option to choose one form of care and reject another. These notions run counter to expectations that still prevail among many medical providers.

Consumers and providers often come to the medical arena with different personal interests. Providers, especially physicians, approach the health care arena seeking prestige, financial gain, and the satisfaction of professional goals, certainly some of which are altruistic. Consumers arrive on the medical care scene desiring accessible, affordable, acceptable, effective care. The differing goals may not be entirely consistent.

In response to the criticism that consumer involvement slows things down, one must ask, What is the goal? Is it expeditiousness or fairness or caring? Should we assume that groups of providers charged with regulating their profession, influencing and setting policy, planning services, or administering medical institutions will have collective interests that parallel those of consumers? The medical care system, although terribly fragmented, is not out of control. A predominant form of control over health care in this country is regulation by health care providers (Waters 1980, 7). Regulation by providers manifests itself by peer review, licensing, accreditation, and other credential-granting programs. Critics charge that these forms of self-control do not sufficiently protect consumers. They argue that the collective interest of health providers, including individuals, groups, and institutions, has been to restrict competition, promote their monopolistic empires, maximize income, and enhance prestige (Cray 1970; Schorr 1970; Harmer 1975; Kotelchuck 1976).

Though providers often discount consumer participation on the grounds that there is no one who can speak for consumers in general, consumers have a fundamental reason for being involved. Consumers believe that medical care should be structured to meet their needs, rather than the aspirations of providers, which may or may not be consistent with consumer desires. Some will argue that the advent of consumer involvement will create conflict. Quite possibly, the more consumerism conflicts with the unreasonable protection of professional dominance, the better the system will be for consumers. The problem, to date, has not been conflict, but the lack of it.

CONSUMER SOVEREIGNTY IN THE MEDICAL MARKETPLACE

The term consumer sovereignty, coined in the 1800s by W. H. Hutt, refers to the potential power of the consumer over the behavior of the producer in the marketplace (Hutt 1936). Over time the term has been refined. According to Creighton (1976, 12), for consumer sovereignty to be a reality the following four conditions must exist:

—Consumer demand must determine the production of goods and provision of services.

—Consumers must have the information necessary to judge the quality, utility, and safety of products and services.

—Consumers must choose products and services that give the greatest utility for the lowest price.

—Both consumers and providers must have free access to the marketplace.

How appropriate is the term in the area of medical care? To what extent is the notion of consumer sovereignty in the medical marketplace viable? For the present at least, the notion of consumer sovereignty appears more mythical than real. In the market for medical care, the balance of power rests with the providers (Vladek 1981, 209–33).

OBSTACLES TO CONSUMER SOVEREIGNTY

Some obstacles have been identified in earlier chapters; thus only brief mention will be made of them here. A major obstacle at present is that the medical care arena does not operate as a typical marketplace. In an excellent analysis, Marmor (1983, 242–43) clearly depicts how the medical care market is hindered by its failure to meet numerous conditions for ideal competition. Unique factors governing both supply and demand have effectively insulated both consumer and provider from those forces that, under a competitive model, would enhance the efficient use of resources. Enthoven (1980, xvi–xvii) and others (Klarman 1977, 215–34; Feldstein 1979) have identified the following features of the current medical scene as those that have reduced competition and contributed to price inflation and inefficient use of resources: (1) the predominance of third-party payers that insulate the individual from sensitivity to cost; (2) cost reimbursement by third-party payers as the basis of payment for medical care, especially to hospitals; and (3) fee-for-service reimbursement of physicians.

The factors are compounded by the role the physician plays in relation to the consumer. Unlike most other goods and services, medical care is characterized by the role of a provider as an agent of the consumer (Fuchs 1978; Wennberg and Lapenas 1980; Gibson 1984, 6). This situation arises from lack of consumer knowledge regarding the diagnosis and treatment of illness and from legal constraints, initiated and reinforced by the providers, on the use of medical care resources. While physicians receive 20 cents of each medical dollar, some estimates indicate that they are responsible for about 70 to 80 percent of all expenditures for medical services and supplies (Somers and Somers 1977). Thus, physicians have a significant effect upon the consumption of medical services. When the physician as agent is combined with fee-for-service and extensive third-party coverage, there is a great potential for excessive and inappropriate use of resources.

Other obstacles to consumer sovereignty include a variety of mechanisms that promote monopolistic practices, such as legal barriers to entry and to input substitutions, and a lack of qualitative and quantitative information for the consumer (U.S. Department of Health and Human Services 1980, 103–4). Certainly, some of the aspects of these mechanisms can be useful. For example, legal requirements such as occupational licensure seek to protect the public by maintaining quality standards, but these same standards may inflate costs by impeding the substitution of lower-priced but equally effective personnel on given tasks. With regard to input substitution, some have advocated greater autonomy of the nurse practitioner to perform specific tasks now reserved for physicians. With respect to the availability of information, state laws and informal prohibitions on advertising by professional associations often make it difficult for consumers to find information on price and quality. Despite some positive policy and legal actions that have loosened constraints on advertising and promoted market information, the medical care market is still resistant to open competition on the basis of cost or qualitative information (Federal Trade Commission 1979). While most hospitals and many clinics now have marketing components, their focus, to date, has been on image promotion. Most of us have seen the advertisement in which a friendly physician hands a lollipop to a child or reassures a senior citizen. Rarely is specific information provided on price or quality of care. It is amazing that Americans can obtain consumer reports on washing machines, but not information on the individuals and institutions that are supposed to be taking care of their lives.

Some of these barriers are weakening, although they still exist. An impetus for change in this area came in the landmark case in which the Federal Trade Commission (FTC) sued the American Medical Association (AMA) and two Connecticut medical societies. After years of testimony citing instance after instance and repeated appeals by the AMA, the FTC ordered the AMA to cease and desist from

> Restricting, regulating, impeding, declaring unethical, interfering with, or advising against the advertising or publishing by a person of the prices, terms or conditions of sale of physicians' services, or of information about physicians' services, facilities or equipment which are offered for sale or made available by physicians or by any organization with which physicians are affiliated. (ibid., 2)

Physicians are by no means the only obstacle. Although medical care providers often claim diehard allegiance to free enterprise, few truly desire the rigors of real competition. Waters (1980) contends that providers have tended to avoid competition and to maximize certainty. For example, hospital associations support rate-setting programs and antitrust exemption laws. Visiting nurse associations, long proponents of geographic franchises, have supported certificates of need for the same protectionist reasons. Because data that reveal quality are usually confidential, the incompetence of some providers and profiteering by some doctors, laboratories, and other parts of the medical industry have been shielded from public scrutiny.[1]

The persistence of these obstacles implies that any significant changes in an improved, cost-conscious, integrated system will not be easy. Health care providers, particularly physicians and hospitals, present a major obstacle. They are well organized and motivated, and they have significant economic and political resources. Introducing effective competition will be difficult.

A last obstacle to consumer sovereignty has been the consumer. Business, labor, government, and individuals have been passive for too long. Part of the problem was understanding the problem. The elements of the problem are now being understood, and there is growing sentiment for change in the way medical care is organized, financed, and delivered (*Business Week* 1984, 138–48; *Newsweek* 1985, 56–58).

CONSUMER SOVEREIGNTY AND COMPETITION

From the outset it should be noted that the competitive approaches being advocated appear to address some of the major limitations of the present medical care system (for example, Enthoven 1978, 650–58). Competitive proposals realize the inherent limitations of open-ended, fee-for-service reimbursement to physicians, cost reimbursement to hospitals, and third-party payment. Proponents also realize the importance of the physician as agent and the lack of cost consciousness by millions of Americans in the selection and use of medical services.

Despite vast differences in their provisions, competitive strategies share several objectives in attempting to meet their goal of letting the marketplace enter the medical care arena (ibid., 709–20). These include:

—Provisions allowing employers, employees, or both to shop around for more cost-effective insurance plans. This cost-conscious shopping may be accomplished through positive incentives such as tax credits, negative incentives such as tax liabilities, or greater cost-sharing provisions by the consumer.

—Fostering competing organized delivery systems. The underlying belief is that, as consumers become more price conscious, insurers and providers will respond by promoting the delivery of more cost-effective medical care.

Ideally, a domino effect is created, by which consumers apply competitive pressure to insurers, who transfer these pressures to providers. Providers who do not develop strategies to compete effectively will wither on the vine. No longer will the existing perverse incentives be rewarded. Rather, as Enthoven (1980, xii) envisions it, providers will form into "competing economic units," as consumers and insurers seek out those who are cost-effective.

While the competitive strategy has a certain basic appeal, whether it is a valuable option, particularly with respect to consumer sovereignty, is questionable. One immediate concern is the feasibility of even introducing a competitive medical care strategy. Groups such as the American Medical Association and the American Hospital Association have shown little inclination to jump on the competitive bandwagon. To the contrary, past history indicates that they can be expected to oppose vigorously any such initiatives and lobby energetically for fee-for-service medicine and cost-based reimbursement as they now exist (Ginzberg 1980, 1112; Roberts 1980, 10). Also, Havighurst (1979, 299) contends that "The greatest obstacle to third-party cost containment is the willingness, even eagerness, of doctors to act collectively to halt, dilute, co-opt, or capture any cost-containment measures that they find objectionable or threatening." It is interesting to note that since the beginning of President Reagan's first term, several bills proposing competition in medical care have been introduced. Now, six years later, in the midst of a deregulatory environment, not one of those bills has been enacted, although in the interim deregulation has occurred in major industries such as airlines and trucking. Even if elements of the competitive approach are introduced, health providers can be expected to resist and "game the system" to thwart competitive initiatives.

In the medical arena there are relatively few sellers. Most providers are not able to sell their services directly to the public. They must work under licensure provisions that restrict the practice of medicine to physicians, who are also limited in supply. Growth of group practice can effectively reduce even further the number of individual sellers and thus have a negative effect on competition. For example, in some communities there may be several hundred physicians but a majority may be affiliated with only one or two group practices. The FTC, in its long-standing case against the AMA, cited numerous instances in which providers conspired to restrain free trade (Federal Trade Commission 1979). Providers, through a county medical society, for example, may agree de facto to avoid competition by either setting rates or maintaining fee-for-service medicine. Sigelman has maintained (1981, 100), "So long as fee-for-service medicine is available as a viable alternative, real competitive market behavior is not likely to occur." To the extent that conventional fee-for-service medicine can operate, it will place inflationary pressure on prepaid group practices. The possibility that competing prepaid group practice plans may not aggressively contain the growth in costs over time is seen in the Federal Employees Health Benefits Program, where over a ten-year period, premiums consistently hovered five to ten dollars per month below those of conventional Blue Cross/Blue Shield (Luft 1980b, 91).

The domino theory of competition assumes that insurers will put pressure on providers to control costs. This assumption is questionable in the light of the historically close relationship between providers and insurers (Law 1974). Quite possibly, some insurers may not act as agents for cost-conscious consumers. Walter J. McNerney, past president of the Blue Cross/Blue Shield Association, acknowledged this possibility, mentioning that insurers can adopt several measures other than negotiating lower reimbursement rates (McNerney 1980). Those measures might include increased reliance on experience rating and preferred risk selection, such as eliminating high-risk groups, to avoid alienating providers.

Another major obstacle to a truly competitive market may be the absence of adequate information. One problem is the very nature of medical care. Unlike many other products, medical care is not a precisely defined good. The treatment associated with a specific set of symptoms or a particular diagnosis can vary significantly. This variability is compounded by the lack of consumer information on cost and quality. The market model assumes that producers compete for consumers on the basis of cost and quality. However, the domino theory imposes insurers between providers and consumers; therefore, consumers may shop for insurers instead of providers. Medical care competition will become a reality only when consumers know more about the cost and performance of different plans and of individual providers. In addition, consumers will need qualitative information about various treatments, as well as the track records not only of individual providers, but also of specific institutions such as hospitals. To date, even in the midst of competitive market forces, providers have exhibited no enthusiasm for efforts to promote public disclosure of qualitative information. It is highly doubtful that they will alter their position.

Consumers, defined broadly as payers, need to know how utilization data compare among doctors and hospitals. They need to know lengths of stay, surgery rates, and diagnosis- and procedure-specific admission rates. Undoubtedly many patients would use this information to pursue the best possible care; this is evidenced by consumers in Washington, D.C., who canceled scheduled heart surgeries at unfavorably reviewed hospitals (*PSRO Letter* 1979). Currently, PSROs collect a wealth of qualitative data (Braverman 1980, 65–90), including mortality and complication rates for individual providers. Ironically, the collection and tabulation of these data are funded by taxes; but opposition from medical providers keeps these data from taxpayer scrutiny. Release of this information could stimulate competition for the consumer's dollars. Roberts (1980, 12) puts it succinctly: "unless competition proponents aggressively support the release of doctor-specific data on surgery complication rates or . . . lists of physicians whom PSROs find to be over-utilizing . . . consumer confusion will blunt the extent to which the market disciplines competitors for poor performance with regard to either quality or price."

Proponents of competition face another formidable problem. To date, competitive delivery systems have yet to prove themselves. Enthoven, like other competitive-market proponents, believes that the noncompetitive cycle can be broken if two or more organized systems compete against each other. Proponents proudly point to the examples of HMO penetration in Minneapolis, California, and Hawaii. However, other economists such as Luft (1980a, 526) recommend caution before jumping on the procompetitive bandwagon. While he readily acknowledges that HMOs can significantly reduce hospital use, Luft finds no convincing evidence that these plans have actually lowered communitywide per capita health care costs, which he considers to be the ultimate measure of cost effectiveness. Also, where there is limited competition, one plan may price itself just under another, reflecting not the lowest possible price but rather a price just slightly less than that of the competition. Though an improvement, the actual cost reduction may not be as substantial as the proponents of competition would prefer.

The competitive strategy assumes that consumers will weigh costs and benefits in the light of their own desires—with costs certainly playing a significant role. However, one feature that distinguishes the purchase of insurance from that of many other goods and services is risk aversion. Whether employees would be willing to trade tax credits for peace of mind is questionable. The experience of members of the Federal Employees Health Benefits Program (FEHBP), a program frequently cited by competitive proponents, suggests that many employees prefer incurring a known insurance premium expense to accepting fewer comprehensive benefits and potentially higher out-of-pocket expenses (Office of Personnel Management 1980). Only a few federal employees choose low-option plans. Of course, this pattern may change, depending upon the incentives, but the experience to date indicates that employees may not simply switch to lower-priced plans that provide fewer benefits.

A potential problem with the competitive approach is that enrollees may shift from high- to low-option plans and back in anticipation of changes in utilization. Proponents of competition argue that because of incentives and disincentives, large blocks of enrollees will choose low-option plans and thus reduce overall demand. But the success of competitive proposals may be jeopardized if enrollees switch regularly between high- and low-option plans. Specifically, analysis by Blue Cross/Blue Shield of use within the FEHBP found that those who switched into high-option plans during the open enrollment period used 45 percent more services than other high-option enrollees (McNerney 1980). Those new enrollees with family coverage used 55 percent more benefits than their other high-option counterparts. Those who switched into low-option plans had 55 percent and 65 percent lower use, respectively, than their low-option counterparts. If employees can anticipate their needs and switch accordingly, the ability of a competitive system to control use is more limited.

One of the most touted advantages of the competitive proposal is that it provides an alternative to regulation of the medical care industry. The Gephardt-Stockman competitive bill clearly states the viewpoint that competition among qualified plans will be based on market incentives and disciplines, thus permitting natural economic forces to work and making regulation unnecessary (*Congressional Record* 1981). This view is reinforced strongly by the President's Commission for a National Agenda for the Eighties, which has asserted "an expansion of the role of competition, consumer choice, and market incentives rather than government control is more likely to create the much-needed stimulus toward greater efficiency, cost consciousness, and responsiveness to consumer preferences so visibly lacking in our present arrangements for providing medical care" (as quoted by Marmor 1983, 240). Proponents of competition see their approach as one that makes health planning, HSAs, and PSROs historical footnotes. Closer examination raises some doubt about these assertions.

While many existing regulations will be eliminated, new regulations will inevitably be formulated; competitive proposals can exist only within their own set of parameters. Although all procompetitive proposals reject present and past regulatory mechanisms, all require "market-correcting" regulation to improve market functioning. In some instances there may be more regulation than there is now. For example, the health insurance industry has traditionally been regulated by the states. Under many competitive proposals federal regulations would supersede existing state provisions. Plans seeking to be certified and marketed would need to become "qualified." To do this, they would have to meet regulations covering minimum benefits for low-option plans and for catastrophic coverage and also meet financial viability standards. Plans would also have an open enrollment period. In essence, the federal government would have to create a regulatory bureaucracy to monitor and evaluate the thousands of plans operating in the marketplace. Detailed monitoring of the tax implications for individuals and employers would also be required, depending upon which plans are offered. The complexities are significant. The resulting regulatory bureaucracy might well result in a de facto full employment bill for a new breed of regulators.

A major criticism of the competitive system is its potential to "blame the victim," which is expressed in several ways. Underlying the promotion of some competitive strategies is the idea that the consumer's misuse of medical care because of price insensitivity needs to be curbed. Making the consumer think twice before using services will curb misuse. One common approach advocated by procompetitive strategists is to raise the price to the consumer through the use of significant deductibles, coinsurance, and copayment. Ignored in the proposal is the fact that physicians, not consumers, are the primary decision makers (*National Health Insurance Report* 1979). Physicians decide if and when to hospitalize, do testing, perform surgery, and discharge. The consumer is relatively passive. It would seem more logical to curb unnecessary use by applying constraints on the decision makers—placing the providers at risk as in an HMO arrangement—rather than by penalizing the consumer. Schneider (1980, 49) sums it up well when he states that to impose consumer restraints "without in any way restraining the pricing power of the physicians . . . is to blame the victim, not to promote 'competition.'" The ultimate merits of a cost-sharing strategy are questionable. As Marmor mentions, the appeal of this approach depends partially on one's view of the elasticity of demand for health services. He contends that the elasticity of demand varies for different types of service. Those services that are low-cost and discretionary have high elasticity, while the elasticity of demand is low for high-cost care, especially with physicians dominating consumption choices. However, low-cost, discretionary services are not necessarily the type to be curtailed. Rather, he maintains that

> High cost, high technology, high intensity services are partially, and perhaps primarily, responsible both for the rapid rise in medical sector expenditures and for the doubts about the worth of such expenditures. Cost sharing would not directly alter the major pressures toward consumption of this type of care since most episodes of high cost care exceed the limit of any feasible deductible. (Marmor 1983, 244)

Not only may competitive proposals "blame the victim," but they have the potential to discriminate against certain employees, such as those who have low incomes, are at high risk, or live and receive their care where medical costs are higher. Workers in high tax brackets now get more tax benefits from employer-paid health insurance premiums than do lower-income workers; but under competitive proposals, which might make insurance benefits taxable, low-income workers may be most vulnerable. This situation may force lower-income workers, who often have greater medical need, to choose between paying higher cost-sharing provisions or foregoing needed care. Depending on its structure, the catastrophic element of most competitive proposals may also aggravate the situation for the lower-paid employee. If the catastrophic component is indexed to an absolute amount, a lower-paid employee may have to pay out several thousand dollars before he can receive coverage. This eventuality could be catastrophic for the low-income person. If the catastrophic component is indexed more equitably to income, monitoring eligibility may present a significant administrative problem.

A sobering perspective on the effects of competition has been offered by Aaron (1984) of the Brookings Institution. In his text, *Painful Prescription: Rationing Health Care,* he agrees that the rapid growth of medical costs is an inevitable consequence of the lack of a free market, but he argues that it is a delusion to think that the cost momentum can be slowed significantly by increasing efficiency, "the hospital version of eliminating waste, fraud and abuse in government." He maintains that greater cost sharing will not have much effect, since "no country has done it—at times of illness people are spared most cost." He is also skeptical about the effect of HMOs on costs, noting that even if every U.S. hospital were to match the alleged 30-percent lower HMO admission rate (presently HMOs cover only 7 percent of the population), the savings would still equal only about 10 percent to 15 percent of the current hospital care budget and cut the health care inflation rate by only 1 percent to 2 percent (ibid.).

One element not often discussed is the rationing of care. The cost of hospital care for a person in Britain, for example, is half that in the United States, primarily because the British are willing to accept rationing of scarce and costly medical resources. According to Aaron (ibid.), even though the United States and Britain train physicians similarly and share common journals and medical research, British physicians necessarily behave differently where treatments have little or no proven effects, especially with expensive procedures for the elderly and terminally ill. The British use one-third less hemodialysis for renal failure and virtually none for persons over age 55. They use one-quarter fewer x-rays per patient and only do one-sixth as many coronary operations as are done in the U.S.

Thurow (1984, 1569–70) argues that we need to reassess medical practice in the United States:

It is traditional medical practice in the United States to employ treatments until they yield no additional payoffs, but with the development of more and more expensive techniques and devices that can slightly improve a diagnosis or marginally prolong life, the expenditures that have to be made before this traditional stopping point is reached have grown to almost unlimited levels. . . . These new medical techniques require a shift in standard medical practice. Instead of stopping treatment when all benefits cease to exist, physicians must stop treatments when marginal benefits are equal to marginal costs. . . . The health-care problem is not a federal or state budget problem. It is a social problem. The expenditure limits are the same regardless of whether the money is spent through the federal budget or private insurance. Our basic problem is that somehow we are going to have to learn to say "no."

Rationing is not a new concept, as some might like to believe. In discussing rationing Fuchs (1984, 1572) mentions that

Although we hear this warning with increasing frequency, taken literally the statement is sheer nonsense. It is nonsense because the United States has always rationed medical care, just as every country always has and always will ration care. No nation is wealthy enough to supply all the care that is technically feasible and desirable; no nation can provide "presidential medicine" for all its citizens. . . . Indeed, there are changes under way—not from no rationing to rationing, but rather in the way rationing takes place—who does the rationing and who is affected by it.

Competitive theorists are well aware of the rationing issue. They suggest that the market is an effective rationing device. This view, of course, raises a whole host of issues, since the poor and uninsured are the most likely to suffer from rationing.

The competitive proposals also need to address the potential problem of what insurers call adverse risk selection. If the incentives built into the competitive proposal work as proponents envision, one would expect that younger, healthier employees will opt for low-premium, low-option plans. That would leave high-risk workers in a pool with a significantly higher premium, which would mean both higher out-of-pocket costs and greater tax liabilities. Historically, group insurance has operated under a community rating system that spreads the medical costs throughout the population. Under a competitive proposal one might anticipate a greater reliance on an experience rating system that would work against the high-risk employees, because of either their poor health status or the nature of their work. Without incorporating some form of subsidy, workers employed in higher-risk workplaces would therefore pay higher premiums.

A major concern frequently expressed is that the poor or nearly poor may not do well under a competitive approach. Critics frequently charge that competitive proposals may restrict the access, choice, and quality of medical care available to the poor and produce a multitiered system. For example, introducing significant cost-sharing provisions in the form of deductibles, coinsurance, or copayments runs counter to the notion of equity of access and consumption. Cost sharing represents a tax or user fee on the sick. If the cost sharing is not indexed to income, it will have a greater effect on lower-income people. Ultimately, it may price people out of the market regardless of need. The regressive nature of cost sharing is clearly described by Barer (1979, 111): "Charges whose aggregate levels for a given family are direct functions of utilization will involve perverse wealth transfers from the ill to the healthy and, to the extent that the poor (including a significant share of the aged) are less healthy than the rich, from low- to high-income classes." Even such a champion of competition as Enthoven (1980, 34–35) argues against cost sharing at the time of need:

> The individual episode of medical care is usually not good material for rational economic calculation. If the patient is in pain or urgent need of care, the transaction is not entirely voluntary. The sick or worried patient is in a poor position to make an economic analysis of treatment alternatives. When my injured child is lying bleeding on the operating table is hardly the time when I want to negotiate with the doctor over fees or the number of sutures that will be used.

Critics also argue that because the poor are less healthy overall, they will, on the average, pay more for treatment. The poor have a greater number of disability days, a higher average length of stay, and higher admission rates than the middle class (Newacheck et al. 1980, 1165). A community-rated, capitation health care plan would have few incentives to enroll the less healthy because they need more medical care. Health plan administrators, like many insurers now, would be hesitant to enroll large numbers of poor people who would reduce their competitive position against other plans that are marketed to healthier groups.

Eder (Touche, Ross, and Co. 1979) reports that the results of Project Health in Multnomah County, Oregon, are not encouraging. There, medically indigent persons were to choose among six comprehensive prepaid health plans with Project Health paying most of the premiums. There was some minor cost sharing based on family income and the cost of a particular plan. One plan withdrew and another was granted a 75-percent rate increase. In turn, the rate increase prompted healthier enrollees to switch plans, resulting in even higher premiums for the remaining clients. What was to be a community-rated plan evolved into an experience-rated one that imposed higher premiums on the poor. Also, 29 percent (many of those with long histories of illness) chose to stay with their personal doctors rather than enroll in the closed-panel alternatives; the greater personal expense to some consumers did not deter their choice of a non-prepaid alternative. Finally, 11 percent of the applicants were not accepted by any plan.

Under several competitive proposals the poor would be given vouchers to purchase medical care. In most instances, the cost of these vouchers would be based on age, marital status, number of dependents, disabilities, and sex, but not on income or health status. Since poor people would need more care, it would be difficult to envision cost-conscious plans competing aggressively to enroll the poor unless, of course, the cost for this additional care was included in the voucher. One counterbalance would be a regulatory element—open enrollment—but that might be softened by provisions allowing plans to limit the number of poor people accepted. The difficulties involved in monitoring and enforcement would be significant.

The voucher system sounds attractive, but it raises a number of issues. Will the premium be sufficient to attract providers, or will physicians process long lines of waiting patients quickly? Will quality standards suffer? Will the voucher system foster a two-tiered or multitiered system of care? Will new limits be imposed on medical care for the very sick, the poor, and the less-fortunate elderly, all of whom are unattractive to HMOs since caring for them costs more than competitively set premiums provide? Reinhardt provides additional insight into the potential problems faced by the poor in a competitive environment. In the past, the seriously ill poor were able to receive some care through a process known to health providers as cost shifting:

> This peculiar and uniquely American approach to indigent care was kept ethically bearable as long as the reimbursement system for paying patients was so open-ended that the cost of treating the uninsured poor could easily be passed on to the paying patients. This now much-maligned process of "cost shifting" actually served as the fig-leaf that covered up what would have otherwise revealed itself to the world as a national disgrace (Reinhardt 1985, 24).

In a competitive environment, Reinhardt (1984, 10) contends,

> All hospitals, however, are likely to find it more difficult in the future to render uncompensated care as the market for hospital services becomes ever more price-competitive. Until now, America has solved this problem in haphazard form through a system of hidden cross subsidies by which paying patients covered the cost of indigent care. This is the process of "cost shifting.". . . It is clear that price-sensitivity among paying patients will eventually squeeze out these hidden subsidies like water out of a sponge. The individual hospital may then simply be unable to carry even a relatively small burden of uncompensated care. Consequently, the underlying social pathos it manifests will be flushed more fully into the open—a disgrace for all to behold.

According to Reinhardt this strategy is just one more example of our low valuation of social peace. He contends that because of such policies Americans incur massive "internal defense expenditures" for police, armed guards, locks, prisons, as well as the crime and vandalism that are not prevented (ibid., 22). In the long run, he maintains, these responses are far more expensive than joining the ranks of the civilized nations.

When we place greater reliance on the market, it becomes extremely difficult to integrate the capitalistic and egalitarian parts of our ethics. The capitalistic element will predominate. The market mechanism's prime virtue is reducing waste or inefficiency, but by saying "no" in a very nonegalitarian way. Since the richest 20 percent of all U.S. households have 11 times as much income as the poorest 20 percent, an efficient market mechanism will give 11 times as much medical care to the top group as it will to the bottom group. Markets are designed to encourage firms to "cream" and "dump" as they search for the most profitable niche, and to avoid low-profit areas (Thurow 1984, 1571). We are already hearing (Kotelchuck 1985) about dumping under diagnosis-related groups, where hospitals receive a fixed prospective payment rather than a cost-based reimbursement, and we certainly can anticipate more such dumping in a competitive environment. Quentin Young, former medical director of Cook County Hospital in Chicago and a staunch opponent of the for-profit enterprise of health care, points out that, in a for-profit environment,

> It is the goal of a prudent manager to reduce losses and to substitute higher profit activity for low yield. In the world of health care, uncompensated or low profit transactions, more often than not, are generated by patients with the greatest health care needs but few resources. Studies indicate that for-profit institutions are skilled in limiting or eliminating the underfunded patient. . . . In an especially bad expression of exclusionary policies, the for-profits exacerbate a long-time practice in American health care delivery. I refer to "dumping." The public sector has traditionally been the place of arbitrary referral of the underfunded patient by the private sector. As government supports have contracted and unemployment-related loss of insurance has risen, "dumping" has increased. The obvious result is to burden, at times to the breaking point, already fiscally-tormented public hospitals. It is ironic that in this situation, for-profit hospital chains have negotiated scores of Faustian pacts with beleaguered county governments to relieve them of their deficit-plagued public hospitals (Young 1984, 450).

PROMOTING CONSUMER SOVEREIGNTY

This chapter has identified a number of obstacles facing competition, and it now advances several strategies to promote consumer sovereignty. These strategies are only partly consistent with currently emerging competitive strategies.

Within the competitive approach, consumer sovereignty could be enhanced by publishing provider-specific information essential for consumers to make informed choices among physicians. This information should include: (1) the training, credentials, accessibility, and practice setting of the physician and the type and availability of the services offered; (2) the cost of the physician's services, in comparison to those of other physicians; and (3) the comparative quality or competence of the physician. To date, consumer directories have had to concentrate almost exclusively on the first category because of the lack of reliable, comparative information about cost and quality.

The availability of cost and quality data for public disclosure should be required by any third-party payer. Not surprisingly, physicians have resisted this disclosure. Consumers must now rely on subjective and frag-mentary information, usually supplied by other patients. In truly competi-tive system, the purchaser has sufficient information to make an informed choice.

Although quality of care is not as easy to quantify, approaches to reviewing and assessing quality have been developed and have been uti-lized for a number of years. Most notable are PSROs, which review the medical necessity and quality of Medicare and Medicaid services. The data collected by PSROs, if properly adjusted for variations in patient mix, could provide consumers with valuable comparative information. Unfor-tunately, to date no provider-specific PSRO information has been publicly accessible under the present policies of the Department of Health and Hu-man Services (HHS), since HHS is unwilling to take any action that would "jeopardize" physician support of the PSRO program (Bogue 1979, 57). Work by Wennberg and Gittelsohn (1982) clearly indicates significant var-iations in medical practice. Knowledge of this information would have sig-nificant cost and quality implications.

The same reasoning can be applied to medical institutions, such as hospitals and nursing homes, and to services such as home health care. Currently, hospitals are required to collect vast amounts of qualitative data that cover elements of structure, process, and outcome. Data from institu-tions (with any explanatory comments the institutions wish to make) should be made available to consumers. Ideally, they should be published along with physician-specific data in the local newspapers in a format simi-lar to that used by *Consumer Reports* in reviewing other products and serv-ices. Quentin Young has commented (1981) that such information "is an invaluable asset for citizens who may need medical care. . . . Health care providers who render quality services at reasonable costs will also benefit." Rather than arguing for this information, it seems rational to have oppo-nents of full disclosure justify their position.

There are a number of other steps that would enhance consumer sovereignty. One is to eliminate current laws or policies that perpetuate a monopolistic approach to medical care. At the institutional level, the cer-tificate of need should be reevaluated. Although the initial CON legislation may have been a well-intentioned attempt to reduce duplication, it has given certain providers a "sole seller" status. To this extent it can inhibit the introduction of more cost-efficient and quality-promoting alternatives. Similarly, regulations that may inhibit the introduction of new delivery

modes (such as requiring significant initial financial reserves for prepayment plans) could be eliminated.

An even bolder approach would be to alter the present licensure
mechanism. Many consumer proponents contend that licensure does more
to protect the provider (especially the physician) than to protect the consumer. Virtually none of the competitive approaches suggests substantive
changes in "who's doing what to whom." Competition would be greatly enhanced if more cost-efficient providers could be substituted for the less
cost-efficient. For example, nurse practitioners might be allowed to work
independently and not under the supervision of a physician; hospital
privileges might be extended to nurse midwives and other medical
providers. Dental hygienists might be permitted to set up their own practices to meet the preventive needs of consumers. The introduction of many
related professionals such as nurse practitioners, physician assistants and
dental hygienists was heralded years ago as a cost-reducing strategy.
Dominance by strong providers has made that notion hollow. If many of
these professionals were allowed to practice, more genuine price competition would probably result, with no loss of quality. Poorer people might
have greater access through more effective sellers and, perhaps, through
lower prices. Of course, any of these new sellers (more accurately, deregu-
lated old sellers) would have to be eligible for insurance reimbursements.

Changes in licensure could be effected in several ways. One way is
licensure review by a group of nationally recognized experts, such as those
in the Institute of Medicine—but not by organized medicine. If this is not
possible, elimination of licensure might be considered. Consumers, as they
do in many other areas, would eventually determine whom they prefer and
who will survive. Under this scenario, one could envision some interesting
joint ventures among various medical providers that are not even imagina-
ble under the present restrictive and hierarchical system. If the goal is a
truly competitive system, we should put the elements of an effective market together, including the introduction of less costly input substitutions.

So far, my suggestions have focused on ways to increase consumer
sovereignty in a competitive market, but there are other ways to promote
consumer sovereignty. Consumer sovereignty implies consumer control.
It is ridiculous to entrust health care to the preferences of groups of medical care providers who control the system. Keisling (1983, 29) clearly summarizes the situation: "The inescapable truth is that the nation has wasted
far too much time and money trying to reform a system that never should
have been allowed to exist in the first place." According to Keisling, to
reduce significantly the rate of growth of our national health care bill,
while keeping our population as healthy—if not making it healthier— we
must make only two basic changes: we must introduce public control of
doctors and hospitals, and changes in medical education.

Keisling maintains that society should decide what it wants, design the appropriate facilities, and determine who will provide those services at what salary. Unlike previous efforts, these initiatives would be planned by consumers for consumers. A salaried health work force is far from a radical suggestion—more than 90 percent of the workers are currently salaried. This proposal would just extend that status to physicians, who should be given a comfortable salary (Keisling suggests about $50,000 a year, adjusted for experience and performance). This salary would keep physicians in the upper 10-percent salary level for U.S. workers. They would also be liberated from the worry of malpractice fees and collecting bills, and thus be able to devote their full energies to the practice of medicine, healing the sick, and promoting health. In other words, a physician "could really be the kind of doctor the AMA conjured up in its recent lobbying efforts for exemption from FTC antitrust review (ibid., 30).

Keisling is not naive, and he expects ferocious opposition—which is where hospitals come in. Hospitals are a major workplace and income source for physicians, but the vast majority of physicians pay virtually nothing toward defraying the costs, such as nurses' salaries and medical equipment, of this workplace. Since the government already pays a significant portion of these costs, the government would offer the physicians a simple deal. Physicians who opt to join the system can continue their present arrangement. Those who do not participate will be assessed a reasonable share of hospital operating expenses; if they refuse, the hospital becomes ineligible for government-financed patients.

Hospitals would come under effective public ownership. Under the present system, they have not demonstrated an enviable record in cost containment but have demonstrated tremendous creativity and ability to maximize income by gaming the reimbursement system. It is ironic that, as evidenced in the recent Institute of Medicine study, the for-profit hospitals have been particularly adept in this regard (Gray 1986). Keisling (1983, 31) contends the knowledge that the physicians can always pick up their black bags and go to the next hospital makes it about as realistic for the hospital administrator to be cost-conscious as it is to ask a retailer to keep people from spending too much money in his store. If hospitals are placed under public ownership, this cycle of wasting money by competing for patients can be broken. Also, society can determine costs instead of leaving the decision to hospitals, which have their own self-serving motives for determining who gets in and who gets what.

A third possible change is greater public involvement in medical education. The public at present subsidizes medical school training but, except for a few programs, has almost no control over the eventual locations or specialties of the trainees. Peters (1977) argues that the public should pay the entire bill for medical education and relieve tomorrow's physicians of the need to earn a six-figure annual salary to repay loans. In urging this reform, Peters suggests that society should

> give every intern and resident a generous salary plus a free Jaguar. This arrangement would deprive them of the last shred of justification for the self-pity that seems to possess all but the most decent doctors in later life, the self-pity that says because I was strapped to pay those tuition bills and because I was exploited as an intern and resident, I am now justified in robbing my patients blind. The doctor who thinks $75,000 a year is his divine right—indeed, a bare minimum from which to advance to ever greater fiscal heights—is the spiritual father of the gross extravagance of our present health-delivery system.

Increased public control over the medical schools would have other advantages. Society could determine the composition of the physician work force. A more rational system might result, with less superspecialization and more levels of care based on consumer needs. Also, free education may offer greater access to less wealthy students, and, when combined with the salary factor, may affect the types of student who apply.

Peters (ibid.) maintains that medical care is too crucial a public concern to be left to those who provide it. In the final analysis, he raises several questions and offers several suggestions:

> Is there any logical reason why medical salaries, specialties and places of work should not be . . . subject to public control? Isn't the assurance of good medical care as important to you as the assurance of adequate protection by the police or the military? Shouldn't doctors be trained in the areas of medicine where they are needed and stationed accordingly? Shouldn't their income be geared, not to what they want, but to what the public can afford? If people don't like public control, they can choose not to become doctors, just as they can choose not to become midshipmen or cadets. If they are already doctors, they can choose not to participate in either the benefits or the restraints of a national health service. In fact, we may want a group of physicians to remain in private practice to provide a competitive measuring rod for the public service.

Sidel (1977) sums up what is necessary for an effective consumer strategy under a competitive system.

> The way to get consumer choice in health care and medical care is by organizing consumers in ways which will force a monopolistic, mystifying professional group to give them the services that they need. If the providers are organized and the people purposely disorganized, and the power to make the system responsive and responsible is thereby dispersed and divided, the power for choice is effectively lost.

The preceding discussion and criticism are not intended to imply that the concept of consumer sovereignty cannot be advanced through a competitive strategy. To the contrary, given our present nonsystem, competitive approaches may well have a positive effect on such issues as cost, quality, and access. It is quite possible that competitive proposals will improve mainstream American medicine. The average American may well benefit. At the same time, this chapter has attempted to identify a number of potentially significant obstacles that must be addressed for sovereignty to become a reality for the entire population.

However, there are more important reservations that transcend the criticism of specific elements of any competitive proposals. The problem with the competitive approaches is their narrow view of sovereignty and, not surprisingly, their correspondingly narrow conception of how sovereignty may be realized. In the present situation consumer sovereignty is perceived within the context of a market mechanism, and strategies are conceived to accommodate this perception. As long as the perception of consumer sovereignty operates within a relatively narrow framework, the gains will also be narrow. What needs to be realized is that what one gets is usually a matter of choice and that there are gains from other types of choice. This chapter suggests a number of additional elements that would promote consumer sovereignty in attempting to obtain accessible, effective, and cost-efficient medical care.

Rather than debate the merits of a competitive approach and rally behind a particular strategy, we need to realize that before making hard choices in health care we should resolve explicitly several significant questions. While many of these were raised long ago, we continue to ignore them or to deal with them in a haphazard manner. For example, is medical care a right? Should we continue to fund most of our health care regressively or promote more progressivity? Should we continue to tie medical care coverage to employment status for the majority of our population? Should we not only openly admit that our present system is at least a three-tier system (get none, get some, get more), but plan accordingly based on a tiered structure? Should we continue to focus on a medical care system or begin to develop a health care system in a broader sense? Should the health care system continue to be dominated by the medical community and medical institutions, or should our system be driven (and controlled) by the needs of the population with public control? What we have is a series of questions rooted in values and ethics. It might be most appropriate to deal with these questions first and develop our responses afterward.

NOTES

1. Data that are collected but not made public include hospital incident reports, infection rates, and mortality and morbidity for various procedures by specific institutions and providers.
2. I refuse to use "paraprofessional," since it denotes something less than a professional.

REFERENCES

Aaron, H., and W. Schwartz. 1984. *The Painful Prescription: Rationing Hospital Care.* Washington, DC: Brookings Institution.

Arnett, Ross H., III, David R. McKusick, Sally T. Sonnefeld, and Carol S. Cowell. 1986. "Projections of Health Care Spending to 1990." *Health Care Financing Review* 7: 1–36.

Barer, M. L., Robert G. Evans, and G. L. Stoddart. 1979. *Controlling Health Care Costs by Direct Charges to Patients: Snare or Delusion?* Ontario Economic Council Occasional Paper No. 10. Toronto: Ontario Economic Council.

Bogue, Ted. 1979. *How to Compile a Consumer's Directory of Doctors and Their Fees.* Washington, DC: Public Citizen Health Research Group.

Boston Women's Health Book Collective. 1972. *Our Bodies Ourselves: A Book by and for Women.* New York: Simon & Schuster.

Braverman, Jordan. 1980. *Crisis in Health Care.* Washington, DC: Acropolis Books.

Business Week. 1984. "The Corporate Rx for Medical Costs." October 15.

Congressional Record. 1981. January 16.

Coniff, J. 1971. "You Can Make a Big Business Care." *Today's Health* 49 (December): 16–19.

Consumers Advisory Council, Executive Office of the President. 1983. *First Report.* Washington, DC: U.S. Government Printing Office.

Corry, James. 1983. *Consumer Health.* Belmont, CA: Wadsworth.

Cray, E. 1970. *In Failing Health: The Medical Crisis and the A.M.A.* Indianapolis: Bobbs-Merrill.

Creighton, Lucy. 1976. *Pretenders to the Throne.* Lexington, MA: Lexington Books.

Duhl, Leonard, and Stephen Blum. 1981. "Health Planning and Social Change: Critique and Alternatives." In *Citizens and Health Care: Participation and Planning for Social Change,* ed. by Barry Checkoway, 271–87. New York: Pergamon Press.

Ehrenreich, Barbara, and John Ehrenreich. 1971. *The American Health Empire.* New York: Vintage Books.

Enthoven, Alain. 1978. "Consumer-Choice Health Plan." *New England Journal of Medicine* 298: 650–58, 709–20.

———. 1980. *Health Plan: The Only Practical Solution to the Soaring Cost of Medical Care.* Reading, MA: Addison-Wesley.

Federal Trade Commission. 1979. Final Order, Docket No. 9064, October 12: 2.

Feldstein, Paul. 1979. *Health Care Economics.* New York: Wiley.

Fuchs, Victor. 1978. "The Supply of Surgeons and the Demand for Operations." *Journal of Human Resources* 13 (Supplement): 35–56.

———. 1984. "The 'Rationing' of Medical Care." *New England Journal of Medicine* 311: 1572–73.

Gibson, Robert M., Katharine R. Levit, Helen Lazenby, and Daniel R. Waldo. 1984. "National Health Expenditures, 1983." *Health Care Financing Review* 6: 1–29.

Ginzberg, Eli. 1980. "Competition and Cost Containment." *New England Journal of Medicine* 303: 1112–15.

Gleen, Karen. 1980. *Planning, Politics, and Power: A User's Guide to Taming the Health Care System.* Washington, DC: Consumer Coalition for Health.

Gray, Bradford, ed. 1983. *The New Health Care for Profit.* Washington, DC: National Academy Press.

———, ed. 1986. *For-Profit Enterprise in Health Care.* Washington, DC: National Academy Press.

Hamilton, Patricia. 1982. *Health Care Consumerism.* Saint Louis: Mosby. 1982.

Harmer, Ruth. 1975. *American Medical Avarice.* New York: Abeland-Schuman.

Havighurst, C. 1978. "The Role of Competition in Cost Containment." In *Competition in the Health Care Sector: Past, Present and Future,* ed. by W. Greenburg, 285–323. Germantown, MD: Aspen Systems.

Hutt, W. 1936. *Economics and the Public.* London: Jonathan Cape.

Keisling, P. 1983. "Radical Surgery: Let's Draft the Doctors." *The Washington Monthly* (February): 26–34.

Kennedy, Edward M. 1972. *In Critical Condition: The Crisis in America's Health Care.* New York: Simon & Schuster.

Klarman, Herbert. 1977. "The Financing of Health Care." In *Doing Better and Feeling Worse: Health in the United States,* ed. John H. Knowles, 215–34. New York: Norton.

Kotelchuck, David, ed. 1976. *Prognosis Negative.* New York: Vintage Books.

Kotelchuck, Ronda, 1985. "Poor Diagnosis, Poor Treatment." *Health/PAC Bulletin* 16: 7–13.

Law, S. A. 1974. *Blue Cross: What Went Wrong?* New Haven: Yale University Press.

Levit, Katharine R., Helen Lazenby, Daniel R. Waldo, and Lawrence M. Davidoff. 1985. "National Health Expenditures, 1984." *Health Care Financing Review* 7: 1–35.

Luft, H. S. 1980a. "Assessing the Evidence on HMO Performance." *Milbank Memorial Fund Quarterly/Health and Society* 58: 501–36.

———. 1980b. "HMOs and the Medical Care Market." In *Socioeconomic Issues of Health 1980,* ed. by Douglas E. Hough and Glen I. Misek, 85–102. Chicago: American Medical Association.

Marmor, Theodore E. 1983. *Political Analysis and American Medical Care.* Cambridge, England: Cambridge University Press.

McGarrah, R. G., Jr. 1974. *A Consumer's Directory of Prince George's County Doctors.* Washington, DC: Health Research Group.

McNerney, Walter J. 1980. "Control of Health Care Costs in the 1980s." *New England Journal of Medicine* 303: 1088–95.

National Health Insurance Report. 1979. "Doctors Play Role in Determining How High Health Costs Climb." November 16.

Newacheck, Paul W., Lewis H. Butler, Aileen K. Harper, Dylan L. Piontkowsky, and Patricia E. Franks. 1980. "Income and Illness." *Medical Care* 18: 1165–76.

Newsweek. 1985. "Southern Baptists in Battle." June 24.

Office of Personnel Management. 1980. *Federal Fringe Benefit Facts, 1979.* Report to Congress.

Peters, Charles. 1977. "A Radical Cure for High Medical Costs." *Newsweek* March 28.

PSRO Letter. 1979. "Study of Cardiac Surgery Raises Quality of Care Issues." 7 (November 15).

Reinhardt, Uwe E. 1984. "The Problem of Uncompensated Care, or, Are Americans Really as Mean as They Look?" In *Uncompensated Care in a Competitive Environment: Whose Problem Is It?* ed. by National Council on Health Planning and Development, 7–30. DHHS Pub. No. HRP-0906304.

———. 1985. "Hard Choices in Health Care: A Matter of Ethics." In *Health Care: How To Improve It and Pay For It,* ed. by Center for National Policy, 19–31. Washington, DC: The Center.

Roberts, M. J. 1980. "Planning and Competition in Health Care Delivery." Paper presented at American Health Planning Association Annual Meeting, San Francisco, June 1.

Schneider, A. G. 1980. *An Advocate's Guide to Health Care Financing.* Washington, DC: Legal Services Corp.

Schorr, Daniel. 1970. *Don't Get Sick in America.* Nashville, TN: Aurora.

Sidel, Victor. 1977. "Comment," In *Effects of the Payment Mechanism on the Health Care Delivery System,* ed. by National Center for Health Services Research, 82. DHEW Pub. No. (PHS) 78-3227.

Sigelman, Daniel. 1981. "The Competitive Prescription for Health Care." *Health Law Project Library Bulletin* 6: 98–122.

Somers, A., and H. Somers. 1977. *Health and Health Care.* Germantown, MD: Aspen Systems.

Touche, Ross and Co. 1979. *Oregon Adult and Family Services Division: Third-Year Evaluation of the Medicaid Demonstration Project in Multnomah County, Final Report.* Portland, OR: Touche, Ross and Co.

Thurow, Lester Carl. 1984. "Learning to Say 'No.'" *New England Journal of Medicine* 311: 1569–72.

U.S. Department of Health and Human Services. 1980. *Health United States 1980.* DHHS Pub. No. (PHS) 81-1232. Hyattsville, MD: National Center for Health Statistics.

Vladeck, Bruce. 1981. "The Market vs. Regulation: The Case for Regulation." *Milbank Memorial Fund Quarterly* 6: 209–23.

The Washington Post. 1969. "Medical System Blasted." July 13: A1–A2.

Waters, William. 1980. "From Rhetoric to Reality in Public Health Policy." *Health Planning Newsletter,* U.S. Department of Health, Education and Welfare, Public Health Service, Health Resources Administration 6 (January): 7.

Wennberg, J. E., and Alan Gittelsohn. 1982. "Variations in Medical Care among Small Areas." *Scientific American* 246: 120–34.

Wennberg, J. E., and J. D. Lapenas. 1980. "On Choosing the Numbers of Needed Physicians." Prepared for the GMENAC Panel on Geographic Variation. Washington, DC: Department of Health, Education, and Welfare, Health Resources Administration.

Young, Quentin. 1981. "Comments Reflect a Critique of *The Doctors/Dentists Directory.*" In *The Doctors/Dentists Directory,* ed. Diane O'Rourke and Thomas O'Rourke. Champaign, IL: Champaign County Health Care Consumers.

———. 1984. "Impact of For-Profit Enterprise on Health Care." *Journal of Public Health Policy* 5: 449–52.

6

Providing Medical Care for the Poor: Medicaid in a Period of Transition

Paul A. Wilson, Pamela K. Bartels, and Dana Rubin

This chapter analyzes the Medicaid program as it is being reshaped by governmental policies and by developments within the health care delivery system. It begins with an overview of the Medicaid program, its major provisions and trends. It then describes attempts to set in operation the New Federalism through the Omnibus Budget Reconciliation Act of 1981 and the Tax Equity and Fiscal Responsibility Act of 1982, delineates several aspects of the competitive environment in health care delivery, and discusses the consequences of these developments for provision of medical care to the poor. The chapter also analyzes several states' experimental attempts to reform their Medicaid programs and concludes with a discussion of major questions and issues for future policy and program development.

The Medicaid program, in operation since 1966, has been one of the mainstays of health care for the poor. Despite persistent and seemingly intractable problems, it has been a major contributor to increased availability and accessibility of good medical care for many of the poor. Many noted improvements in the health status of the poor are attributable in large part to Medicaid provisions (Davis and Schoen 1978). Alarm over the escalation of health care costs in concert with other developments can seriously weaken the commitment and capacity to provide good medical care to those with limited financial resources.

Three interrelated developments pose a threat to the gains of earlier years. First, the New Federalism, which seeks to place increased program and fiscal responsibilities on already burdened state and local governments, is altering the federal-state relationships that have supported the Medicaid program traditionally. For example, attempts to limit federal spending, as one expression of the New Federalism, include the tightening of eligibility criteria for welfare, which automatically excludes tens of thousands of people from Medicaid benefits. Second, the current emphasis on "competitive strategies" for health care delivery is creating an environment in which it is disadvantageous for hospitals and other providers to engage in cost shifting, and unprofitable for them to provide services to those who lack the means to pay their full charges. The third and most pervasive influence on current developments in health care delivery is concern over dramatic cost increases. The goal of controlling escalating costs has eclipsed that of ensuring availability and accessibility of health care. Thus, at the same time that governments eliminate or limit the financial access of many poor people to medical care, health care providers operate under conditions that make it increasingly difficult to offer charity care.

Several states are attempting to reform their Medicaid programs in response to the conflicting responsibilities they face. A major feature of some experiments is abandonment of retrospective payment on the basis of "customary and reasonable charges" for each service delivered. This fee-for-service reimbursement method offers little incentive to providers to constrain overall costs. A number of states not only are experimenting with alternative approaches to reimbursement but also are attempting to create alternative service delivery systems. These experiments, with new program developments and reimbursement methods, may yield results that will make it possible to provide quality care at manageable cost levels.

MEDICAID: AN OVERVIEW

Medicaid was passed as Title XIX of the Social Security Act in 1965 and began providing benefits in 1966. The program is financed jointly by federal and state funds and is state administered. It was intended to finance medical care for low-income persons in two specific categories: children and adults eligible for Aid to Families with Dependent Children (AFDC) under Title IV-A, and those eligible for benefits under the Supplemental Security Income (SSI) Program for the aged, blind, and disabled as provided in Title XVI of the Social Security Act. Those who qualify for either of these cash transfer programs are identified as categorically needy, and are automatically entitled to Medicaid benefits.

States also have the option of offering coverage to the medically needy, who are defined as those who fall into one of the categories of persons receiving cash assistance (i.e., the aged, blind, or disabled, and members of families with one parent dead, absent, incapacitated or—at state discretion—unemployed) but do not receive cash assistance because their incomes are above the threshold for such assistance. The criterion for eligibility as medically needy is an income not exceeding 133⅓ percent of the state's AFDC income standard for a family of the same size. States also may include low-income persons for whom federal matching funds are not provided regardless of how low their income, such as single adults, childless couples under 65 years of age, and most two-parent families. Finally, states may also elect to provide "buy-in" coverage for the aged, in which Medicaid pays Medicare premiums and copayments. About 12 percent of Medicare recipients were also covered by Medicaid through Supplemental Medical Insurance in 1980 (Health Care Financing Administration 1983, 3).

Service Coverage and Use

Every state program is required to provide inpatient and outpatient hospital services, laboratory and x-ray services, skilled nursing facility (SNF) services for individuals 21 years old or over, home health services for those eligible for skilled nursing services, physician services, family planning services, rural health clinic services, and early, periodic screening, diagnosis, and treatment (EPSDT) for persons under an age determined by the state (21, 20, 19, or 18 years). States also may elect to provide other services such as eyeglasses, prescription drugs, intermediate care facilities (ICFs), physical therapy, and dental care.

The numbers and kinds of elective service differ widely among the states. For example, as of September 1, 1981, Wyoming provided 7 elective services beyond those federally mandated, and these were available to the categorically needy only. South Carolina offered 14 additional services to the categorically needy only. In contrast, Illinois provided 29 and Michigan provided 24 additional services to both the categorically needy and the medically needy.

The use of services varies considerably among the states as well. The proportion of recipients using general hospital services in Minnesota in fiscal year (FY) 1980, for example, was 13.4 percent, whereas in the District of Columbia it was 56.6 percent. Skilled nursing facility use varied in this same period from a low of 0.05 percent in Maryland and Oklahoma to a high of 41.6 percent in Connecticut. Intermediate care facilities were used by 2.1 percent of recipients in California and by 63.2 percent in South Dakota (ibid., 118). These variations reflect both differential benefit offerings among the states and differences in population needs.

Trends in Numbers of Recipients and in Payments: 1973–80

The scope of the Medicaid program is extremely broad. The program provides access to medical care to almost one of every ten persons in the nation. There were approximately 19.6 million Medicaid recipients in 1973, and 22.9 million in 1977. This number declined by 3.1 percent per year in 1978 and 1979, rising a modest 0.2 percent in 1980 to a total of 21.6 million, or 10.1 percent over the 1973 figure. Of this total, the aged, blind, and disabled accounted for 6.2 million or 28.8 percent; AFDC recipients totaled 14.1 million or 65.1 percent; and other Title XIX medically needy persons made up the remaining 7 percent (ibid., 85–86, tables 4.4, 4.5).

Despite the large numbers of persons served, only about half of the poor are covered nationwide. However, the ratio of recipients to the total number of poor persons varies widely among the states. In 1980 South Dakota provided benefits to only 23 percent of the poor, while California served 97 percent of the poor. Thirty-one states in 1980 provided Medicaid to 50 percent or less of those under the poverty line. The overall average was 54 percent, compared with 59 percent in 1970 (ibid., 81–82, table 4.2).

The disabled, both categorically and medically needy, increased in number between 1973 and 1980 at rates of 5.9 and 7.3 percent per year, respectively. Medically needy adults in AFDC increased by 7.1 percent per year. All other groups increased at very modest annual rates (between 1.5 percent and 1.9 percent) or declined in number. For example, the number of blind and elderly decreased by 1.2 percent annually, and the number of children in AFDC decreased by 3.5 percent per year or 22 percent over the period between 1973 and 1980 (ibid., 20, table 2.4).

The costs of the program, in absolute dollar amounts and in rates of increase, continue to cause grave concern. The federal government's matching formula is open-ended, and the federal dollar contribution is based on costs incurred by the states.

States are also burdened. In 1980 their share was $10.61 billion or 44.4 percent of the total $23.3 billion for that year. In many states Medicaid costs represented almost half of the total state health expenditures. The other half of those states' health dollars had to provide for mental health facilities, public health programs, municipal and county hospitals, and state-owned university hospitals, all of which require substantial levels of support (Altman and Hearn 1982).

From 1973 to 1980 expenditures increased from $8.64 billion to $23.3 billion, an annual growth rate of 15.5 percent. However, expenditures for the various recipient groups increased at different rates. The percentage of total 1980 expenditures represented by the amount spent on each group was disproportionate to the percentage of total recipients constituted by that group. The payments for the aged, blind, and disabled increased at a rate of 17.3 percent annually. This group, making up 28.8 percent of total recipients in 1980, accounted for 68 percent of all Medicaid payments in that year (Health Care Financing Administration 1983, 23). Payments for services for those covered under AFDC, on the other hand, increased at a rate of 12.1 percent. This group, constituting over 65 percent of all recipients, received services representing 28.1 percent of total expenditures in 1980 (ibid., 29). The differential growth rates in the amounts spent on the aged, blind, and disabled and on those eligible under AFDC reflect a tendency to limit the Medicaid eligibility of the latter group.

While such a strategy may impede the rate of cost increases in the short term, it is doubtful that it will prove an effective or satisfactory cost-containment strategy. It will not be effective because, like medical costs generally, it is the increase in cost per unit of service, not overall volume of use, that is a more potent contributor to inflation. It is not satisfactory because those whose eligibility is terminated may not receive necessary care and may eventually need services for more serious and costly medical conditions.

Response to specific needs of select population groups, principally the aged and disabled, has resulted in a program emphasis on institutional services (i.e., SNFs and ICFs). This trend cannot be ignored in addressing issues of cost, nor can it continue without limiting the capacity of states to provide adequate care for the poor other than the aged and disabled.

The bias of Medicaid toward long-term care is evidenced by the fact that Medicaid pays for approximately half of all nursing home expenditures nationally (Blendon and Moloney 1982). Moreover, skilled nursing facility and intermediate care facility services accounted for 42.5 percent of all Medicaid payments in 1980. From 1973 to 1980 the number of days of care in SNFs declined slightly, while expenditures for these services increased at an annual rate of 9.5 percent. The rate of increase in days of care in ICFs was 4.3 percent, while the annual expenditure increase averaged 17.7 percent (Health Care Financing Administration 1983, 43). However, these average national figures disguise the magnitude of costs in individual states. For example, since Medicaid began to cover ICF services in 1973, the cost of these services increased 89.7 percent in Georgia, 270 percent in Kentucky, and 127.9 percent in Wisconsin (Holahan, Scanlon, and Spitz 1977, 19–21). By 1975 ICF services were absorbing from 18 percent to 52 percent of all program expenditures in selected states. By 1980, inpatient hospital services and nursing home care combined accounted for over 70 percent of all Medicaid expenditures nationally.

Efforts to provide support services that preclude or delay more costly institutional care are reflected in the 20 percent annual increase in the use of home health services. Expenditures for home health services grew at a rate of 44.4 percent per year between 1973 and 1980 (Health Care Financing Administration 1983, 43). The relatively large growth rate in outpatient hospital services may also reflect attempts to limit or find alternatives to nursing home care. Table 6:1 shows the various rates of growth in selected service categories, the rate of growth of payment levels, and the proportion of total expenditures each service category claimed in 1980.

Table 6:1—Rates of Growth in Selected Service Categories and Expenditures (1973–1980) and Percent Total Expenditures in 1980

Service Category	Annual Rate of Growth in Use	Annual Rate of Growth in Expenditures	Percent of Total Payments
Inpatient Hospital	# days of care 1.6%	13.4%	27.8%
SNF	# days of care 0.7%	9.5%	15.9%
ICF	# days of care 4.3%	17.7%	26.7%
Outpatient Hospital	# recipients 8.8%	22.4%	4.7%
Home Health Services	# recipients 20.0%	44.4%	1.4%
All Other Services			23.5%

Source: HCFA, Medicare and Medicaid Data Book. Washington, DC, 1983, Tables 2.9, 2.15, 2.16, 2.17, 2.18.

THE NEW FEDERALISM AND COMPETITIVE FORCES IN HEALTH CARE DELIVERY

The election of Ronald Reagan in 1980 brought a radical shift in federal policy formulation and direction generally and in health care policy specifically. The New Federalism consists of ideological, political, and social principles that were translated into efforts to limit the role of the federal government; immediate steps to offer business and industry relief from regulation; and early proposals for tax relief for business, industry, and individuals. Costs of big government were to be drastically reduced for economic stability and growth.

Domestic programs were, and continue to be, the prime targets for cuts to accommodate the shifts in policy and program directions. According to the New Federalism, these programs and their contributions to overall governmental expenditures are serious detriments to economic and social progress.

The meaning of this approach for health policy and programs was well expressed in a 1981 publication by Edward N. Brandt, Jr., Assistant Secretary of the Department of Health and Human Services. He pointed out that the service programs within the Public Health Service were to be cut by 25 percent, and he suggested that "we might not be getting all our federal money's worth from these many service programs." The states, he observed, were already doing a great deal in developing and maintaining programs related to communicable diseases and maternal and child health services, as well as criminal justice, housing, employment, public works, and social services. The net result of such efforts, he suggested, was "to exact a very high cost in both economic and social terms" (Brandt 1981, 6). There was the additional cost of regulations, which inhibited state and county "movement and judgment." The policy agenda, therefore, was to "redress the balance of authority, and begin to ease the fiscal, social, and service burdens, too."

It is not clear from Brandt's statement precisely whose burdens were to be eased. As noted above, the states carry major responsibility for health programs and facilities, some of which are not federally supported or have limited federal support. The New Federalism increased the financial and administrative responsibilities borne by the states. Perhaps of more long-term significance, the Reagan administration also succeeded in accomplishing what other administrations had failed to do—namely, alter the basic federal-state relationship in operating programs such as Medicaid.[1]

Provisions of 1981 and 1982 Legislation: Eligibility and Service Restrictions

States made repeated attempts to reduce, or at least to control, escalating Medicaid costs from very early in the life of the program (Wing 1983). The most readily available means for cost containment is to restrict the number of those eligible. This can be done directly by restricting eligibility of optional groups for Medicaid services or indirectly by limiting AFDC eligibility. The latter strategy involves reducing or freezing the state's payment standards, in which case inflation, rather than direct political action, limits eligibility. In 1979, for example, only 11 states were within 90 percent or more of their comparable 1970 standard levels. In other words, adjusting for inflation, these states were paying amounts almost comparable to their 1970 payment levels. Many of the remaining states were well below this level. The result is that families have to be increasingly poorer to qualify for AFDC and Medicaid (Budetti, Butler, and McManus 1982).

The Omnibus Budget Reconciliation Act of 1981 (PL 97–35) reinforced this strategy by imposing a nationwide asset limit for eligibility, limiting the amounts that can be disregarded for income determination for AFDC eligibility, increasing "workfare" requirements, and counting as income such resources as food stamps and housing subsidies (American Public Welfare Association 1981).

It was more difficult for the states to limit the Medicaid eligibility of SSI recipients because federal SSI eligibility standards had to be applied. However, states could apply 1972 income eligibility standards and thus effectively eliminate some SSI recipients who would otherwise be Medicaid-eligible. Those rendered ineligible would nevertheless receive benefits if their medical expenses reduced their incomes below the standard. As of February 1982 36 states covered all SSI recipients (Rowland and Gaus 1982, 34).

States also employed the direct method of simply restricting eligibility for Medicaid, especially of the medically needy. Prior to 1981, states that covered the medically needy were required to provide services that were comparable to those for the categorically needy. The Omnibus Budget Reconciliation Act redefined "comparability" and restricted it to such services as ambulatory care for children, prenatal and childbirth services, and ambulatory care for those receiving institutional care. Second, states were no longer required to cover persons under 21 years of age who would be eligible for AFDC if they were attending school. Coverage of these persons was left to state discretion. States could also discontinue coverage of some or all optional groups (Davis 1981; Rowland and Gaus 1982, 31).

These strategies for reducing eligibility exclude select groups from program benefits, as the trends in total numbers of recipients show. Richard Schweiker, Secretary of the Department of Health and Human Services at that time, estimated that 115,000 persons would lose benefits because of the 1981 changes in SSI eligibility criteria and 500,000 would be ineligible by virtue of changes in AFDC (Iglehart 1982). About half of the states have general assistance programs, and some of these programs provide support to families who become ineligible. However, medical care provisions are not available through general assistance. The institutions of last resort for those ineligibles needing medical care are county and municipal hospitals or, if available and accessible, private hospitals and other providers willing to provide charity care.

Federal Expenditure Reductions

The federal strategy for controlling Medicaid expenditures also included a 3-percent reduction in federal outlays for fiscal year 1982 and reductions of 4 percent and 4.5 percent for 1983 and 1984, respectively. A state could recoup one percentage point for having a hospital cost rate review system in place, an unemployment rate equal to or greater than 150 percent of the national average, or a recovery rate on fraud and abuse that amounted to 1 percent of the quarterly federal Medicaid share—a possible total of three percentage points (Davis 1981).

Creation of Health Care Block Grants

Federal reduction of Medicaid funds, restriction of AFDC and SSI eligibility requirements, and lessening of federal requirements for service provision were intended primarily to reduce federal spending. However, a strategy to give the states greater discretion in running their Medicaid programs was included. The strategy was to attempt consolidation of related categorical health programs into a single "block" with funding levels set for each block.

The Reconciliation Act of 1981 created four block grants to cover some 24 programs at an aggregate funding level 25 percent below 1981

levels for all programs taken individually (Brown 1983). The Maternal and
Child Health Block Grant replaced seven earlier programs, such as crip-
pled children's services, genetic counseling, and adolescent pregnancy services. The Preventive and Health Services Block Grant also consolidated 7
earlier categorical programs, including hypertension control, home health,
health education, and emergency medical services. A block grant was also
created to include mental health center services and alcohol- and drug-
abuse programs, and a single block was created for community health
centers. Other programs, such as family planning, immunization, tuberculosis and venereal disease detection and treatment, and migrant health
center programs, were left as categorical, but their funding was reduced below 1981 levels.

Administrative Changes: State Discretion in Program Management

The most significant influence on future developments in the Medicaid
program may prove to be the administrative changes that were either required or allowed by the 1981 and 1982 legislation. Several of these
changes, such as allowing states to require copayments from certain groups
of the categorically needy, were clearly restrictive in nature, representing
attempts to save on expenditures by limiting "unnecessary" utilization. A
somewhat similar provision allowed states to "lock in" recipients who were
identified as overutilizers. These persons were to be assigned to a specific
provider for the management and monitoring of all care. Similarly, states
were permitted to "lock out" providers who abused the program.

Another set of provisions permitted administrative flexibility in running the state programs. States were given much greater latitude in their
choice of service delivery mechanisms. The first such change was the elimination, in 1981, of the requirement that health maintenance organizations,
which contracted with the state for delivery of care to Medicaid recipients,
had to be federally qualified. The requirement was immediately reinstated
in 1982. Legislators were apparently fearful of a repetition, on a national
scale, of California's experiment of the 1970s with a statewide network of
prepaid health plans. That experiment resulted in attempts at profiteering,
as some providers pressured eligible persons into enrolling, collected their
state capitation fees, and provided very little health care (Iglehart 1983;
Ensminger 1982).

However, the general principles of HMO-like service delivery arrangements did prove attractive to federal legislators, who directed their
attention to administrative provisions for more state experimentation with
delivery systems as well as reimbursement mechanisms. States had been required to pay "reasonable" costs for all allowable services after the services
were delivered, following the Medicare principles of reimbursement. As in-

dicated above, this cost-based retrospective payment system placed the states in a passive position. It also prevented them from knowing what their final costs would be until the end of the year (when they determined the balance between what the state had paid on an interim basis and what the providers had actually delivered in services). This arrangement is a perverse incentive for providers, since reduction in the volume of services rendered translates into a direct reduction of revenues (Feuerhard 1981).

The Reconciliation Act of 1981 eliminated the requirement that states reimburse on the basis of provider-defined reasonable costs. This change enabled states to reimburse on the basis of rates they established, so long as these rates were adequate to meet costs that any efficient facility would incur. States were also required to give special consideration to facilities serving disproportionate numbers of the poor when setting their rates. Whatever reimbursement scheme was adopted, access to inpatient hospital services of adequate quality was required. Many states moved to one of five general approaches: prospective rate setting, budget review, budget review by exception, rate increase control, or charges, or to a combination of these approaches.[2]

Waivers of Federal Requirements

Waivers provided under section 2175 of the Omnibus Budget Reconciliation Act and through Section 1115 of the Social Security Act allow states to experiment with various methods of delivering services. These waivers are of two types. The first allows for the lock-in and lock-out provisions discussed above, but also allows waivers of "freedom of choice" and of the "state wideness" requirement. Under these waivers, consumers' freedom of choice of a provider can be limited to a single provider. This limitation permits the states to experiment with case management and preferred provider agreements for select groups of recipients. In these experiments, eligible persons are assigned to a provider who is responsible for and manages all of their medical care. Providers accepting responsibility and agreed-upon rates are "preferred." Waiver of the statewideness requirement makes it possible for experiments to be conducted on a limited, local basis without consideration of the comparability of the services received by those in the experiment and the services received by other recipients in the state. It also offers the opportunity to experiment in localities where providers are both available and interested in participating. As of August 1982, 30 requests for waivers of freedom of choice had been received from 15 states; 18 of these requests were submitted under authority of a primary care network (Iglehart 1983).

A second set of waivers allows states to set aside requirements that

Medicaid funds be expended for medical services only. These waivers allow for reimbursement for home health care and community-based long-term care services. This kind of waiver is obviously a response to the high cost of institutional care. It reflects a determination to maintain patients in their own homes when possible. There is a risk, however, that costs could run higher than institutional care under such arrangements, primarily because more people are likely to make use of the services (Holahan 1983). Legislators were sensitive to this possibility and stipulated that costs under the waivers could not exceed costs that would have been incurred without the waivers. Iglehart (1983) reports that by February 1983, 52 such waivers had been applied for. Homemaker services, home health aides, adult day health care, and respite care services for family caretakers were the most prominent among the requests.

Congressional Modifications of Administration Proposals

Before leaving this discussion of the ways in which the New Federalism affected Medicaid provisions, it is worth noting three significant modifications that were made in original administration proposals. First, the administration had called for a "cap" on total federal Medicaid expenditures of 5 percent over the total 1981 expenditures. This cap was to be adjusted for inflation in subsequent years. The effect of such a cap would be to restrict the states' programs severely; Medicaid costs had been rising at an annual rate in excess of 15 percent. Alternatively, states could simply assume a much greater proportion of program costs. However, if passed, the cap might in fact have jeopardized the viability of the programs in some states. Second, the original administration proposals called for a much more extensive application of the block grant mechanism. In combination with the budget reductions that were applied to the grants, this would also have had the effect of putting increased financial burdens on the states if they were to maintain their levels of programming. Congress rejected both proposals but met the administration's overall budget reductions (Wing 1983, 37–41).

Another administration proposal was advanced in 1982 that offered an exchange of programs between the federal and state governments. The federal government was to assume full responsibility for Medicaid, and the states were to run their own AFDC and food stamp programs. This federalizing of Medicaid had been proposed as early as 1977 as a means of increasing the equity and efficiency of the program (Schultze 1977). The proposal was rejected in part because of the ambiguity surrounding what was to be exchanged, under what conditions, and with what expected consequences (Brown 1983; Wing 1983).

IMPACT OF THE 1981–82 LEGISLATION:
ENROLLMENT AND EXPENDITURE TRENDS

The immediate and expected result of the legislation discussed above was a decrease in the overall numbers of Medicaid recipients. Current figures indicate that there were 21.6 million persons enrolled in 1983 (the last year for which statistics are complete), 426,000 fewer than in 1981 (Health Care Financing Administration 1985). There were more than 754,000 fewer persons under the age of 21 enrolled in 1983 and 235,000 fewer Title XIX recipients other than AFDC-eligibles. The number of adults under age 65 increased by 211,000, and adults over 65 had a net increase of almost 500,000 by 1983. Not only were there fewer recipients, but those who received services under the program represented only 45 percent of the national poverty population in 1982 (Health Care Financing Administration 1984), whereas the figure was 54 percent in 1980 and 59 percent in 1970. This downward trend in the proportion of poor enrolled undoubtedly reflects increasing numbers of poor during the recession of the early 1980s as well as cuts in eligibility.

The proportions of recipients in the various eligibility categories and their respective claims on overall expenditures stayed about the same as in the 1973–80 period. The aged, blind, and disabled (combined) made up 28 percent of the total number of recipients and claimed 72 percent of the total 1983 expenditures of $32.4 billion. AFDC adults and children made up 69 percent of the total number of recipients and received services amounting to 25 percent of the total expenditures. Other Title XIX recipients (3 percent of all recipients) received the remaining 3 percent of service expenditures. These figures reflect both the restriction of eligibility criteria for program participation and the pressure on states to cut back on expenditures.

The bias toward services to the elderly and disabled is also reflected in the proportion of expenditures for selected medical services. SNF and ICF services were provided to 23 percent of all recipients but consumed 43.6 percent of all expenditures. When hospital inpatient services are included in these calculations, 40.2 percent of recipients received services from the three sources and accounted for over 70 percent of all expenditures (ibid.).

State Responses: Service Limitations

As indicated earlier, states had continuously struggled with increasing budgetary pressures generated by Medicaid expenditures. States attempted to reduce costs by limiting eligibility, reducing the scope and duration of services, and extending the requirement of "minimal" copayments from recipients. The Tax Equity Act extended this last strategy to include certain groups of categorically needy.

Virginia and California provide examples of the kinds of limit placed on services. Virginia limited services for medically needy adults to prenatal and delivery services for pregnant women. Medically needy children were limited to ambulatory services only. All services for AFDC dependents 18 years old and over as well as their caretakers (if there were no children under 18 in the household) were discontinued. These limitations corresponded to the federal AFDC eligibility changes in the Reconciliation Act of 1981 (Gibson 1983). California limited coverage of the medically indigent to persons under age 21 and to adults in SNFs and ICFs. Responsibility for the care of all other medically indigent adults in California was shifted to the counties, but with only 70 percent of the funds for which these persons would have been eligible under MediCal in fiscal year 1983 (Brown 1984).

Most states also instituted or expanded the limitations to be placed on other services. By 1983, 12 states had set limits of from 12 to 45 inpatient hospital days per year. Five other states placed limits on the number of in-hospital days "per spell of illness." Twelve states limited the number of hospital outpatient visits per year. Other limits, imposed by most states, included limits on the number of drug prescriptions one could fill per month, or the number of reimburseable prescriptions one could fill within a specified time period (Health Care Financing Administration 1984, 17–18).

"Reform" of Reimbursement Methods

Another state response that has serious implications for many providers is alteration of reimbursement rates and revision of reimbursement mechanisms. As early as 1981, for example, Maryland faced a $39 million Medicaid deficit and attempted to save $12 to $15 million by refusing to pay hospital bills for recipients whose hospital stays were in excess of 20 days (Passett 1981). Illinois, in response to similar kinds of budgetary pressure in 1981, reduced reimbursement for Medicaid recipients' hospital stays to a maximum of $500, regardless of duration of stay or types of service rendered. Other states have avoided such drastic action, but all have significantly lower rates for Medicaid services than providers receive for privately insured patients.

California's experience illustrates well the "ripple effect" created by such reductions in reimbursement rates (Schoen 1984). When medically indigent adults were declared ineligible for MediCal, county inpatient and outpatient facilities were inundated with patients. However, in addition to the indigents who were transferred from MediCal to the county facilities, it was discovered in at least one county that the number of MediCal clients increased by 20 percent above what earlier experience would have indicated. Presumably, this was due to their having difficulty getting care privately. Fearful that the costs of indigent care might be shifted to their charges, private insurance companies requested that they be allowed to negotiate contract prices with the state as well. Private insurers were authorized to form preferred provider organizations, negotiate acceptable rates with those providers, and pass any savings on to subscribers in the form of lower premiums (Brown 1984). This California experience also reflects two general developments in the evolution of a competitive health care system—economic transfers of patients from one provider to another, and cost shifting from publicly insured and charity patients to the privately insured.

Economic Transfer of Patients

Economic transfers of patients or, what is less elegantly called dumping, occurs with increasing frequency, burdening those facilities upon which patients are dumped. Cook County Hospital in Illinois, for example, experienced a fivefold increase in the rate of emergency room transfers from other hospitals in the Chicago area within a two-year period.[3] This change corresponded with the advent of limitations on Medicaid reimbursements.

It is not altogether clear how many patients are being transferred, from what facilities they are coming, or what conditions they have, but the practice is widespread, and the major reason for it is clear. The more its proportion of uninsured patients rises, the more tenuous a hospital's financial position becomes. As Medicaid reimbursement decreases relative to reimbursements from private insurers, the hospital's vulnerability is increased. Jewish Hospital and Medical Center of Brooklyn treated all the indigent who came for treatment and ended in bankruptcy—an increasing threat for hospitals, some of which are being purchased by for-profit chains or entering into contracts with hospital management companies (Townsend 1983). Some degree of inefficient management must be considered in assessing these cases, but the financial liability that poor and uninsured patients represent to particular providers such as municipal hospitals cannot be overestimated (Hadley and Feder 1983).[4]

One significant aspect of this issue is the relative disadvantage experienced by providers of care to the poor in the face of competitive bidding for state contracts. Reimbursement on the basis of diagnosis-related groups and competitive bidding generally compensates on the basis of the established cost of an average case in the category. Patients with predictably more expensive illnesses than the average, particularly if they do not have the resources to pay their bills in full, become candidates for "referral" (Schwartz 1985). Municipal or other hospitals that receive such patients in disproportionate numbers are at a severe disadvantage in competitive bidding. This disadvantage is one of the major forces encouraging market segmentation by income and type of insurance criteria, rather than by health needs. The result is the "demarketing"—a more generalized form of dumping—of undesirable patients whose medical conditions and financial status push a facility's bid prices higher than those of its competitors (Schoen 1983).

Some teaching hospitals and other municipal hospitals that sell out to for-profit chains try to preserve their social responsibilities to the poor through the creation of trust funds from the proceeds of the sale. Anderson and his colleagues (1985, 204) observe, however, "that teaching hospitals sold in the next ten years, even at the prevailing premium prices, will not secure endowments large enough to maintain their social contributions much beyond the year 2000."[5]

Cost Sharing Limited

Cost sharing has traditionally been one way of dealing with charity care or limitations on Medicaid reimbursements. The shortfall from uninsured or charity patients is shifted to the charges of privately insured patients. This hidden tax was estimated to be $59 billion in 1981 (Health Insurance Association of America 1982). In this period of competitive health care, however, the extent to which hospitals and other providers can shift the costs of the indigent and publicly insured patients onto others is diminishing. Corporations and businesses that pay health benefits for employees are also seeking respite from escalating health care costs. They are attempting to use their individual and joint purchasing power to negotiate better prices through coalitions, utilization controls, restructured benefit packages, and negotiated payments. Other examples of these attempts to reduce costs include negotiated caps on hospital payments and discounts to employees who agree to use preferred providers with whom more favorable, lower rates have been negotiated (Feder 1982). The obvious result is that providers must limit or even eliminate cost shifting to compete successfully for these privately insured patients.

IMPACT OF RECENT TRENDS: EFFECT ON HEALTH STATUS

Improvements in the health status of the poor since Medicaid became operational in 1966 have been widely observed. Utilization of health care services by the poor, particularly physician services, has improved dramatically, and access to hospitals has increased (Davis and Schoen 1978).

Infant mortality rates among blacks dropped from a staggering 44 deaths per 1,000 live births in 1960 to 23 per 1,000 in 1978. In this same period, the infant mortality rates among whites dropped from 23 deaths per 1,000 live births to 12 per 1,000. It was also observed that there were significantly fewer deaths among low-income women who received prenatal care during their first pregnancy through Medicaid benefits than among women without these services in other states (Congressional Budget Office 1981). The number of deaths from pneumonia and tuberculosis, as well as maternal death rates, dropped precipitously (Schoen 1983).

These and other gains in the health status of the poor cannot be attributed solely to Medicaid, but the program has made a major contribution to these advances as a critical element in a broader set of health care initiatives for the poor. The developments outlined above threaten to erase or seriously impede further progress. Copayments are reported to be limiting use of basic health services (Axelrod 1983). Preliminary reports from a number of urban centers indicate that infant mortality rates are on the rise. Reports of malnutrition among increasing numbers of children are appearing, and the Boston City Hospital Pediatrics Department observed greater numbers of children failing to thrive after mothers lost their AFDC and Women, Infant, and Children program eligibility (Rosenbloom 1983). A General Accounting Office study of 11,550 cases of working poor in five cities revealed that between 14 and 24 percent of those dropped from Medicaid have either foregone or been refused medical treatment (American Public Health Association 1984).

Medically indigent adults who lost their MediCal benefits in 1981 were assessed after six months without benefits. In contrast with a comparison group of patients whose program benefits had continued, those who lost benefits showed significant declines in measures of access to care, satisfaction with care, and overall health status. Those with hypertension showed elevated blood pressures, and diabetics had higher or uncontrolled blood sugars (Lurie et al., 1984).

Other reports indicate that patients are seeking care belatedly or not at all because of lack of resources. Patients are either not obtaining needed medications or are taking them less often to make them last longer (Guttmacher 1984). Guttmacher also cites a survey by the Legal Services Corporation of Iowa ("Health Care Needs of Low Income Iowans," January 1984), which revealed that over 36 percent of all respondents needed physician and dental services that they could not afford. Thirty-three percent of the disabled and the elderly and 21 percent of those under age 21 reported that they could not obtain needed prescription drugs.

The financial cuts and other restrictions in the Medicaid program, however, are only part of the threat to the health status of the poor. David Axelrod, commissioner of health for the state of New York, pointed to the broader impact of cuts in other health programs through adoption of the block grant mechanism (Axelrod 1983, esp. pp. 77, 80). In New York alone, an estimated 24,000 to 44,000 fewer persons would be screened for hypertension. Reductions in the child nutrition and school lunch programs affect the nutritional requirements of millions of children. In New York it was estimated that as many as 57,000 poor women and their children could lose access to supplemental food, and in 1981 (before reductions) the program reached only an estimated 36 percent of those in need. The threat to the health status of women and their children is clear in the face of the convincing medical evidence that a pregnant woman's nutritional intake has a strong effect on her infant's health (ibid., 80).

A report issued by an interdenominational research group shows that, in addition to the three-quarters of a million children dropped from the Medicaid rolls, another 290,000 fewer children would have health services available through community health centers because of reductions in their programs. In addition, close to half a million fewer children were screened for lead poisoning in 1983 (Interfaith Action for Economic Justice 1984, 13–16).

It is not possible to predict with precision the long-term consequences of the developments outlined above. Insofar as access to needed medical care is being limited, it is fair to say that the health status and life chances of millions of poor Americans are being jeopardized. Given the extent to which barriers to health and medical care are being created, it is reasonable to assume that costly medical conditions are accumulating. The concerted efforts of Congress to maintain the Medicaid program, and the willingness of some states to attempt genuine reforms, indicate that there continues to be a commitment to provide necessary care. The Intergovernmental Health Policy Project, in the 11th edition of *Major Changes in State Medicaid and Indigent Care Program* (December 1985), reported that 28 states had expanded eligibility, extended service coverage, and created limited medically needy programs. No state reduced eligibility in 1985 (American Public Health Association 1986). The nature and extent of future service provision will depend in large part on lessons learned from current state experiments with Medicaid reforms.

STATE EXPERIMENTS: ATTEMPTS TO RESTRUCTURE MEDICAID

The foregoing discussion makes clear that the Medicaid program faces several conflicting demands. The goal of providing the poor with accessible health care of high quality, while at the same time containing escalating costs, poses the basic and most serious dilemma. Congressional attempts to maintain federal spending levels and the states' apparent unwillingness to make even more drastic cuts indicate a commitment to health care for the poor. If cost containment and good care for the poor are to be realized, however, basic changes must be made in the organization and structure of the program. This need has become increasingly evident as cost-containment strategies such as utilization review, peer review, and certificate-of-need regulations have proved disappointing (Steinwald and Sloan 1981).

Means by which the Medicaid program can be restructured were provided by the Budget Reconciliation and Tax Equity legislation. In addition to using waivers that permit case management systems, states can also enter into prepaid risk contracts with provider organizations and can share with recipients any resulting cost saving (in the form of additional services or direct payment). To encourage the participation of health maintenance organizations and other prepaid providers in the program, the previous limit of fewer than 50 percent Medicare and Medicaid enrollees was raised to 75 percent. States are required to continue Medicaid eligibility to the end of an HMO's minimum enrollment period for Medicaid-covered enrollees who would otherwise lose their eligibility. This provision affords HMOs more predictability and stability in subscriber turnover. Brokering services to assist recipients in choosing among competing health care organizations can also be provided.

As of 30 June 1985, 28 states had submitted a total of 116 waiver requests to the Department of Health and Human Services. Eighteen states had 54 approved waivers by that date (Sanders 1985, 1–13). All of these requests were for implementation of various case management or primary care network programs. The remainder of this section will discuss several salient features of these programs. Most of the programs have operated for a relatively short period, but several studies are reflecting outcome trends and issues, which will also be discussed.

Program Goals and Rationale

The stated goals of the programs are expressed in similar terms, regardless of differences in the origin or evolution of states' efforts. Among the most salient are the goals of providing access to good health care services for the poor; continuity of care; provider control of use of services with reduction or elimination of inappropriate, unnecessary, and expensive care, such as use of hospital emergency rooms for nonemergency acute care needs; increased physician participation in provision of care to the poor; and reduction in costs. The ways in which these goals are being pursued, like those of the Medicaid program generally, vary from state to state and often within a state. However, there are features common to all the programs.

The recipients' choice of provider is restricted to provider participants who are part of a primary care network (PCN) or a provider group or organization such as an individual practice association (IPA), or an HMO. In this way, both access to care and continuity of care are to be assured.

The providers whom recipients select (or to whom they are assigned) have responsibility for the recipients' care, and preauthorization by these providers is necessary for recipients to receive specialty or other services, such as inpatient hospital care, medical tests, or prescription drugs. Thus, emphasis is placed on primary care and improved ambulatory care, with decreased reliance on emergency rooms and inpatient services (Brezenoff 1983). The case manager assumes some financial risk, although both the kind and degree of risk vary throughout the programs.[6]

Scope of Programs

Beyond the basic principles and general parameters of the programs, the differences are great. First, the scope of the PCN and case management programs varies from relatively small county efforts to statewide programs. In Utah, for example, 75 percent of the Medicaid population of 55,000 lives in three counties, and 18,000 were enrolled with a case manager early in the program (Freund 1984). Wayne County, Michigan (which includes the city of Detroit), on the other hand, had 280,000 Medicaid-eligibles at the beginning of the program in 1982, but enrollments had reached only 38,000 by March 1984 (ibid., 70). Only California and Arizona have statewide programs, although California has different individual county programs operating within its overall MediCal program (Sullivan 1984; Kern 1984). New Jersey has designed a statewide program that is to be implemented in four phases (Haynes and Kern 1984).

Reimbursement Mechanisms

The reimbursement rates and procedures vary from the traditional fee-for-service to prepaid capitation and competitive bidding. Massachusetts's Commonwealth Health Care Corporation (CHCC) negotiates rates with the state on a per capita basis for each provider plan, and financial risk is shared across providers within the entire corporation. New Jersey's voluntary program also reimburses on a capitation rate based on recipient groups' age, sex, county of residence, and eligibility category. The Michigan Physician Primary Sponsor Plan, the Utah Choice of Health Care Program, and California's Monterey County have all maintained fee-for-service for primary care physicians. Utah considered contracting with hospitals for separate reimbursement rates. However, hospitals serving high proportions of the poor that did not win contracts with the state were seen to be financially vulnerable, and a prospective payment mechanism for hospital services was adopted. It should be noted that differentiated payment arrangements between primary care physicians and hospitals compromise the utilization control objective of case management, in that the primary care physician bears no risk in recipients' use of hospital services (Freund 1984). Other variations on the reimbursement procedures include monthly case management fees of three dollars per recipient in Michigan and two dollars per recipient in New Jersey paid to providers in addition to the service fees. Colorado raised its Medicaid reimbursement rate by 5 percent and offered an additional 5 percent reimbursement bonus as an incentive to physicians to join the plan (West 1983).

In California, the state department of health services can contract with individual and group providers (e.g., HMOs) or with primary care physicians to organize case management plans. Prepaid contracts are also drawn up with individual hospitals, with groups of hospitals, and with counties that run their own programs. The state can establish rate differentials to cost-effective HMOs to encourage prepayment plans. In 1982, the 245 hospitals with state contracts covered 72 percent of the historical Medi-Cal expenditures (Johns, Derzon, and Anderson 1985).

Arizona, which did not have a Medicaid program until 1982, also reimburses on the basis of a competitive bidding process with private and county hospitals, HMOs, and other provider groups. Services are thereby provided on a countywide basis with at least two competitive bids sought from each county. Arizona also requires copayments for services, established on a sliding scale (Freund 1984).

California's early experience with unscrupulous providers who contracted with the state and then underserved recipients (a danger in any prepaid plan) prompted that state to establish a quality assurance program. Arizona seeks to assure quality through program monitoring by the state's contract administrator. Patients also have the option of choosing a different provider, although in many cases this option may be limited due to lack of transportation or knowledge. In part as a quality assurance measure, privately insured persons and state employees are given the opportunity to enroll in the programs. The expectation is that this group of patients would be more vocal in their complaints if services were not adequate or were otherwise unsatisfactory. In the first year of the program, however, none of these groups had chosen any of the plans (Vogel 1984).

Patient Mix and Enrollment

Many programs, particularly in the early periods of development, have tended to limit enrollment to AFDC-eligibles who make up the relatively healthy segment of the Medicaid population. As the programs become operational and experience accumulates, other eligible groups, including

SSI, those on old age assistance (OAA), and the medically needy, have been enrolled. However, there is the danger of adverse selection of clients. Oregon, for example, began Project Health in 1976 and found that the least healthy, highest risk patients gravitated toward particular provider plans. Many provider groups withdrew from the program as a consequence, and one plan subsequently negotiated a rate increase on the basis of the disadvantageous patient mix. The state later created county PCNs into which the highest risk patients were screened (Gibson 1983). Colorado enrolls all Medicaid eligibles, as does Arizona and New Jersey (where the medically indigent are also included). Those who do not choose a primary care physician receive authorization cards for coverage of emergency medical care only (West 1983). Programs have had varying degrees of success in enrollment, and most include only a fraction of the total Medicaid population.

Outcome Evaluations

Programs are being evaluated for effectiveness and cost efficiency. The five-year experience of the Arizona program, for example, is being assessed by the Health Care Financing Administration (HCFA). Preliminary evidence on contract bidding in both California and Arizona has been positive, although problems and dangers have been noted, such as the disadvantageous position of providers serving large numbers of the poor and the vulnerability of some facilities that do not receive contracts. Attempts at cost saving by reducing inpatient hospital services also pose a threat to more rural hospitals (Vogel 1984; Johns, Derzon, and Anderson 1985; Christianson 1984).

Michigan's plan is undergoing extensive evaluation. Preliminary results indicate that there are dramatic declines in service use among recipients. Payments to physicians, for example, were reduced over a period of nine months by 35.4 percent for enrollees, in contrast with a 0.1 percent decrease among a control group. Outpatient hospital encounters decreased 79.8 percent in comparison with a decline of 32.1 percent for the control group. Inappropriate or excessive use of prescription drugs declined among enrollees by 21.7 percent, in contrast with an increase among the control group of 41.7 percent (Bachleda 1984).

CONTINUING ISSUES AND QUESTIONS

The lessons learned and the experience gained in the brief period of state experimentation will be more evident as the HCFA completes its assessments and the states proceed with their evaluations. The state experiments provide the basis for consideration of continuing and emerging issues with the experimental programs, as well as consideration of Medicaid generally.

Several aspects of the state reforms will require continued attention. First, freedom of choice will be the subject of debate. Whatever general philosophical and value questions are involved in restriction of choice, there are pragmatic issues to consider. The patient may be the best judge of the adequacy of provider performance, and the positive health consequences of a good relationship between patient and provider may dictate that clients have wider ranges of choice. On the other hand, as provider groups offer increasingly diverse packages of health care services at varying price levels, privately insured persons may also find their range of choice narrowed; that is, lower-priced packages may restrict choice of physician, as well as range of services. Cost containment may restrict the choices of all consumers.

The freedom-of-choice question is also to be considered in relation to the influence of stigma that is attached to the poor. If the middle and upper classes exercise their freedom of choice by avoiding facilities that serve significant numbers of the poor, freedom of choice for the poor will have to be reexamined. The results of stigma, together with the market segmentation trends noted earlier, may result in a highly differentiated health care delivery system or, more accurately, group of separate systems. Freedom of choice will be negligible in this situation. In short, the poor will be barred from participation in the mainstream of American health care.

Choice is closely related to providers' availability and proximity to concentrated populations of the poor. Adequate supply of physicians and provider organizations remains a perennial problem in inner-city areas. The concept of freedom of choice is reduced to empty rhetoric in such situations. The likely persistence of this problem should prompt serious consideration of proposals for increased development and support of community health centers as basic providers of care in these areas (Davis 1982).

As indicated above, continuity of care has been emphasized as a goal of the Medicaid experiments. Experience with the experimental programs may indicate that this goal will have to be balanced with an equal emphasis on comprehensiveness of care. This balance will become particularly critical if, in response to rising costs, reduced use of services becomes overemphasized. There is no doubt that unnecessary and inappropriate use of services must be avoided, but *unnecessary* and *inappropriate* are not precisely defined, nor can they be. An alternative approach to reducing use that commends itself from a cost-effectiveness standpoint, is increased attention to preventive care and health promotion. Such a focus could minimize the danger of a counterproductive emphasis on reduced utilization.

PCNs require extensive relationships among administrative units, providers, and state and county health and welfare departments. Iglehart (1983, 980) points out in reference to the Massachusetts program that

"Designing the CHCC system has been an exercise in diplomacy, community organizing, and political intrigue. . . . The process involves teaching hospitals and community health centers, whose respective stewards rarely spoke before, and other social-welfare interests that have competed in the past."

The concept of case management is simple, but its implementation and operation are not. Attention will have to be given to the various interorganizational and interprofessional relationships that influence program operation and service delivery. For example, the relationship between those social workers who are responsible for welfare eligibility determination and those social workers or health workers who are responsible for health program enrollment could have significant consequences for clients. Misunderstanding or lack of communication between these workers could deprive some clients of needed services. Continuing professional experience with clients who are related to both welfare and health programs will offer opportunity for increased coordination.

The variations in reimbursement mechanisms used by the states and counties offer the opportunity to assess the service delivery consequences as well as the cost effects of various reimbursement schemes. This assessment will be facilitated considerably as improved data collection and information processing requirements are met by those who monitor and assess eligibility groups to determine prepayment rates. Continued experience with and refinement of information management systems can shed light on possible alternative strategies for overcoming the disadvantages faced by facilities that serve disproportionate numbers of the poor.

In many respects, the issues raised by Medicaid reform programs mirror those raised by the Medicaid program generally, but they also hold the promise of policy and program change. The reform programs, for example, have given priority to participation by AFDC recipients. If the programs reveal improved health status among this group, the potential long-term benefits of concentrating on mothers and children may receive renewed attention and support. So long as Medicaid bears the burden of the absence of a viable long-term care policy and effective development of long-term care programs, the danger persists that AFDC recipients will be underserved and their health care needs unrecognized.

Finally, federal-state-local governmental relationships and the respective responsibilities of each governmental level must be continually assessed, defined, and redefined. The state experiments may reveal constructive program approaches that can be adopted nationally. The specific role of the federal government in relation to the variety of state programs is in transition and needs to be clearly defined. Many current developments suggest that the original Medicaid goal of bringing the poor into the mainstream of American medicine has been abandoned. If that is the case, then new approaches to delivery of health care to the poor must be devised and implemented. Concentrated efforts at all levels of government and within the private sector are needed for such a task.

NOTES

1. Wing 1983 gives a detailed political history and analysis of this achievement.
2. For details about the advantages and disadvantages of these approaches, see Feuerhard 1981.
3. The number of transfers per month increased from 122 in June 1981 to 618 in June 1983 (Kinzer 1984).
4. See also Sloan, Valvona, and Mullner 1982.
5. For case studies of the sale of municipal hospitals, see Townsend 1983.
6. The basic characteristics and principles guiding PCNs or case management programs and the cost-containment goals of these approaches are detailed in Sullivan et al. 1983.

REFERENCES

Altman, D., and R. Hearn. 1982. "Strengthening Public Hospitals and Local Health Departments." In *New Approaches to the Medicaid Crisis*, ed. by R. J. Blendon and T. W. Moloney, 219–46. New York: F and S Press.

American Public Health Association. 1985, 1986. *The Nation's Health*. Washington, DC: The Association.

American Public Welfare Association. 1981. *Washington Report*. 16 (6).

Anderson, G., C. Schramm, C. Rapoza, S. Renn, and G. Pillari. 1985. "Investor Owned Chains and Teaching Hospitals: The Implications of Acquisition." *New England Journal of Medicine* 313: 201–4.

Axelrod, D. 1983. "State Government: Block Grants in Health." *Bulletin of the New York Academy of Medicine* 59: 75–81.

Bachleda, S. 1984. "Medicaid's PPSP—Is It Working?" *Michigan Medicine* (May): 234–36.

Blendon, R. J., and T. W. Moloney, eds. 1982. "Perspectives on the Medicaid Crisis." In *New Approaches to the Medicaid Crisis*, ed. by R. J. Blendon and T. W. Moloney, 3–18. New York: F and S Press.

Brandt, E. N. 1981. *Health Services: A Shared Responsibility, Reconsideration of the Federal Role*. Washington, DC: Institute of Medicine.

Brezenoff, S. 1983. "Remarks on the 1982 Annual Health Conference." *Bulletin of the New York Academy of Medicine* 59: 82–86.

Brown, E. R. 1984. "Shifting the Burden of Illness: The Impact of the 1982 Medi-Cal Reforms." *Health/PAC Bulletin* 15 (1): 25–30.

Brown, L. D. 1983. "Health Policy and the Reagan Administration: A Critical Appraisal." *Bulletin of the New York Academy of Medicine* 59: 31–40.

Budetti, P., J. Butler, and P. McManus. 1982. "Federal Health Program Reforms: Implications for Child Health Care." *Milbank Memorial Fund Quarterly/Health and Society* 60: 155–81.

Christianson, J. B. 1984. "Provider Participation in Competitive Bidding for Indigent Patients." *Inquiry* 21: 161–77.

Congressional Budget Office. 1981. *Medicaid: Choices for 1982 and Beyond.* Washington, DC: U.S. Government Printing Office.

Davis, C. K. 1981. "Season of Change for Health Services." *HCFA Forum:* 22–29.

Davis, K. 1982. "Contracting with Community Health Centers." In *New Approaches to the Medicaid Crisis,* ed. by R. J. Blendon and T. W. Moloney, 199–218. New York: F and S Press.

Davis, K., and C. Schoen. 1978. *Health and the War on Poverty: A Ten-Year Appraisal.* Washington, DC: Brookings Institution.

Ensminger, C. 1982. "Beware the Medicaid Cap: Ronald Reagan Wants to Sell His California Turkey." *Health/PAC Bulletin* 12 (8): 12–16.

Feder, J. 1983. "Effects of Changing Federal Health Policies on the General Public, the Aged, and Disabled." *Bulletin of the New York Academy of Medicine* 59: 41–49.

Feuerherd, K. M. 1981. "New Strategies for Containing Hospital Costs under Medicaid." *HCFA Forum:* 18–21.

Freund, D. A. 1984. *Medicaid Reform: Four Studies of Case Management.* Washington, DC: American Enterprise Institute, 28–36.

Gibson, R. 1983. "Quiet Revolutions in Medicaid." In *Market Reforms in Health Care: Current Issues, New Directions, Strategic Decisions,* ed. by J. A. Meyer, 75–102. Washington, DC: American Enterprise Institute.

Guttmacher, S. 1984. "Poor People, Poor Care." *Health/PAC Bulletin* 15 (4): 15–17.

Hadley, J., and J. Feder. 1983. "Hospitals' Financial Status and Care of the Poor in 1980." Executive Summary, Working Paper 3179-02. Washington, DC, Urban Institute.

Haynes, P. L., and R. G. Kern. 1984. *Evaluation of Medicaid Competition Demonstrations: The New Jersey Medical Personal Physician Plan.* Washington, DC: Research Triangle Institute.

Health Care Financing Administration. 1983, 1984. *Medicare and Medicaid Data Book.* Washington, DC: U.S. Government Printing Office.

Health Insurance Association of America. 1982. *Hospital Cost Shifting: The Hidden Tax.* Washington, DC: The Association.

Holahan, J. T. 1983. "The Medically Needy and Needy." *Bulletin of the New York Academy of Medicine* 59: 59–68.

Holahan, J., W. Scanlon, and B. Spitz. 1977. *Restructuring Medicaid Controls and Incentives.* Washington, DC: Urban Institute.

Iglehart, J. K. 1982. "Health Policy Report: Federal Policies and the Poor." *New England Journal of Medicine* 307: 836–40.

———. 1983. "Health Policy Report: Medicaid Turns to Prepaid Managed Care." *New England Journal of Medicine* 308: 976–80.

Interfaith Action for Economic Justice, Center on Budget and Policy Priorities. 1984. "End Results: The Impact of Federal Policies Since 1980 on Low Income Americans." Washington, DC: Interfaith Action for Economic Justice.

Johns, L., R. Derzon, and M. Anderson. 1985. "Selective Contracting in California: Early Effects and Policy Implications." *Inquiry* 22: 24–32.

Kern, R. G. 1984. *Evaluation of Medicaid Competition Demonstrations: The Santa Barbara County Health Initiative.* Washington, DC: Research Triangle Institute.

Kinzer, D. M. 1984. "Care of the Poor Revisited." *Inquiry* 21: 5–16.

Lurie, N., N. Ward, M. Shapiro, and R. Brook. 1984. "Termination from MediCal— Does it Affect Health?" *The New England Journal of Medicine* 311: 480–84.

Passett, B. 1981. "Reform Medicaid? The View from a Community Hospital." *HCFA Forum:* 31–34.

Rosenbloom, D. C. 1983. "New Ways to Keep Old Promises." *Health Affairs* 2: 44–55.

Rowland, D., and C. R. Gaus. 1982. "Reducing Eligibility and Benefits: Current Policies and Alternatives." In *New Approaches to the Medicaid Crisis,* ed. by R. J. Blendon and T. W. Moloney, 19–46. New York: F and S Press.

Sanders, M. 1985. "Summary of Freedom of Choice Waiver Requests." Washington, DC: Health Care Financing Administration.

Schoen, C. 1984. "Medicaid and the Poor: Medicaid Myths and Reality and the Impact of Recent Legislative Changes." *Bulletin of the New York Academy of Medicine* 60: 54–65.

Schultze, C. L. 1977. *The Public Use of Private Interest.* Washington, DC: Brookings Institution.

Schwartz, W. B., J. Newhouse, and A. Williams. 1985. "Is the Teaching Hospital an Endangered Species?" *New England Journal of Medicine* 313: 157–62.

Sloan, T., J. Valvona, and R. Mullner. 1982. *American Hospital Association Survey of Medical Care for the Poor and Hospitals' Financial Status.* Chicago: American Hospital Association.

Steinwald, B., and T. Sloan. 1981. "Regulatory Approaches to Hospital Cost Containment: A Synthesis of the Empirical Evidence." In *A New Approach to the Economics of Health Care,* ed. by M. Olson, 273–307. Washington, DC: American Enterprise Institute.

Sullivan, S. 1984. *Evaluation of Medicaid Competition Demonstrations: The Monterey County Health Initiatives,* Washington, DC: Research Triangle Institute.

Sullivan, S., R. Gibson, P. Samors, J. Meyer, and R. McKinnon. 1983. *Restructuring Medicaid: A Survey of State and Local Initiatives.* Washington, DC: American Enterprise Institute.

Townsend, J. 1983. "When Investor-Owned Corporations Buy Hospitals: Some Issues and Concerns." In *The New Health Care for Profit: Doctors and Hospitals in a Competitive Environment,* ed. by B. Gray, 51–72. Washington, DC: National Academy Press.

Vogel, R. 1984. "AHCCCS: A New Medicare-Medicaid Model in Arizona." *New England Journal of Medicine* 310: 533.

West, D. R. 1983. "Update: Colorado Medicaid Primary Care Physician Program." *Colorado Medicine* (July): 182–83.

Wing, K. R. 1983. "The Impact of Reagan-Era Politics on the Federal Medicaid Program." *Catholic University Law Review* 33: 1–91.

7

The Sentimental Marketplace:
Who Controls Child Health Care?

James E. Black

This chapter provides a description and analysis of dramatic changes in American pediatrics from the 1880s to the 1930s.[1] Pediatrics originated in the late nineteenth century as the specialty of a small, elite group of academic physicians dedicated to research. Although these physicians had some private practice and administered a few children's hospitals, their share of child health care services was quite small. More children were treated by general practitioners, and a large number of children, most of them urban poor or rural, received no professional health care at all. During this period, a new market for child health care was established by a "child welfare movement" led principally by women. Funded by state and federal programs, the movement won national acclaim for its innovative and effective approaches to child saving. The pediatric community gradually adopted the values and practices of the child welfare movement, eventually taking over its leadership. By the 1930s, pediatricians had established themselves as the principal defenders of poor children as well as the scientific authorities on childhood.

The history of American pediatrics was shaped by both classical market forces and a desire for professional recognition. Pediatricians sought to improve their low status within the medical profession by vigorously investigating childhood illness. Their early research efforts went unrecognized by the public, however, which applauded instead the humanitarian and practical work of the child welfare movement. Jones (1983, 214) has described pediatricians of this period as following the lead of their patients' mothers largely out of economic necessity. The mothers drew

Supported by a SmithKline-Beckman Medical Perspectives Fellowship. I thank Evan M. Melhado and Paula A. Treichler for help with all phases of this work.

legitimacy and power for themselves from scientific disciplines, and pediatricians found it financially expedient to provide the mothers with the tools and authority of "rational motherhood." In addition, pediatricians' participation in publicly acclaimed child welfare programs served to advertise their therapeutic skills and the importance of employing them routinely, providing the means for thousands of pediatricians to expand pediatrics into a primary care specialty by the 1940s (Stevens 1971, 200).[2]

Though plausible, the economic argument is limited. Pediatricians may have gained more psychologically than financially by adopting a popular ideology as their own. They were able to improve their cultural authority within the profession through their research in charity hospitals for poor children. (This research eventually enabled pediatricians to shed the image of mere "baby feeders" and gain respect as practitioners of high-technology subspecialties like neonatology.) The broad scope of the child welfare movement also allowed pediatricians to claim some authority in many scientific fields, such as developmental psychology and nutrition, previously ignored by physicians. Furthermore, the pediatricians who took over leadership positions in the child welfare movement were able to redirect substantial public favor and attention toward themselves, augmenting their credentials as scientific experts by becoming compassionate guardians of children as well.

Pediatricians did not adopt the progressive values of the child welfare movement as a temporary ruse to acquire prestige and larger practices. After they had gained control of the movement and installed their research and educational interests, they formed in 1930 the American Academy of Pediatrics, the first medical organization that placed political and social concerns about children's health on the same level as scientific research. The progressive values in pediatrics have been retained into the 1980s, and pediatrics is now often regarded as one of the most "liberal" specialties (Faber and MacIntosh 1966, 299–300).[3] Although classic market forces can explain much of the early behavior of pediatricians, their enduring interest in both progressive and academic aspects of medicine suggests that psychological needs like self-esteem are still significantly influencing the ideological character of pediatrics.

EARLY PEDIATRICS

The first American pediatricians were members of a small medical elite, their status usually resting on research rather than on practice. Abraham Jacobi (1830–1919), the first eminent American pediatrician, established this research orientation for pediatrics by encouraging the careful observation of children by clinical investigators in special hospitals rather than at home (Jacobi 1890, 10). Pediatricians believed that research and teaching were the proper work for pediatricians and expressed little interest in social or political issues related to children. Their central interest in improving and extending pediatric theory and research is evidenced by the statement that the first major pediatric society in the United States, the American Pediatric Society, was formed in 1888 to "place the study of pediatrics on the same elevated plane that has been established for adult life" (Rotch 1891, 6). The second major pediatric organization, the Association of American Teachers of Diseases of Children, formed in 1906 as a small group similarly devoted to teaching and research (Faber and MacIntosh 1966).

Underlying this interest and possibly motivating it was some anxiety about the quality of pediatric teaching and research. Such concerns were voiced by Thomas Morgan Rotch (1849–1914) of Boston, who told the American Pediatric Society in 1891 that careful research could "break down and sweep away these misleading structures" of old pediatric theory and then "build up a new fabric on a stable basis" (Rotch 1891, 7). A. C. Cotton of Chicago told the Illinois Medical Society in 1898 that "the monographs and lectures on the care and management of the infant and a good portion of our textbooks on pediatrics resembled more the popular cookbooks . . . than scientific treatises based upon known physiologic and clinic data (Cotton 1898, 225).

Pediatrics faced some difficulties in becoming a specialty because it had very few members, lacked dramatic research findings in the basic sciences, and suffered from neglect in the medical schools. In 1900 there were fewer than 6 full-time pediatricians in the United States among some 50 academic physicians interested in childhood illness (Smith 1951, 176). By 1914 the number of pediatricians had increased to only 138 nationwide, nearly all of them male academics (Faber and MacIntosh, 1966, 11). By 1934 the ranks of pediatricians had grown to 1,734, but they included only a small percentage of nonacademic practitioners in large cities (Veeder 1935). Because pediatricians were so few, almost all health care of children was in the hands of general practitioners, women physicians, midwives, and, most important, the mothers themselves.

Most of the powerful therapeutic and diagnostic arsenal of modern pediatrics was unavailable to early pediatricians. While infectious diseases were the major threat to children's health, public health laboratories for diseases of children were developed relatively late. In 1900 lumbar puncture and x-rays were still unavailable for diagnosis. The chief killer of children, infantile diarrhea, was treated with barley water and sea air. Venipuncture in infants was not generally successful until 1915. Furthermore, pediatricians in 1925 were practicing without sulfa drugs, steroids, antibiotics, or electrolyte therapy (Smith 1951, Gamble 1953). No American medical school put even the "least stress" on pediatric methods in 1890 (Jacobi 1890, 7), and no medical school had a department of pediatrics in

1898 (Holt 1923, 11). Langley Porter of San Francisco acknowledged that he had "a hard time to convince students that babies don't bite" and stated that pediatricians needed to instill in their students more enthusiasm about babies (discussion following Christison 1918, 33). Perhaps worst of all for these specialists, the public had somehow gained the impression that the gentler methods of homeopathy were more appropriate for children than those of pediatrics (Grotham 1902, 341).

In spite of these difficulties, pediatricians argued that the care offered by mothers and health professionals was intolerably poor and therefore justified additional pediatric teaching and research. Such efforts would help the "large number of sick infants and young children through-out the land who are suffering from the vigorous treatment of their zealous medical attendants" (Rotch 1891, 9). In addition, pediatricians felt that the general practitioner must "be forced to understand that he has but a lim-ited knowledge of what he has been in the habit of considering simple questions" (ibid.). Mothers, rather than pediatricians, were corresponding-ly expected to perform most of the actual care of children, but only under the enlightened guidance of the pediatricians. Jacobi (1889, 15) described the pediatrician as a "pedagogue by profession" who teaches child care methods to mothers. L. Emmett Holt (1855–1924) of New York told the Mothers Convention in 1899 that the burden of preventing and treating childhood illness was theirs, but he expected that their scientific training would come from pediatricians (Holt 1899, 233). Although mothers were considered ignorant, pediatricians recognized that "the mother's care, af-fection, and milk are essential" to the infant's survival (Smith 1896, 96). Thus pedagogy defined the early partnership between mothers and pedi-atricians.

From the beginnings of their specialty in the 1880s, pediatricians felt that infant feeding was their major clinical problem. Recognizing its enor-mous public health potential, pediatricians felt that the problem of infant feeding should "incite to research" anyone interested in early life (Rotch 1893, 505). Unfortunately, their efforts led to ever more complex formu-lations for infant feeding, severely taxing the arithmetic abilities of many general practitioners, who eventually turned back to old-fashioned methods or commercial formulations instead.[5] Rotch, whose reputation was based upon some of the more complex formulations, found it "hu-miliating" that "non-medical capitalists," rather than physicians were preparing infant formulas (Rotch 1893, 506). Infant feeding was barely a clinical issue at all for medical students, who were "apt to pass it by as per-taining to the nurse and not the doctor" (Keating 1884, 88).[6] Furthermore, lay activists like Nathan Strauss were leading, with no substantive help from pediatricians, effective and popular campaigns for clean milk.[7]

Despite their self-justifying claim of authority regarding child health care, the early pediatricians declined to enter the sphere of public health.

Many presidents of the American Pediatric Society recommended that pediatricians make their authority felt in every home throughout America, but little action ever came of the rhetoric. Henry Coit of New Jersey claimed that "the physician is the proper custodian of matters affecting public health," but he recommended that physicans not become involved in political questions of health care (Blackfan 1938; Coit 1893, 11). Most pediatricians probably agreed that, because of public indifference, it would be a "useless task" for pediatricians to try to alter public opinion (Coit 1893, 10). While pediatricians were interested in charity hospitals for children, the wards were also considered an essential source of training or research material. For example, J. T. Christison of Saint Paul, Minnesota noted the value of charity cases in pediatric instruction, and he added that "there is nothing I think so important in pediatric teaching as this social work" (Christison 1918, 31).[8] Concerned that obstetricians might also desire such patients for teaching, he noted that "the baby becomes the property of the pediatrician the moment it is severed from the mother" (ibid.). Although pediatricians got relatively little of the respect they felt they deserved, they were inclined to pursue their specialty quietly within the traditional arena of teaching and research.

THE CHILD WELFARE MOVEMENT

The problem of children living amidst disease and poverty became a major public scandal in the 1880s. Newspapers reported outbreaks of cholera, typhoid, diphtheria, yellow fever, and infantile diarrhea among children. Compounded by malnutrition, infectious diseases produced very high mortality rates for young children nationwide. The press also illustrated the hazards of industrialization and urbanization, telling graphic stories of children working 14-hour shifts in dangerous sweatshops, living in tenement slums with little ventilation or sewerage, and eating inadequate or contaminated food. Poor children had little access to professional health care, surviving with only the help of maternal care and patent remedies. Rural children faced epidemics every season and often suffered from malnutrition. Professional medical care was frequently too distant, and families relied chiefly on domestic remedies and health manuals. Popular magazines often linked the health problems of these children to scandals of immorality, "hoodlumism," illiteracy, and poverty.[9]

The strongest advocates for children's health came primarily from several closely related social movements, each composed of women who claimed superiority over male physicians in the care of women and children.[10] The earlier belief in infant depravity, a quality that led children necessarily to unhappiness and filth, was transformed into the newer belief in the malleability of young minds, and in the potential of enlightened effort in nurturing happy and prosperous children. High standards of morality and decorum and the romanticization of children and childhood evolved in the early nineteenth century as a central part of the "cult of domesticity." From this cult the "mother's movement" emerged, in the last part of the nineteenth century, to claim a divinely ordained role for mothers as the sanitation and public health officers in the home and as the principal healers of children. These mothers celebrated traditional maternal qualities, while simultaneously embracing the rationality and empiricism of regular medicine and claiming "mothercraft" as one of the sciences that could be analyzed, refined, and taught outside the home. Physiology and hygiene were encoded in the major principles of nineteenth-century feminism and became proper study for women of all classes. As an editorial in an 1868 issue of *Mother's Magazine and Family Circle* put it, "the mother must study her duty" ("Mothers Should Learn to Think" 1868, 136).

Confidently asserting that the best defense of the home is a strong offense, the mother's movement attempted to clean up society in its entirety. The pride taken by these women in their efforts is evident in the 1914 report in *Child Welfare Magazine* of a rural teacher who single-handedly organized her small Oregon community to provide a hot-lunch program for the schoolchildren (Williams 1914). Their optimism even extended to the daring recommendation by Winifred Stoner (1914, 232) that all mothers of the world carefully raise their children so that they would never fight another war. The National Kindergarten and Elementary College, established to demonstrate that "as goes the child, so goes civilization," would help to strengthen democracy and eliminate selfish nationalism ("A New School for Mothercraft" 1922, 262).

The initial interest in the 1880s in child welfare, however, was not entirely an unselfish concern for the health and happiness of poor children. The humanitarian and liberal values of the child welfare movement were accompanied by fears that poor children would spread disease or grow up to be paupers, criminals, or even anarchists (Ehrenreich and English 1973). Enlightened selfishness was apparent, for example, when W. Almont Gates told a 1909 conference on children that keeping poor children with their mothers, instead of removing them to an institution, was preferable because it would produce good homemakers and prevent future generations of paupers (Gates 1909, 8). Another motivation for the protection of poor children was the cultural linkage of sin and disease in the late nineteenth century. For example, the third annual report of the California Society for the Prevention of Cruelty to Children in 1881 stated that hoodlumism was spreading in San Francisco like a pestilence (p. 3), and a Chicago charity journal in 1888 defined pauperism as a disease (Child Welfare Council of Chicago 1888, frontispiece).[11]

The child welfare movement was deeply influenced by women physicians and healers who adopted values from the earlier popular health

movement. That movement had included many women healers who rejected the harsh purges and emetics of regular medicine in favor of
naturopathic, holistic, and preventive methods.[12] These healers argued that
female physicians could treat women and children more humanely and effectively than male physicians. Many women practitioners of regular medicine in the late nineteenth century adopted clinical values from the
popular health movement and played leading roles in campaigns to improve child health. Women physicians were the "new force in medicine"
that linked mental, moral, and physical aspects of child care by working
closely with teachers and mothers (Rutherford 1893). One of the most notable of women physicians, Elizabeth Blackwell (1821–1910), wrote that wom-
en physicians with the "essential qualities of maternity" could reach into
the home, where scientific research "had little direct effect on domestic
life" and where men could not do well in the care of women and children
(Blackwell 1902, 12).

From 1900 to 1926 approximately 1,000 women were graduated as
physicians each year (Morantz 1978). In contrast to the academic pediatrician, the female doctor was the "born foe of cruelty and injustice," deliberately fighting on the broader public front of reform groups, social purity
groups, temperance organizations, mothers' clubs, and women's colleges
(Blackwell 1902, 26).[13] These physicians wrote numerous articles and
pamphlets, believing that educating the public was a major part of their
clinical function. They skillfully managed the mass media. For example, a
baby-saving campaign in Chicago had the *Daily Tribune* run favorable stories on it each day, eventually leading to a long-running advisory column
on child-rearing methods (Kingsley 1914, 13–18).

Even at the early stages of the child welfare movement it was apparent that these women wanted to claim a new area of health care that had
been largely ignored by other health care workers, a market extending
from the home to federal programs for mothers and children (Morantz
1978; Rothman 1981, 178–80). The child welfare advocates had economic, as well as ethical, incentives to spur on their efforts. Besides serving as
the political expression of cherished moral principles, the child welfare
programs also provided a wide-open market for women, one of the very
few professional markets open to them at the time. This market was
claimed by arguing that women could best provide care for themselves and
their children. Emphasizing the mother as the primary caretaker, these
women emphatically rejected the passive student role the academic pediatricians had given them.

Women physicians set up charitable health care programs across the
country; these programs featured many innovations that were eventually
incorporated into mainstream medicine. Among the approaches first put
into wide practice by women health activists were pediatric nursing, public health nursing, medical social work, patient education, preventive medi-

cine, outpatient clinics, and nutrition programs. The New York Infirmary for Women and Children established the Sanitary Visitor program, through which women medical graduates would go out into the working-class community to obtain clinical experience and to teach preventive measures to families (Antler 1976). The sanitary visitors gained a practical appreciation of how their patients lived, and emphasized in their teaching the most practical and effective of self-care measures.

The teaching of cleanliness, ventilation, nutrition, and mental hygiene was also apparent in other charity hospitals run by women physicians. For example, the California Women's Hospital in 1887 provided "the comforts of home," and the Hospital for Children in San Francisco provided outreach services for the poor with an emphasis on preventive medicine, even to the extent of keeping their own cow to provide the freshest milk for babies (California Women's Hospital 1887; Hospital for Children 1890).[14] Women physicians also administered the first governmental programs to aid mothers and children. S. Josephine Baker was the principal agent behind efforts in New York City, organizing, for example, the medical examination of 24,000 schoolchildren in 1906. The exams, including tests of sight, hearing, teeth, nutrition, and intelligence, showed that 75 percent of the children were in need of some medical care (Baker 1906, 450).

One feature of the child welfare movement challenged the authority of pediatricians—the implicit assumption that women could be autonomous, effective, and even powerful in their child-saving work. Parenting manuals recommended that children grow up without ever seeing a physician (Blake 1883, 84). Education of mothers played the central role in governmental programs to improve the nutrition of mothers and children (Langworthy 1912). Articles exposing the poisons in patent medicines and children's candy stressed the importance of educating mothers rather than establishing pure food and drug laws (for example, see Bok 1904). Lucy Dairs, one of the first public health nurses, claimed in 1903 that the public health nurse, holding "a little clinic all by herself" with the tenement families, would keep children out of hospitals (Dairs 1903, 339).[15] Lilian Wald (1915, 40) explained why mothers did not want to bring their children to hospitals by pointing out that her Henry Street public health nursing program had only 9 percent infant mortality while some New York hospitals, where children were under the care of regular physicians, averaged 38 percent.

Although pediatricians found fault with them for their sentimentality, the leaders of the child welfare movement firmly believed that they were using the most effective and scientific clinical approaches. In 1903 the managers of the San Francisco Ladies Protection and Relief Society reported (1903, 7) that "charity has become less sentimental and more reflective.

We are more scientific in methods without being . . . less sympathetic. . . . Our belief in the germ theory and sanitary science may be entirely compatible with the truest charity."

The women health activists achieved some important legislative successes, gathering the eager cooperation of private philanthropy, state and municipal agencies, and the press to lobby successfully for the U.S. Children's Bureau, established in 1912 to evaluate and protect the health of American children. By dominating the children's charities and governmental agencies for children, the women activists were able to push through the first legislation requiring compulsory immunization, improved housing, better sanitation, legalized contraception, restricted child labor, clean food and water, city parks, and free public education.[16]

The activists then worked to secure passage of the first federally funded health care program for women and children, the Sheppard-Towner Act of 1921, "a stunning victory for women reformers, who saw in its passage the first result of female suffrage" (Rothman 1981, 177). Julia Lathrop, chief of the U.S. Children's Bureau, had proposed federal aid for mothers and children in 1917 (Lemons 1973, 154–55). In the widespread favorable publicity for the child welfare movement, the bill was submitted by Senator Morris Sheppard (D-Texas) and Representative Horace Towner (R-Iowa) in the 66th Congress. Florence Kelley, who worked with the Women's Joint Congressional Committee to lobby for the bill, was joined by other politically experienced groups like the League of Women Voters. The media, most notably *Good Housekeeping,* published strong editorials favoring passage and vigorously condemning any politician who stood in its way (U.S. Children's Bureau 1926, 20). After the Sheppard-Towner Act was passed, an editorial in *Journal of the American Medical Association* (1921) gave credit for its passage to the strength of the women's political lobby, which had even engineered support for the bill in the 1920 Democratic party platform.

Over its term (1921–29), the act required the federal government to allocate a little over one million dollars for five years of work (Rothman 1981, 184). The act granted women a large public health domain that had been previously neglected as a market for health care, unequivocally placing women in control of most child welfare activity in the country.

The mandate of the program was to reduce infant and maternal mortality by giving the states matching funds to establish prenatal and child health centers. These centers were to be staffed primarily by women professionals, who taught personal hygiene and infant care and gave advice on child rearing. Supporters of the act promised that educating mothers about maintaining a clean home, examining children periodically, and providing good milk and food would substantially improve the health of all American children. With the aid of matching funds (and few expensive

Figure 7:1—A "Little Mothers" Class in Chicago. From Kingsley 1914, 14.

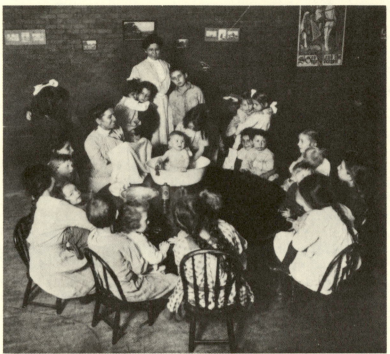

physician salaries or construction costs), nearly 3,000 clinics were established nationwide between 1924 and 1929.

The agency controlling these projects, the U.S. Children's Bureau,
proudly noted in 1931 that it had sponsored 3 million home visits by
nurses, the examination of 4 million patients in the clinics, and the distribution of 22 million pieces of educational literature (ibid., 185). A survey
of American cities in 1925 revealed that nearly all provided regular medical examinations and nursing services for schoolchildren, suggesting that
the efforts in the schools were similarly successful (American Child Health
Association 1925).

Most of the 812 public health nurses employed under the Sheppard-
Towner Act in 1926 were teaching "little mothers" classes (see fig. 7:1), an
effort to educate the older sisters who provided the only day care services
available to poor families at the time (U.S. Children's Bureau 1926, 20).
Baker (1926, 330) affirmed that "the infant welfare station is as much a part
of the public function as the public baths, public playgrounds, libraries,
and schools." These clinics were apparently effective, for clinics in Portland, Oregon reported in 1922 a death rate for babies less than one-seventh

that of the city overall (Ulysses Moore of Portland, discussion following Heunekens 1923, 49), and the Detroit clinics reported a death rate for one-month-old infants about half that of the city overall (Rand 1926, 30).

IDEOLOGICAL TRANSFORMATION OF PEDIATRICS

Supporters of the Sheppard-Towner Act had purposely left pediatric research and actual medical treatment of poor children within the respective domains of pediatricians and general practitioners. Descriptions by women health professionals active in the movement (for example, Rand 1926; Baker 1959) usually emphasized that the movement was a cooperative effort of pediatricians working alongside nurses, social workers, educators, and (significantly) the mothers themselves.

Compromise with the pediatricians was encouraged because their research and academic status were sources of authority and legitimacy for the women health activists. In this sense, the leaders of the child welfare movement had excluded pediatricians from any substantial role in the actual care of children, but their scientific stature as experts and consultants lent the movement a powerful political tool. Because the established power of the American Medical Association (AMA) posed the only substantive threat of competition in this new market of child health care, the women activists avoided the section of the market already dominated by general practitioners. Instead, the clinical sphere of the movement was restricted to nonremunerated, preventive measures like immunizations and hygiene instruction, and to medical care of only the very poorest children in charity hospitals.

The pediatricians, however, began to worry that the child welfare movement was leaving them behind. The conflict was a matter of unfortunate timing: academic pediatricians could not appeal to any glamorous research breakthrough to gain respect among their peers (as other specialties could), and the public fascination with child welfare was heaping power and respect on the women activists. The hope of pediatric research had begun to fade, and some pediatricians reluctantly began gambling on social activism to get them out in front of the women activists and practitioners. Once in charge, perhaps they could gain respect from their colleagues and the public, and perhaps even turn the public fancy toward pediatric research.[17]

This change in attitude among pediatricians appeared gradually and with some ambivalence, perhaps because the women activists did not pose an immediate or direct challenge to the income or professional status of the pediatricians. At an American Pediatric Society meeting in 1909, Holt suggested that the child welfare problem publicized in the newspapers "is not so much along the line of work of most of us as other matters more strictly medical. I believe we can do our best along lines of research" (discussion following Rotch 1909). Isaac Abt of Chicago spoke of the pediatrician's "mission to stimulate and encourage scientific work to the highest degree. It should be farthest from our purpose to become entangled in political or legislative questions" (ibid.). At the same meeting, however, Rotch (1909, 8) acknowledged the substantial contributions of women in child health care and added, "We physicians, however, whose mission it really is to guide the progress of various reforms connected with early life and see that they do not go astray, should interest ourselves in curbing exaggerated ideas." Rotch argued against child labor laws because they would deprive cotton pickers in the South "of the very outdoor work which is best for them" (ibid., 9) and stated that "the laity, however earnest and enthusiastic it may be, is in no way fitted to deal with what is really an intricate scientific study." Furthermore, pediatricians should not "allow the ignorant though humane laity to take charge of this duty to the young. . . . This army of self-sacrificing, indomitable, and philanthropic women should submit to the guidance of generals who possess the necessary knowledge for best dealing with the situation" (ibid., 12).

Many pediatricians shared Rotch's belief that the child welfare movement was led by "enthusiastic laymen whose arguments are often unwittingly handicapped by sentiment" (ibid., 9). S. M. Hammill of Philadelphia claimed in 1914 (p. 13) that the child welfare movement was guided by women, who were unwise, irrational, and "often swayed by sentiment." He urged the American Pediatric Society to take over the helm of the child welfare movement instead. The pediatrician "has withheld his assistance and influence so long that the lay organizations have learned to do without him" (ibid., 16). Hollopeter of Philadelphia acknowledged (1900, 18) the advances already made in child health by women activists and belatedly recommended that pediatricians also speak up in the child health debate.

Eventually, however, the pediatricians began adopting many of the values of the women health activists. By 1917, the University of California pediatrics department claimed the lead from "largely sentimental" lay people in recognizing progressive aspects of child health care, seeking to become "a center for the education of the public along child hygiene lines" (Bolt 1917, 61). The pediatrics department was progressing from "a lack of knowledge of the social and economic needs of the patient" to "a distinct recognition of the social as well as medical aspects of child life" (ibid., 60, 65). Abt suggested in 1919 that infant mortality could be substantially reduced by educating mothers on child care and feeding. Contemporary therapeutics, he argued, was ineffective at improving children's health, so pediatricians would do better to focus on well-baby management, nursing, and parent education. He further suggested that medical students should be compelled to do public service in the child welfare movement, in order "to learn of the appalling death rate among infants, the great waste of human life, and the basic loss to the world caused by this infant slaughter." This training of medical students in preventive medicine was also expected to produce the future leaders of the child welfare movement (Abt 1919, 33).

Medical inspection of schools, a type of practice previously lacking prestige (ranking alongside working for insurance companies), now took on a central public health mission. Abt predicted (1919, 36) that much progress in child health would be made by these school physicians, and he recommended that they receive even more specialized training in child psychology, education, nutrition, and sociology. Harold Mitchell (1924, 283) claimed that this kind of practice provided "for every child a chance to achieve the limit of his endowed capacity for wellbeing."

In the 1920s, pediatricians continued to uphold their view that preventive medicine and parental education played a primary role in pediatrics. Holt (1923, 13) still favored pediatric research, but he suggested that the future of pediatrics lay in preventive medicine and in teaching health care to the public; Hammill (1914, 15) acknowledged a great debt to sociologists for helping pediatric care; and Rene Sand (1919, 38) maintained that "there is no fixed boundary between medicine and sociology, between social work and medical work." Sand also stated that although social workers, teachers, and nurses were rapidly outdistancing pediatricians, the leadership of pediatricians would be appreciated because grants would be better funded and because medicine could serve as an unbiased, scientific mediator in social disputes. Lester Evans of Fargo, North Dakota, stated (1926, 3) that "this newer emphasis on the educational aspects of our programs is of utmost importance."

The pediatricians' support of the child welfare programs extended even to criticism of the medical profession. In 1923 H. M. McClanahan of Omaha suggested that doctors were generally reluctant to do much public service because they had been turned against it while in medical school; physicians were "too conservative or too self-centered to carry to the public that valuable information concerning public health that we as a profession almost alone possess" (discussion following Abt 1919, 37). The indifference of physicians deserved much of the blame for governmental intervention in child health care, according to Julian Hess of Chicago (discussion following Heunekens 1923, 47). On the practical side, E. J. Heunekens of Minneapolis stated in 1923 (p. 46) that the child welfare stations in his city had cut into the practices of local physicians, but he recommended that doctors in private practice provide the public with similar services, and he criticized "backward physicians" who opposed public health efforts for infants.

The pediatricians also seemed to appreciate their economic stake in the child-saving programs. Lester J. Evans (1926, 8) pointed out that "mothers are greatly impressed to learn that a physician can tell them what kinds of shoes their children should wear." Oscar Reiss of Los Angeles, though disapproving of the so-called charity cases who drove up to the baby-saving stations in motor cars, still believed the services were worthwhile, since once parents learn the "necessity of this service, they will soon seek this attention from their physicians" (discussion following Heunekens 1923, 48). A national survey in 1930 found that 63 percent of pediatricians were satisfied with the child welfare programs, only 5 percent claiming the programs had hurt their practices (White House Conference on Child Health and Protection 1931).

REPRISAL FROM GENERAL PRACTITIONERS

The larger group of general practitioners, on the other hand, were worried that the child welfare programs were stealing away some of their patients. These general practitioners worked in a crowded and highly competitive market in which careless charity could substantially diminish a physician's already marginal income.[18] Although they later realized that the new methods of preventive medicine could be co-opted to gain more patients, their early opposition led to the dismantling of many child welfare programs. Their motivations and perceptions of the child welfare movement were so different from those of the pediatricians that a remarkable factional crack appeared in the usually solid front of the AMA.

Most general practitioners cared little about public health programs during the late nineteenth and early twentieth centuries. Control of public health programs in the domains of water purity, sewerage, and clean milk had been quietly conceded to states and municipalities (Rothman 1981, 180). So long as they left the traditional doctor-patient relationship undisturbed, public health campaigns met only the benevolent disinterest of general practitioners. These physicians saw the charitable projects of public-spirited men in medicine as mainly serving vanity and power. Their own charity was more private than political. Even the charity of filling out birth records for the state was accepted by general practitioners in 1897 only after long debate.[19] Private charity often consisted of reducing a fee or extending more credit to a patient, but even these practices were regarded with suspicion. James Walk of Philadelphia condemned casual charity because it would be abused by "the sponging horde, who have plenty of money for the theatre, the ballgame, and the saloon; but none for the physician" (Walk 1897, 78). He decried as "wrong and unjust" the popular belief that physicians should provide more charity than other trades (ibid., 83). I. N. Pickett of Odell, Nebraska also disliked the "false idea" that medical practice is a work of charity, noting that "philanthropy does not pay our bills or charity fill our stomachs" (Pickett 1902, 225). E. K. Williams (1904) encouraged physicians of the Arkansas Medical Society to establish a reputation of getting their fees by fair means or foul, and A. McCurry of Texarkana, Arkansas suggested that the best outcome of a case was getting the money (discussion following Williams 1904, 166).

Such pragmatic and business-minded physicians were very sensitive about the child welfare programs. A child whose parents could pay was a highly prized patient, because a physician who successfully attended a child from birth could secure the entire family's lifetime patronage (Donegan 1972, 23). Public health officials knew that family physicians welcomed the new patients referred to them by child welfare programs. However, family physicians considered clinical treatment of children to be strictly a private matter between doctor and patient. When Boston began free inspections of schoolchildren in 1894, Samuel Durgin took great care not to offend local physicians by cutting into their practices (Durgin 1897, 10). Although the Rhode Island school inspection program primarily referred children to local doctors, Charles Chapin still had to defend his program against charges of medical socialism made by suspicious family practitioners in 1909. C. H. Hughes, editor of *Alienist and Neurologist,* was mildly supportive of the child welfare movement in 1910, suggesting, for example, that physicians should teach hygiene and neurology in the schools. By 1914, however, when the programs were rapidly expanding, the editorial tone became stridently critical of the "socialist agenda" hidden in the child welfare programs (Hughes 1910, 126; 1914, 189).

The successful campaigns to establish the U.S. Children's Bureau and related municipal and charitable programs had been controversial, but the Sheppard-Towner Act provoked a major political crisis among general practitioners. An unusual alliance, including the AMA, chiropractors, antivaccinationists, and antisuffragists, adopted a virulently misogynistic tone in their opposition to the act (Lemons 1973, 172–75). For example, the *Illinois Medical Journal* claimed in 1921 that the sponsors of the bill were *"endocrine perverts, derailed menopausics,* and a lot of other men and women who have been bitten by that fatal parasite, the *upliftus putrifaciens,* in the guise of uplifters, all of whom are working overtime to devise means to destroy the country" (p. 143). In the floor debate, Senator James Reed of Missouri was worried that "all the medical doctors who have been concerned in the preparation of literature or the work of the [U.S. Children's] Bureau are women, and are, I believe, with one exception unmarried." He found it amusing that the provisions of the bill were designed by "an aggregation composed almost exclusively of spinsters," especially if the bill was merely "the fulminations of propaganda and the imagination of superannuated single ladies." More bothersome, however, was his suspicion that the Children's Bureau was steered by "fantastic doctrines of the European socialist and bolshevist" (*Congressional Record* 1921, 8760, 8765, 8767).

The women activists, however, were apparently confident that their efforts could overcome any obstacles imposed by physicians or conservatives. Anne Rude of the Children's Bureau wrote (1921) that the Sheppard-Towner Act "belongs in its health aspect to that field of hygiene which doctors have long since turned over to the laity to practice." She described opponents of the act as a "reactionary group of medical men who are not progressive and have no public health point of view (Rude 1922). Women physicians were noticeably outspoken in their support of the act, especially in the *Medical Woman's Journal.* Ella Oppenheimer (1921) even criticized the AMA in its own journal for aligning itself with long-time foes like chiropractors, herbalists, and antivaccinationists.

Some members of the AMA began to see the value of some aspects of the Sheppard-Towner Act in their own practices. A nationwide survey of physicians asked nonpediatricians in 1931 about the public health campaign to educate parents in the health needs of their children and the necessity of periodic examination. Only 3 percent of the physicians said it had hurt their practice, while 51 percent said it helped (White House Conference 1931, 80). An interesting feature of the Sheppard-Towner Act required many communities to gain approval from the local medical society before any matching funds could be dispersed. While this was intended to prevent any direct conflict with the county medical societies, it had the effect of inducing physicians to come out publicly in favor of what they might not have liked in private (Rothman 1981, 191–93). Periodic health examinations had been in use previously, but the AMA endorsed them only after they gained popularity in the public health programs. Haven Emerson, for example, recommended (1923, 1381) that practitioners should begin instructing their patients in matters of personal hygiene, although many physicians might "not find themselves at once prepared" for this new service. Although the AMA saw the public popularity of the child welfare programs as one of their most threatening characteristics, physicians began to exploit these programs by claiming that they required medical expertise and should never be turned over to lay organizations or mothers (Rothman 1981, 191–93).

In spite of these benefits, the AMA never wavered in its public opposition to the Sheppard-Towner Act. The association complained that federal intervention in health affairs infringed on states' rights, cost too much, and supported centralized medicine. In its 1922 meeting the AMA House of Delegates passed a resolution stating that the Sheppard-Towner Act was an "imported socialist scheme," an opinion that caused a major split between the academic pediatricians and the general practitioners in the AMA.[20] At the same meeting in Saint Louis, the Pediatrics Section had passed a resolution of its own approving of the Sheppard-Towner Act. Although the AMA House of Delegates had condemned the act the very same day, it was the resolution of the Pediatrics Section that was splashed across the Saint Louis papers the next morning. Pediatric historian Marshall Pease (1952, 15–17) described the resulting hot tempers: "A commit-tee of wrath was sent by the House of Delegates to reprimand the Pediatric Section. They were met with unrepentance and jeers." Because by this time physicians rarely engaged in public criticism of their peers in other special-ties, these events suggest that the pediatricians were motivated by more than a need for respect. Public advocacy on behalf of poor children like-ly caused pediatricians to internalize their professed progressive values, even to the extent that these physicians became the eager radicals of their profession.

PEDIATRICIANS AT THE HELM

While the AMA and its strange allies inflicted considerable damage in their fight against child welfare programs, the alliance between the Children's Bureau and the pediatricians may also have contributed to the failure of Congress to renew the Sheppard-Towner Act in 1929 (Rothman 1981, 195). With coaching from the pediatric and obstetric specialists, the Children's Bureau gradually shifted away from the feminist assumption that mothers would be the central source of health care for children. The concern of the child welfare workers that their work be reflective and scientific, rather than sentimental, encouraged the new assumption that only highly trained specialists could understand the complexity of childhood illness. The baby clinics were therefore perceived to be less valuable because they did not employ experts, and the education of mothers became irrelevant with mothers' loss of autonomy.

The moral tone assimilated from the public health movement be-came a bit strained among the pediatricians who gained control of the 1931 White House Conference for Child Health and Protection. These an-nual meetings had been dominated previously by women activists pursu-ing goals that gave mothers and women health professionals center stage in child health programs. Their exclusion of pediatricians from all but a nominal role as experts still bothered Adrian Lambert of New York in 1931, who commented that "if one might judge from reading the papers and popular magazines, he would think that . . . the doctor is here [in child welfare work] a kind of necessary evil, he must be used, but that is about all" (p. 99). Lambert went on to say that it took courage to emphasize in the conference report "the fact that the child is in reality the work of the phy-sician, when the salons of our legislature usurp our power " (ibid.).

The first pediatricians insisted that mothers perform most health care activities for children, making use of expert advice based on labora-tory research. The academic pediatricians won control of the child protec-tion movement, gaining seats on many of the important governmental and charitable committees that were previously occupied by women. Thus they were able to turn once more to their previous interests in research.[21] They also expected mothers now to ask general practitioners and pediatricians for help in actual care because these services were now too complex for the layperson. The Subcommittee on Medical Education, part of the 1931 White House Conference on Child Health and Protection, concluded that the welfare nurse, nutrition worker, psychologist, and medical social worker are all ultimately dependent on medicine, thus justifying the "new" interest in medical research and education. The conference of 1931 focused the attention of the child welfare movement for the first time on the education of physicians (White House Conference 1931, 79). Lambert (1931, 99) described the committee report as a "declaration of independence" for pediatricians. He agreed with the committee that physician education was the crux of solving the child welfare problem.

However, with this victory of the old agenda there remained some self-doubt about pediatricians' efforts to improve the health of poor children. At a meeting of the American Child Health Association, largely controlled by physicians in 1928, Carl Henry Davis (1928, 36) asked, since "the medical profession has not attempted to correct the situation which caused the Sheppard-Towner legislation . . . what have we to offer as a substitute?" This question reflects a lasting internalization of social values in this specialty that is still expressed in the "liberal" efforts of contemporary pediatrics. While pediatrics is now a mix of primary care and glamorous, high-technology subspecialties, pediatricians have mostly retained their earlier social role of advocates for children.

Explanation of the ideological transformation of pediatrics from the 1880s to the 1930s apparently requires consideration of both economic and psychological factors. As Jones has pointed out, those pediatricians needing income from private practice would have some interest in supporting the political aspirations of their patients' mothers. Because the well-baby approach to child care vastly expanded the number of visits by children to doctors in the 1940s, financial interests can also help explain the popularity of preventive medicine in contemporary pediatrics. However, pediatricians conspicuously resented the popularity of the women activists, and their willingness to become rebels in the AMA suggests that needs for social recognition and self-esteem have also played substantial roles in this transformation. Additional evidence for this theory lies in the motivations of the women physicians, who established both careers and self-worth by their efforts, and those of the general practitioners, who expressed their economic anxieties about competition in terms of a socialist-feminist threat.

The ideological transformation of pediatrics early in this century can provide a model of how social and psychological factors can interact with economic ones in determining the future of health care. Self-concept will be an important factor, for example, in how physicians decide ethical questions about financial self-interest in and control of health care corporations. Influence over health care can be gained by shaping public attitudes about the trustworthiness, reliability, and motivation of doctors, nurses, and hospitals. Public expectations of the doctor-patient relationship, the funding of charity, and even what constitutes health care can have direct impact on such issues as the survival of private practice and an expanded role for nursing. In predicting the direction of medical care, therefore, it seems quite important to consider social and psychological factors as well as those traditionally considered purely economic.

NOTES

1. Some general references on the history of American pediatrics are Pease 1952, Faber and Macintosh 1966, and Cone 1979.
2. Advertisers of children's products made the pediatrician and family doctor into quite popular images of expertise and authority at this time (e.g., in *Parent's Magazine*).
3. Kunitz 1983 has explored the connections between the early progressive and contemporary liberal values of pediatricians. The textbook by Allmond 1979 is a good example of progressive values that have been transmitted to the present generation of pediatricians.
4. See also Holt 1923 and Van Ingen 1914 for contemporary perspectives.
5. See Apple 1980 for a discussion of how infant feeding influenced pediatric practice.
6. Apple 1980 and Jones 1983 showed that infant feeding, although clinically uninspiring, was a central economic pillar of many medical practices.
7. See Freeman 1897 for a contemporary description of pure milk campaigns.
8. See also Holt 1898 for an early rationale for pediatric hospitals. Holt's career started in the Babies' Hospital of New York, first established by women physicians (see McNutt 1889).
9. See Cone 1979, 99–129, or articles reprinted in Bremner 1970.
10. Some general references are Leach 1980 and Morantz 1977.
11. Attributed to R. T. Paine.
12. For a general discussion, see Leach 1980.
13. Louise Harvey 1898 of Los Angeles, for example, outlined this sort of ambitious program.
14. Both were funded and run by women as charity hospitals "open to all," but fewer than 2 percent of the patients were of non-European origin. However, W. W. Murphy 1904 reported that Mothers Clubs in California did try to help some Chinese and Mexican children.
15. The nurses had a new self-confidence and independence that was in sharp contrast to the servility prescribed to them a few decades earlier by Hughes 1887.
16. See Lemons 1973 for a description of the establishment of the U.S. Children's Bureau and related political work of these women. Details of some of these programs can be found in United States Children's Bureau 1913, 1915.
17. Pediatricians like Caille 1904 and Shaw 1938 usually attributed their involvement in the child welfare movement to an acute awareness of the tragic

amount of childhood suffering and of how easily it could be prevented. Although their support of progressive reforms was described as a simple matter of conscience, the leading pediatricians of the period nearly always neglected to mention the role of women activists in their reviews of how pediatrics became involved in the child welfare movement. Two exceptions are Abt 1919, who referred to the movement's leadership as "professional men and women" (p. 33), and Cone 1979, who acknowledged the central role of the women's movement.

18. See Starr 1982, book 1, chap. 5, about practitioners' attitudes toward charity work and public health.

19. Supported by Emma Lucas 1897, 376, but other physicians felt that the state of Illinois should be billed for services rendered.

20. Women physicians did not have enough representation in the AMA House of Delegates even to negotiate a compromise with regard to the Sheppard-Towner Act ("No Medical Women in House of Delegates of AMA" 1921).

21. See Cone 1979 and Faber and MacIntosh 1966 for descriptions of the mature character of American pediatrics.

REFERENCES

Abt, Isaac. 1919. "Teaching of Medical Students to Meet the Requirements for Various Civil Activities of His Community." *The Association of American Teachers of the Diseases of Children* 13: 30–35.

Allmond, Bayard W. 1979. *The Family Is the Patient: An Approach to Behavioral Pediatrics for the Clinician.* Saint Louis: Mosby.

American Child Health Association. 1925. *A Health Survey of 86 Cities.* New York: The Association.

Antler, Joyce. 1976. "Medical Women and Social Reform—A History of the New York Infirmary for Women and Children." *Women and Medicine* 1: 11–18.

Apple, Rima D. 1980. "'To Be Used Only under the Direction of a Physician': Commercial Infant Feeding and Medical Practice, 1870–1940," *Bulletin of the History of Medicine* 54: 402–17.

Baker, S. Josephine. 1906. "The Medical Inspection and Examination of School Children in New York." *Annals of Gynecology and Pediatry* 19: 450–51.

———. 1922. "Why Do Our Mothers and Babies Die?" *The Ladies Home Journal* 39 (April): 32.

———. 1926. "Problems in Connection with the Administration of Well Baby Clinics." *Public Health Nurse* 18: 329–32.

———. 1959. *Fighting for Life.* New York: Macmillan.

Blackfan, Kenneth D. 1938. "Past Presidents of the American Pediatric Society." *American Journal of Diseases of Children* 56: 1–13.

Blackwell, Elizabeth. 1902. "The Influence of Women in the Profession of Medicine." In *Essays in Medical Sociology.* New York: Bell. Reprint. London: Arno Press, 1972.

Blake, Mary. 1883. *Twenty-six Hours a Day.* Boston: D. Lothrup.

Bok, Edward. 1904. "The Patent Medicine Curse." *The Ladies Home Journal* (May): 18.

Bolt, Richard A. 1917. *Problems Presented to the Children's Department of a University Hospital in Meeting the Social Needs of a Cosmopolitan City.* Master's thesis, University of California.

Bremner, R. H., ed. 1970. *Children and Youth in America.* Vol. I. Cambridge, MA: Harvard University Press.

Caille, A. 1904. "The Influence of the American Pediatric Society in Promoting the Welfare of American Children." *Transactions of the American Pediatric Society* 16: 6–10.

California Society for Prevention of Cruelty to Children. 1881. *Third Annual Report.* San Francisco: The Society.

California Woman's Hospital. 1887. *20th Annual Report.* San Francisco: The Hospital.

Chapin, Charles V. 1934. "The Medical Inspection of Schools in Providence." In *Papers of Charles V. Chapin, M.D.* New York: Commonwealth Fund.

Child Welfare Council of Chicago. 1888. *Council* 1 (April): 1.

Christison, J. T. 1918. "The Modern Pediatric Teaching." *The Association of American Teachers of the Diseases of Children* 12: 30–32.

Coit, Henry L. 1893. *A Plan to Procure Cow's Milk Designed for Clinical Purposes.* Reprinted in *Children and Youth in America,* ed. by R. H. Bremner, Vol. I. Cambridge, MA: Harvard University Press, 1970.

Cone, Thomas E., Jr. 1979. *History of American Pediatrics.* Boston: Little, Brown.

———. 1976. *200 Years of Feeding Infants in America.* Columbus, OH: Ross Laboratories.

Congressional Record. 1921. 67th Cong., 1st Sess., Vol. 61, pt. 9.

Cotton, A. C. 1898. "Infant Feeding at Home and Abroad." *Transactions of the Illinois State Medical Society*: 225–32.

Dairs, Lucy W. 1903. "The Outdoor Relief of the Children's Hospital, Boston." *American Journal of Nursing* 4: 337–39.

Davis, Carl Henry. 1928. "Report of the Section of Obstetrics, Gynecology, and Abdominal Surgery." *Transactions of the American Child Health Association*: 36.

Donegan, Jane Bauer. 1972. *Midwifery in America, 1760–1860: A Study in Medicine and Morality.* Doctoral dissertation, Syracuse University.

Durgin, Samuel H. 1897. *Medical Inspection of the Schools.* Boston.

Ehrenreich, Barbara, and Deidre English. 1973. *Complaints and Disorders: The Sexual Politics of Sickness.* Old Westbury, NY: Feminist Press.

Emerson, Haven. 1923. "Periodic Medical Examination of Apparently Healthy Persons." *Journal of the American Medical Association* 80: 1376–78.

Evans, Lester J. 1926. "The Physician's Way of Securing the Parent's Cooperation." *Transactions of the American Child Health Association* 2: 3–9.

Faber, Harold, and Rustin MacIntosh. 1966. *History of the American Pediatric Society.* New York: McGraw-Hill.

Faegre, Marion L. 1931. "A New Understanding of Childhood." *Public Health Nurse* 25: 210–11.

Freeman, R. G. 1897. "The Strauss Milk Charity of New York City." *Archives of Pediatrics* 14: 838.

Gamble, J. L. 1953. "Early History of Fluid Replacement Therapy." *Pediatrics* 11: 554.

Gates, W. Almont. 1909. "The Dependent Children of California." *Proceedings of the Children's Conference.* San Francisco.

Grotham, Georgiana. 1902. "Progress in Therapeutics in the Diseases of Children." *Proceedings of the Nebraska State Medical Society* 34: 340–45.

Hammill, S. M. 1914. "Responsibility of the Pediatrist toward the Problems of Public Health." *Transactions of the American Pediatric Society* 26: 12–16.

Harvey, Louise. 1898. "Home Sanitation." *Transactions of the Medical Society of the State of California* 28: 102–8.

Heunekens, E. J. 1923. "Methods of Using Child Welfare Stations in the Teaching of Pediatrics." *The Association of American Teachers of the Diseases of Children* 17: 44–46.

Hollopeter, W. C. 1900. "The Pediatric Outlook." *Transactions of the Section on the Diseases of Children, American Medical Association* 16: 15–18.

Holt, L. Emmett, Jr. 1898. "Scope and Limitations of Hospitals for Infants." *Transactions of the American Pediatric Society* 10: 147.

———. 1899. "Physical Care of Children." *Proceedings of the Third National Congress of Mothers.* Philadelphia.

———. 1923. "American Pediatrics—A Retrospect and Forecast." *Transactions of the American Pediatric Society* 35: 9–18.

Hospital for Children and Training School for Nurses. 1890. *Annual Report.* San Francisco: The Hospital.

Hughes, C. H. 1887. "Don'ts for Hospital and Private Nurses of the Sick." *Peoria Medical Monthly* 7: 606–8.

———. 1910. "School Reforms Needed." *Alienist and Neurologist* 31: 126.

———. 1914. "The Physician's Duty in Forming Public Opinion." *Alienist and Neurologist* 35: 189.

Illinois Medical Journal. 1921. 39: 143.

Jacobi, Abraham. 1889. "The Relations of Pediatrics to General Medicine." *Transactions of the American Pediatric Society* 1: 15–17.

———. 1890. "Introductory." In *Cyclopedia of the Diseases of Children,* ed. by J. M. Keating, I, 1–14. Philadelphia: J. P. Lippincott.

Jones, Kathleen. 1983. "Sentiment and Science: The Late Nineteenth Century Pediatrician as Mother's Advisor." *Journal of Social History* 17: 79–96.

Journal of the American Medical Association 1921. 77: 1913–14.

Keating, John. 1884. "Infant Feeding." *Archives of Pediatrics* 1: 88–95.

Kingsley, Sherman C. 1914. *Steps in the Evolution of Baby Welfare Work in Chicago.* Chicago: Elizabeth McCormick Fund.

Kunitz, Stephen J. 1983. "The Historical Roots of Ideological Functions of Disease Concepts in Three Primary Care Specialties." *Bulletin of the History of Medicine* 53: 412–32.

Lambert, Adrian V. S. 1931. "Report of the Medical Section." In *Pediatrics: Education and Practice,* White House Conference on Child Health and Protection, 1–8. Washington, DC: U.S. Government Printing Office.

Langworthy, C. F. 1912. "Standards for Home Management in Relation to Food Problems." *Home Progress* 2: 8–18.

Leach, William. 1980. *True Love and Perfect Union: The Feminist Reform of Sex and Society.* New York: Basic Books.

Lemons, J. Stanley. 1973. *The Woman Citizen.* Urbana: University of Illinois Press.

Lucas, Emma J. 1897. "The Physician's Duty to the State in Relation to Sanitary Affairs." *Transactions of the Illinois State Medical Society*: 373–78.

Martin, Anne. 1920. "Every Woman's Charge to Serve Humanity." *Good Housekeeping* 70 (February): 20–21.

McNutt, S. A. 1889. "The Babies' Hospital—A Summer's Work." *Medical Record of New York* 35: 234.

Mitchell, Harold H. 1924. "Organization of School Medical Inspection." *Transactions of the American Child Health Association* 2: 233–37.

Morantz, Regina. 1977. "Making Women Modern: Middle Class Women and Health Reform in 19th Century America." *Journal of Social History* 10: 490–507.

———. 1978. "The 'Connecting Link': The Case for the Woman Doctor in Nineteenth-Century America." In *Sickness and Health in America,* ed. by R. Numbers and J. Leavitt, 117–28. Madison: University of Wisconsin Press.

"Mothers Should Learn to Think." 1868. *Mother's Magazine and Family Circle* 36: 136–37.

Murphy, W. W. 1904. "Reports of State Presidents." *Proceedings of the National Congress of Mothers*: 47–48.

"A New School for Mothercraft." 1922. *Child Welfare Magazine* 117: 262–64.

"No Medical Women in House of Delegates of AMA." 1921. *Medical Woman's Journal* 28: 22.

Oppenheimer, Ella. 1921. Letter. *Journal of the American Medical Association* 76: 1418–19.

Pease, Marshall Carlton. 1952. *American Academy of Pediatrics, 1930–1951*. Evanston, IL: American Academy of Pediatrics.

Pickett, I. N. 1902. "The Business Side of Our Daily Work." *Proceedings of the Nebraska Medical Society*: 225–33.

Rand, Winifred. 1926. "How Public Health Nursing May Contribute to the Normal Development of the Child." *Transactions of the American Child Health Association*: 27–35.

Rotch, Thomas Morgan. 1891. "Iconoclasm and Original Thought in the Study of Pediatrics." *Transactions of the American Pediatric Society* 3: 6–9.

––––––. 1893. "The General Principles Underlying All Good Methods of Infant Feeding." *Boston Medical and Surgical Journal* 129: 505–6.

––––––. 1909. "The Position and the Work of the American Pediatric Society toward Public Questions." *Transactions of the American Pediatric Society* 21: 7–39.

Rothman, Sheila M. 1981. "Women's Clinics or Doctors' Offices: The Sheppard-Towner Act and the Promotion of Preventive Health Care." In *Social History and Social Policy*, ed. by D. Rothman and S. Wheeler. New York: Academic Press.

Rude, Anne E. 1921. Letter to Gertrude Lane, June 25. Quoted by Sheila M. Rothman, "Women's Clinics or Doctors' Offices: The Sheppard-Towner Act and the Promotion of Health Care," in *Social History and Social Policy*, ed. by D. Rothman and S. Wheeler, 186. New York: Academic Press, 1981.

––––––. 1922. Letter to Senator Sheppard, July 7. Quoted by Sheila M. Rothman, 1981, "Women's Clinics or Doctors' Offices: The Sheppard-Towner Act and the Promotion of Health Care," in *Social History and Social Policy*, ed. by D. Rothman and S. Wheeler, 180. New York: Academic Press, 1981.

Rutherford, Frances. 1893. "The New Force in Medicine and Surgery." *Proceedings of the Michigan State Medical Society*: 41–48.

San Francisco Ladies Protection and Relief Society. 1903. *48th Annual Report*. San Francisco: The Society.

Sand, Rene. 1919. "Why the Pediatrician Should be the Leader in Infant and Child Welfare." *The Association of American Teachers of the Diseases of Children* 13: 38–39.

Shaw, Henry L. K. 1938. "The American Pediatric Society and the Child Welfare Movement." *Transactions of the American Pediatric Society* 50: 74–79.

Smith, J. Lewis. 1896. "Hindrance to the Successful Treatment of Disease of Infancy and Childhood." *Transactions of the New York State Medical Society* 13: 95–96.

Smith, R. M. 1951. "Medicine as Science: Pediatrics." *New England Journal of Medicine* 244: 176.

Stafford, Henry E. 1936. "The Changing Pediatric Practice." *Journal of Pediatrics* 8: 376.

Starr, Paul. 1982. *The Social Transformation of American Medicine: The Rise of a Sovereign Profession and the Making of a Vast Industry*. New York: Basic Books.

Stevens, Rosemary. 1971. *American Medicine and the Public Interest*. New Haven, CT: Yale University Press.

Stoner, Winifred Sackville. 1914. "War the Result of Improper Child Rearing." *Child*

Welfare Magazine 9: 232–33.

Townsend, Charles W. 1899. "Remarks on Infant Feeding, with Special Reference to the Home Modification of Milk." *Boston Medical and Surgical Journal* 140: 275–77.

United States Children's Bureau. 1913. *A Preliminary Report on What American Cities are Doing to Prevent Infant Mortality.* Washington, DC: U.S. Government Printing Office.

———. 1915. *Baby-Week Campaigns. Suggestions for Communities of Varying Sizes.* Washington, DC: U.S. Government Printing Office.

Van Ingen, Phillip. 1914. "Recent Progress in Infant Welfare Work." *American Journal of the Diseases of Children* 7: 471.

Veeder, Borden S. 1935. "Trends of Pediatric Education and Practice." *American Journal of the Diseases of Children* 50: 1–10.

Wald, Lilian D. 1915. *The House on Henry Street.* New York: Holt, Rinehart & Winston.

Walk, James W. 1897. "The Limits of the Physician's Duty to the Dependent Classes." *Bulletin of the American Academy of Medicine* 2: 75–85.

White House Conference on Child Health and Protection. 1931. *Pediatrics: Education and Practice.* Washington, DC: U.S. Government Printing Office.

Williams, E. K. 1904. "The Business Side of Our Profession." *Transactions of the Arkansas State Medical Society*: 158–65.

Williams, W. 1914. "A History of the Hot Lunch Program at Dexter, Oregon." *Child Welfare Magazine* 9: 202–03.

8

The Other Face of Competition: Nursing's Struggle for Autonomy

Walter Feinberg and Suzanne R. Langner

In this chapter, we articulate an argument for greater autonomy for the nursing profession and examine the way in which some medical and nursing students have incorporated features of the argument into their own day-to-day understanding of their future professional roles. We begin by sketching central aspects of the mature, well-formulated arguments about professional status that have been developed in both medicine and nursing. We then examine the way in which the nursing argument, as an ideal type, is represented in the subjective understandings of students who are training to become nurses and physicians. We do this by analyzing interviews with students. To the extent that medical and nursing students are able to perceive health care on a structural level—one that addresses the needs of the health care system—they will assess an argument for or against a particular professional view on its own merits. To the extent that professional autonomy is not understood in terms of its implications for the system of health care, important aspects of arguments will be deflected and misunderstood. Because we find that students, medical and nursing, have a number of difficulties in incorporating nursing's argument into their day-to-day understanding of health care, we return at the end of the chapter to examine some of the reasons for these problems.

While the two positions that we characterize as the medical and nursing arguments address the difference in status between the two professional groups, the labels that we have chosen are not intended to imply that a majority of physicians or a majority of nurses hold the position that we have associated with their profession. Many nurses continue to believe that their proper role is to act as handmaidens to physicians, and a number of physicians recognize the important, independent function that professional nurses can serve. We simply wish to make the point that there are two reasonably coherent, and somewhat conflicting, arguments for the status of these two health care groups. We call one the medical argument because it implicitly supports the elevated status of the physician, and we call the other the nursing argument because it seeks to raise the status of the nurse.

THE PHILOSOPHY OF MODERN MEDICINE

The argument for the autonomy of nursing has been developed in the context of a long-standing belief that the domination of medicine in the health care field is a legitimate result of extended training and superior knowledge. A rationale for this belief, established very early in this century, is strongly associated with the writings of Abraham Flexner (1910). In many respects, Flexner's argument still provides the soundest rationale for the dominance of the medical profession, and it is therefore against the backdrop of his concerns that the argument for nursing can be most clearly presented.

Writing for the Carnegie Foundation on the reform of medical education, Flexner expressed two primary objectives. The first was to establish medicine as a science, with the same rigorous standards as any other science. The second was to create the educational climate that would enable medical researchers and practitioners to maximize the growth of medical knowledge. He proposed that the basic biological sciences form the foundation of medical practice; as scientists, doctors must understand the laws governing the normal functioning of the human organism and the various abnormalities that interfere with such functioning. After mapping these biological spheres, medicine would then be in a better position to develop the procedures for successfully intervening to alter the course of disease and return the body to normality. Much of this work would be taught during the clinical years.

In proposing that medicine become more scientific, Flexner was also proposing that it become more specialized. He believed that specialization was essential if the developing gap between medical research and medical practice was to be narrowed and if both research and practice were to progress at a faster pace. Specialization was Flexner's response to both the actual and the potential acceleration in the growth of medical knowledge. It was the way in which medical research and practice needed to be organized as the body of available medical knowledge became too vast for any single individual to comprehend. While Flexner did not extend his remarks to the proper relationship between the medical profession and other health care providers, his views have provided a principal source for justifying the dominance of the physician. The superior training of the physician would provide the leadership required to achieve improvements in health.

The implications of Flexner's argument for medical education were many. First, medical students were to be selected for training because of their demonstrated proficiency in the relevant sciences. Second, medical education was to be attached to university research. Third, the proprietary medical schools were to be closed down. Fourth, the number of practitioners was to be reduced in order to remove destructive competition and to protect the quality of medical practice. Last, the time required to obtain a medical degree was to be significantly extended.

In making his case for reform in medical education, Flexner was addressing the needs of the medical system as a whole and proposing educational mechanisms that he considered necessary to the maximization of the growth and effective utilization of medical knowledge. In this sense the medical argument, much like the nursing argument we will examine below, was addressing the needs of the health care system as a system.

If we fail to appreciate that the rationale for elevating the status of physicians is the effective development and use of medical knowledge on the system level, we will misperceive certain issues. Questions such as why physicians tend to have high salaries, or why the medical profession maintains its dominance over the health care field, will be addressed as if they were questions about the relative moral worth of different individuals (doctors make a lot of money because they sacrifice a lot and work hard) rather than as questions about the goals and priorities of the system of health care.

NURSING'S CHALLENGE TO THE PHILOSOPHY OF MEDICINE

While nursing has not developed a report that can match the prominance of Flexner's,[1] it is developing a coherent argument for advancing its status as a profession. The reconstruction of this argument presented here is drawn from the literature in the field and from discussions with nursing faculty members at four-year, university-based nursing programs. Much like the argument that Flexner advanced for improving medical education, the argument for nursing is built on an understanding and a vision of the health care system as a system. However, it emphasizes different features of that system and gives priority to different goals. For example, instead of placing the highest priority on the growth of medical knowledge, more concern is given to the distribution of health care services (for an example, see "Equal Access to Care is Nursing's Challenge" 1985). Moreover, nursing would like more emphasis to be placed on preventing and coping with disease and less on crisis intervention (American Nurses' Association 1965). Since advocates of the nursing argument believe that medical doctors are primarily concerned with crisis intervention, and nurses with prevention and coping, and that these two goals are of equal merit, they conclude that some adjustment in the relationship between the two professional groups is required. In other words, medicine and nursing are two equal professional groups, each serving to further the cause of health care, and they should be treated as such.

The advocates of this newer conception of health care point out that crisis intervention is but one aspect of the management of health and disease. Equally important is promoting disease prevention,[2] on the one side, and helping patients and their families cope with chronic illness, on the other. It is averred that meeting these goals requires a thorough understanding of a patient's daily life, an understanding that includes knowledge of family and cultural attitudes, of the economic situation of the patient, and of the patient's habits and dispositions. It is further pointed out that medicine's response to the need for specialists has created a gap in primary health care, and that too often the extraclinical factors that affect disease prevention and wellness go unattended. Through training that would join the biological, behavioral, and social sciences in clinical application, and through continuous and direct contact with patients, it is concluded that nursing could stand in the best position to close this gap.[3]

Just as the biological sciences form the foundation of the medical profession, so, it is claimed, the behavioral and social sciences, linked to a general understanding of the biological sciences, should form the foundation of the nursing profession. Therefore, if health care is to progress, the nurse must no longer accept the role of physician's handmaiden. The knowledge that makes an effective nurse, while different from that which makes an effective physician, is equally important. The focus of concern is not medicine as such, but health care, and health care is a field in which both medicine and nursing must play a part. Thus, the argument continues, both nurses and physicians must have their own sphere of authority grounded in their own unique knowledge base.

The nursing argument grants that the knowledge base of the physician does indeed rest on the biological and clinical sciences, just as Flexner proposed. However, it adds that the knowledge base of the nurse rests upon a more general understanding of the above areas as they are appropriately integrated with the social and behavioral sciences. When these areas are taught appropriately, they are intended to lead to an understanding of the social and cultural factors influencing the health of people from different economic and cultural groups (Fawcett 1984). Nursing is therefore ready to close the gap created by overspecialization in medicine and to extend important health care services to many underserved segments of the population. The implications are many. Among the most significant is the view that the tenure of nursing education should be extended to a minimum of four years of university training with a heavy emphasis on social science work, and that graduate education should be required for many nursing functions (American Nurses' Association 1965). With an upgraded and more uniform education, nurses should be accepted as equal members of a health care team.

Although this argument differs significantly from that advanced by Flexner, it too addresses health care as a system. However, whereas the medical model has emphasized the growth of knowledge, nursing emphasizes its distribution. Whereas the medical model has accepted specialization as a necessary feature of medical development, nursing has noted the gaps created in the health care system by an unbalanced emphasis on specialization. Finally, whereas medicine has improved its ability to cure disease, nursing is calling for stronger efforts in prevention and coping. For many this means that traditional ideas about the location of health care services need to be revised, and that, for example, the hospital should be seen as but one of a number of places where health care services can be delivered. Community or neighborhood clinics, hospices, and home visits are a few of the alternative arrangements that might become available as health care services are extended.

It is important to note that this argument has not only an abstract philosophical appeal, but also an influence on the subjective understanding of both nursing and medical students as members of each group think about their own professional role. However, as we will see, the nature of this understanding differs both within and between these two groups.

NURSING'S PERCEPTIONS OF MEDICAL DOMINATION

While the medical profession has tended to look upon the subordinate status of nurses as necessary for effective medical care, arguing that the superior training of physicians warrants greater authority, some advocates of the nursing argument are beginning to view medical dominance from a political standpoint. There are two essential aspects to the political side of nursing's argument. The first aspect places the struggle between nursing and medicine within the framework of the struggle between men and women (Ashley 1976; Melosh 1982, 7; Gibson 1984). The second views the difference in authority, rewards, and status as a function of the relationship that the two professional groups have to the market in general. This relationship is said to have resulted from the political success that physicians achieved in controlling the training and placement of nurses, especially during the early part of this century.[4] By emphasizing the political aspects of the physician-nurse relationship, nursing has issued an important challenge to the view that medical dominance is necessarily in the interest of better health. Nursing has challenged medicine's argument on political grounds and in so doing has initiated a reexamination of the nature of its own profession.

In classifying the conflict between medicine and nursing as an aspect of the struggle between men and women, nursing is confronting both the expectations of the medical profession and the historical inability of many nurses to strive for professional autonomy. In other words, this perspective helps explain not only the subordinate status of the nursing profession, but also the submissive attitude of many nurses. According to this view, the fact that the ranks of nursing have been filled with women with very different motivations, many of whom saw nursing as secondary to their role as wives and mothers, has historically diluted the influence of those who have viewed it as a primary career. Moreover, a long-standing conflict between the professional and humanitarian roles of nurses has placed nursing at a disadvantage in relationship to medicine. It is not that the two goals are inherently in tension; after all, doctors are expected to be both professional and humane. However, as Melosh (1982, 24) points out, for many traditional nurses, the professionalization of nursing, with its call for higher education and the development of a specific body of knowledge toward the pursuit of autonomy, was viewed as unwomanly and as depreciating the work that nurses performed.

The lower status given to woman's work provided a very difficult climate for those nurses with higher professional aspirations. While both medicine and nursing require the performance of a number of routine tasks, medicine has managed to associate itself with less routine, more discretionary tasks.[5] Nursing, however, has been identified with routine tasks such as bathing and cleansing. According to the nursing argument, the identification of nursing with these tasks was consistent with the general perception of the caring, nurturing role of women. While such work in and of itself is extremely important for health care, it does not carry with it any special status in societies that give high priority to technological medicine.

From the standpoint of the nursing argument, the association of nursing with routine tasks has been successfully enforced through physicians' historical ability to control the health care market and the training of other providers. Some evidence for this view has come from sources that are relatively disinterested regarding the legitimacy of the status difference between doctors and nurses. As Starr points out, until the late 1800s and early 1900s, physicians perceived themselves to be in a precarious professional state, one that they felt required considerable protection against lay healers and unscrupulous colleagues who would cut fees to attract a share of the market. Many physicians perceived nurses as an additional threat, suspecting that, given the opportunity, nurses would usurp physicians' prerogatives in caring for the sick. Thus, to enhance their own professional status, physicians placed artificial constraints on the training and activity of nurses (Starr 1982, 78–145).

Proponents of the political interpretation point out that the development of the modern hospital gave physicians a strong influence over the nursing profession (Kalisch and Kalisch 1978, 131–66; Ashley 1976, 9; Bullough and Bullough 1978, 297). Since hospitals were dependent upon physicians for business, the nurses hospitals employed were required to be especially attentive to the physicians' desires. Moreover, since physicians initially owned or controlled many hospitals, they held direct authority over the hospital nursing staff. Finally, many of the training schools founded to teach young women to become nurses were financially dependent upon the hospitals with which they were affiliated. In return, schools provided the hospitals with a continuous flow of inexpensive labor. This arrangement enabled physicians and their hospitals to exert a strong influence over the available pool of nurses, and hence to control wages.[6]

A NOTE ON METHODOLOGY

In the following sections we look at some of the ways in which some medical and nursing students hold the medical and nursing arguments. We do not know if this sample is representative of opinions of students in these fields as a whole, and it is not our aim to conduct a survey, a research method that has some limitations in relation to our purpose. Opinions on a given topic may be extremely fluid, and what counts as representative one day may not be representative the next. More important, because the topic studied by survey research is predefined by the researcher, little can be done to understand how the topic shapes the subject's life and thoughts. Survey researchers can ask a person to rate the importance of an issue, but they cannot explore the themes of everyday discourse to understand how a certain topic is incorporated into the routine of practical thought. Finally, opinions tapped by survey methods may be grounded to different degrees in rational justifications, but the survey does not test the strength or the rationality of the justifications.

The method used in these interviews probes the justifications people give for their views about the proper sphere of authority for nurses and physicians. The project may be conceived of as an exploration of applied philosophy. By probing the justifications for professional authority that different students provide, the project aims to understand the points of tension and conflict that exist both within one person's scheme of justification and among the justifications held by different people. In that way we can better locate the differences between the expression of a well-formulated argument and its reception by those training to be professionals. We asked participants to voice their own thoughts and to respond to counterarguments. The interviewer developed some of these arguments.

However, many were developed by earlier subjects, and the interviewer introduced them to reflect an opposing point of view.

Subjects included medical and nursing students representing a variety of backgrounds and perspectives. In addition, both the medical students and the university-trained nursing students had been exposed to
issues relating to medicine and society, and thus many of the issues raised
in the interviews were not completely new to them. We expected that the
students would differ in their ideas about the proper relationship between
doctors and nurses. By probing their responses to questions about the
authority and autonomy of the various health professions, we hoped to see
the different ways in which a point of view is held and the way in which
different students react when their own favored view is presented with certain obstacles. We can also see the tensions that might exist between the formal arguments for medicine or nursing and the subjective understandings
that students have, both of these arguments and of their implications for
professional autonomy.

STUDENTS' SUBJECTIVE UNDERSTANDINGS
OF PROFESSIONAL AUTONOMY

Ultimately the argument for providing greater autonomy to the nursing
profession rests upon two premises. The first is that doing so will close the
gap created by specialization in medicine and will thereby improve the
quality of health care and make it available to an increasing number of people. The second is that knowledge of social and behavioral sciences will
provide a necessary complement to the physician's greater training in the
physical and biological sciences, and thereby mandate a reconsideration
of the boundaries between professional groups. We treat each of these issues in turn. Then we explore the extent to which students in both medicine and nursing understand the arguments for professional authority.

The Distribution of Health Care

While both medical and nursing students frequently addressed issues relating to the quality of health care on an individual level with little prodding,
medical students often had more trouble perceiving issues relating to the
social distribution of health care. While there were notable exceptions in
these interviews, university-trained nursing students, perhaps because of
exposure to a certain faculty point of view and their distance from the
hospital, tended to respond to the issue of distribution more spontaneously
than either medical students or hospital-trained nursing students.[7] Even as
the initially open-ended questions were narrowed to help the respondent
focus on problems of distribution, medical students frequently found other

modes in which to respond. It was not that they were consciously avoiding the question; it was simply that other thematic structures seemed to dominate these students' concerns.

For example, the interview with Ann, a fourth-year medical student, was held in her office while she was on clerkship duty in a primary care unit of a teaching hospital. In the early part of the interview Ann had expressed strong respect for, and dependency on, the nursing staff. The discussion was interrupted by a patient who had returned to the hospital to keep her second appointment. The patient had originally visited the primary care unit complaining of a cold and back pains. It was also found that her blood pressure was high. By the time of the second visit the first two problems had improved, and Ann spent the session talking to the woman about her blood pressure and recommending some simple changes in diet.

When the patient left, the interview continued. Ann was asked whether anything that she had done could not have been done equally well by a trained nurse. Ann responded that she wondered about that herself, especially within the field of pediatrics, her anticipated specialty, where, she reported, much of the work is routine. She also observed that, because of the routine nature of that kind of medicine, many pediatricians seem to leave the field for more technical subspecialties. The interviewer then asked whether this meant that Ann's own education might gradually induce her to leave an area of need because of the routine nature of the practice. The question was intended to leave an opening for a discussion about the priorities and the distribution of medical service, without necessarily pushing the conversation in that direction. However, Ann's response took the question in another reasonable direction. She spoke of her own interests, responding that she intended to work with adolescents because she enjoyed the social contact more than most medical students.

The questioning then became more direct. Ann was asked whether it is appropriate for medical schools to put high achievers through intensive programs in order to do routine work. Again her response was on a personal level: she loved this kind of work. The interviewer then asked, in reference to the session with the patient, whether this kind of counseling was an efficient use of personnel. Her response continued within the same mode that she had set previously. She considered it a real triumph that the patient, who was black, had returned to the hospital because "among the population [poor and black] the attrition is very high." The interviewer then became quite direct, speaking first about the projected oversupply of physicians and asking whether it was truly a problem of oversupply or whether it was an oversupply only in the context of the present structure of medicine, in which patients must come to the physician located in a hospital. Ann responded within an individual-medical mode, stressing the consequences, such as possible stroke or heart attacks, should the patient not come back. She did not address the political or the economic implications of the question. Nor did she address these problems for the many patients who, as she had noted earlier, do not come back.

A few days later, a response in an interview with three graduate students in nursing provided a sharp contrast to Ann's. One of the nurses, Nancy, was black and worked in a community facility. The interviewer reported on the session between Ann and her patient and on the interview with Ann that followed. Nancy responded that "in terms of the black community [she] could not envisage an oversupply of physicians or nurses," and she wondered why the physician was in a hospital rather than in a neighborhood health center.

Ann's response was not unusual. The tendency to deflect questions having political and structural implications and to perceive them as simply questions involving either personal inclinations or individual medical judgments was quite common in the interviews with medical students. The links between medical education, medical practice, the distribution of medical services, and the general health of the society were not easy for some of these students to perceive. Even beginning medical students, who, unlike Ann, were not already socialized into the thought patterns of the profession, gave similar responses.

Maria was a 26-year-old, first-year medical student. She was born in Puerto Rico but had lived on the mainland since she was 2 years old. Maria's educational background was unusual for a medical student. Like many medical students she had graduated with a major in chemistry and biology, but before entering medical school she trained for an additional 3 years to become a physician assistant with a specialty in pediatrics. She described her physician assistant training as very rigorous, observing that it was narrower in scope than medical school but of greater depth. Clinical experience began in the first year and continued through parts of the second and third years. She said that within a few months after she began practice she became frustrated with the limitations placed on physician assistants and decided to apply to medical school. She now planned to continue her medical training for 10 more years and to practice in obstetrics. During the course of her training as a physician assistant, she had spent some months working in clinics in both Puerto Rico and Colombia, and she intended to practice in Puerto Rico when her medical training was complete.

Perhaps because of her clinical experience, Maria was especially sensitive to certain unnecessary procedures that resulted in higher cost for medical treatment. Describing her present part-time job as a blood/gas technician in a local teaching hospital, she went into great detail about physicians who order routine tests on an emergency basis, thereby increasing the cost. She was critical also of the medical school for not teaching its students about cost containment. She reported that the training program for physician assistants paid considerable attention to this issue.

As Maria concluded her comments on cost effectiveness she conjectured whether she would be likely to change the situation after her 10 years of medical training. This off-the-cuff comment was significant, because we had earlier discussed her interest in rural and Third World medicine as well as her work in Colombia and Puerto Rico. The interviewer now tried to connect these interests to Maria's concern for cost effectiveness.

> **Interviewer:** If you had your choice, and given the training you had before this . . . and given a different perception by doctors and patients, especially doctors, would you have felt comfortable with the knowledge you have as a physician's assistant in doing what you feel needs to be done in rural medicine and Third World medicine?
>
> **Maria:** When I was there, when I was in Colombia, I'd say about 95 percent of what walked into the office was . . . just acute illness that anybody who had a little bit of training in infectious disease or pharmacology could have handled. I don't think it needed a physician to handle it and so I, myself, would have felt comfortable doing that. Most of the chronic cases . . . were so bad they went someplace else and they wouldn't even bother coming to the clinic because they were very bad off. But most of the day-to-day people who came in were just acute care things that I could have handled. Yes. They've even done studies on that and most of the auxiliary people in Africa and South America can do almost 100 percent of what walked into the clinic and 90 to 95 percent of what goes into the clinic. I was talking to a pediatrician when I was working in [a large U.S. city]—you know it's a big city and general pediatrics people were very bored with what they did. . . . In cities like ——— I don't think it's very challenging to work just in general pediatrics.
>
> **Interviewer:** Given your goal, which is to work in these [Third World] areas, given that there are legal limitations on what you can do, putting that aside for the moment, what are you getting here that is adding to your ability to perform?
>
> **Maria:** I guess if I didn't have the law to contend with . . . if I needed to learn anything else, I could have done it on my own rather than come here.

While Maria showed considerable sensitivity to issues of cost on an individual level, she had more difficulty addressing this problem on a structural level. Although she believed that most of her training would be irrelevant for the kind of work that she wanted to pursue, she did not address the issue of cost effectiveness as she responded to questions about the additional 10 years of medical education that she projected.

A number of classical studies (for example, Becker et al. 1961) have pointed out that during the course of medical education subtle pressures develop propelling students toward specialization. Although the interview with Maria was conducted at the end of her first year, these pressures were already visible as she began to make plans for pursuing her residency after graduation.

Maria: When I came here I didn't know how difficult it was . . . to get a residency. . . . We had a talk on how to choose a residency program, and you know some hospitals are really wanted by students, so it's very hard. You can get 500 applications for three slots or six . . . and there's a lot of competition out there, too. It just seems even worse when you get here.

Interviewer: What do you do to make yourself . . .

Maria: More . . .

Interviewer: More desirable?

Maria: They told us to write a paper and they said to do research. Get into research; everybody should get interested in research. I've never been interested in research, and then lately I've been thinking what could I do that, you know, might be a good little project.

While Maria has not abandoned her original goal of serving areas of need in Third World countries, she is already feeling other influences that may alter that goal. Unlike Ann, however, when pressed, Maria was able to address the issue of physician dominance. Indeed, as a physician assistant, she experienced the frustration of having her own training underused. Yet even for Maria these are largely issues of personal import, having to do with her own sense of frustration. Her sensitivities are clearly consistent with the nursing argument. She is aware of problems of inefficiency and cost. She has a real interest and a demonstrated commitment to providing a more equitable distribution of medical services. Yet her sensitivities to these issues do not lead to a critical analysis of the health care system itself or the priorities it represents. She is aware of some of the changes she is undergoing as she ponders ways to become more attractive to residency programs. She does not see these changes as a response to the way health care is structured socially or politically.

When questions that could lead to an examination of the location and distribution of health care are continuously deflected and interpreted as questions about the personal inclinations of practitioners, the boundaries between professional groups are likely to be perceived as fixed by some natural order. When they are viewed in this way, the jurisdictions of different professional groups are unlikely to be seen as matters for conscious choice and deliberation. Since the nursing argument is primarily an argument about professional jurisdiction, we can expect that some forms of resistance to it can be traced to a conflict over the nature of professional boundaries.

Professional Boundaries

While the role of the physician occupied a central focus of the nursing student's discourse, some medical students had to be reminded that the nurse played any role at all in health care issues. For example, Michael, a first-year medical student, was asked to describe what he had just referred to as "the rungs of the ladder." He began with the "lowly premedical student" and ended with the surgeon. When he finished, the interviewer remarked that Michael did not mention the roles of other health professionals such as the nurse, and asked Michael how he viewed these people. Michael replied,

> Unfortunately this may seem arrogant to you, but they are basically all subordinate to the physician. The physician is the one who makes the rules, he's the one who makes it go, he's the reason the others have jobs.

Until this point in the interview Michael had not mentioned other professional groups. Rather, he seemed to regard them as a taken-for-granted part of the medical environment and, as the above quotation indicates, had little inclination to question the hierarchical relationship that he described. Nevertheless, Michael was very quick to pick up on interview cues and to shift his response when it seemed appropriate to do so. When asked whether the situation that he had just described was to be thought of as "a natural characteristic of medicine or the result of the way it happens to be structured," he entered into a lengthy and critical analysis of the role of the AMA and of the inherent value of nurses. In response to this question he seemed to offer a view of existing professional boundaries that is more consistent with the nursing argument:

> I think it is more of a characteristic of American medicine, because the education that the nurse gets puts her in a position where she could easily make many of the simple diagnoses and certainly carry out most of the interventions that are necessary. Unfortunately she has little authority or autonomy. So she is legally subordinate to the physician. So it's partly cultural, partly legal.

Here Michael shifted his emphasis, stressing the cultural and legal components of medical dominance. As the interview continued, the focus shifted further, and Michael began to highlight the political aspects of medical dominance. He appeared to echo some of the more radical expressions of what we have called the nursing argument. The interviewer began by asking why Michael thought that the nurse is culturally and legally subordinate. Michael answered,

> Doctors want authority. Basically it's a situation where any person in power will do anything that he can to attempt to hold that power and expand upon it. About the turn of the century the physician became one of the most respected and powerful beings in this country, and with that respect came corruption which is almost inherent in any form of power. The physician is susceptible to that and is almost into that arrogance or power-seeking nature, and I think the situation has come about partly through the efforts of the AMA to increase the power of the physician.

In contrast to the corruption and quest for power used to characterize the medical establishment, Michael described the nurse as well qualified to take on more responsibility. "The nurse knows the patient better than the physician does, and the nurse sees the patient more on a day-to-day basis than the physician does and interacts more with the patient's family, so that the nurse is probably more qualified to make a diagnosis on the basis of these criteria." At this point Michael had essentially recapitulated the nursing argument in his own terms and, perhaps in response to his perception of the attitude of the interview, had moved from suggesting that the borders between professional groups are fixed by some inexorable force to suggesting that the boundaries are political constructs established to serve the interests of the medical profession. At this point Michael's response is not much different from that of Nancy who, when speaking of the role of the hospital and the subordinate position of the nursing staff, responded, "Well, hospitals were established for the convenience of the physician. All the patients, laboratories, x-rays, libraries, etc., are there for the convenience of the physician to do his little thing and leave."

However, in contrast to Nancy, Michael's response did not appear spontaneous. Rather, it seemed to be molded as he tried to read the interviewer. Following Michael's depreciation of the motives of the medical profession and praise of the nursing profession, the interviewer pressed him with a concrete example. "What if a nurse told a dying patient that he was dying when the patient asks, even though you disagree that the patient should be told. What kind of reaction would you have?" The question asks for a decision about a problem that, given the implications of the nursing argument, should come under the nurse's domain. The clinical judgment has already been made by the physician—the patient is going to die. The question to be answered is who will have authority to decide whether the patient should be told that death is imminent? If, consistent with the reasoning of the nursing argument, the nurse knows the patient better than the doctor does, one would expect that the nurse's jurisdiction would be granted in this case. At the very least one might expect some hesitation, since the moral implications of the nursing argument seem to lead in one direction, while legal reality may lead in another. It was therefore somewhat surprising when Michael responded without hesitation, "I'd probably have her fired. She does not have the responsibility to act that way."

In Michael's initial response, the structure, boundaries, and authority relations are not challenged and are seemingly viewed as a part of the natural order of medicine. The doctor is "the one who makes it go." He is "the reason the others have jobs." Nancy viewed the structure as contrived, as established by and for the convenience of a small interest group—the physicians. While Michael arrived at this view after considerable prodding, he did not incorporate it into his ideas about the daily practice of health care.

There are differences in the way various students hold both frameworks: "the hierarchy is natural" and "the hierarchy is contrived." Some students, like Michael, are considerably flexible and are able to adapt to the other point of view without seeming to feel the tension. Others hold onto their preferred framework with considerable tenacity and regard every challenge as an occasion to plant their feet more firmly than before. We will see this kind of response in the next section, as we probe another aspect of the argument for professional authority—the claim of a specialized body of knowledge.

Professional Authority

Considerable disagreement and confusion seem to exist within the ranks of both medical and nursing students about the grounds for their claim to professional authority. Both the traditional argument for the dominance of the medical profession and the newer argument for the autonomy of the nursing profession rest upon the premise that a specialized body of knowledge places practitioners of the profession in a uniquely important position. There is a serious conflict within nursing about the appropriateness of this conception of the profession. This conflict is expressed in the struggle between university- and hospital-based nursing programs and is reflected in the responses of students in these programs to questions about the basis of professional authority. Similarly, there are considerable differences among medical students about the role that basic science courses are intended to serve in medicine. We found significant disagreement, uncertainty, and confusion about the overall relevance and utility of these courses. We will address these two conflicts in turn.

Within the nursing profession, there is considerable debate about the value of theoretical coursework as opposed to practical clinical experience. However, even students trained in the university, who accepted the importance of coursework in the social and behavioral sciences, expressed a strong need for more clinical work. An example appears in an interview with one of the more militant university nursing students. The interview ended when she had to leave for a clinical session. The student was attending the clinical class with considerable hesitation, because it was to be held in a hospital whose workers were striking, and the student did not want to cross the picket line. However, she felt that she could not afford to relinquish the clinical training and had therefore decided to attend the session, even though it meant crossing the line. Despite her doubt about the sufficiency of her own clinical training, the nursing argument maintained a strong influence over this student's perception of her future competence. She expressed concern that university-trained nurses would start their nursing careers with an initial clinical disadvantage when compared to students trained in a hospital-based program, but she also believed that this deficiency would be quickly overcome on the job. In the long run, she believed that the theoretical underpinnings of her training would better equip her for a professional role.

This feeling was not shared by students who were training in a hospital-based program. The students from the three-year, hospital-based program appeared to have been influenced by some aspects of the nursing argument, but they did not give much credibility to the training of the university students, which they considered clinically deficient. Even though their own training in the social and behavioral sciences was very limited, they did not express the view that they had missed something important by not attending a university-based program. In other words, these students accepted aspects of the nursing argument while ignoring some of its fundamental features. Much like their counterparts in the university, they expressed dissatisfaction about the dominance of medicine over nursing and did not see themselves as simply handmaidens to physicians.

Nevertheless, because their program in the social and behavioral sciences was very limited, and because no other credible case for an independent knowledge base was developed, the basis for their claim to a more independent role was unclear. With the exception of a few courses taken at a local four-year college, most of their time was spent in actual clinical work in the hospital and coursework directly related to this clinical apprenticeship.

To some extent the students in this program echoed the views of their counterparts at the university, voicing the opinion that nursing is an independent profession having its own diagnostic focus and procedures. As one of the seniors put it, "I see [nurses] struggling now to get free from under the doctor's control and . . . establishing their own professionalism." Yet these students granted that the physician must inevitably maintain greater authority and responsibility, and they did not counterpoise this concession with an insistence on a sphere for their own authority. "I think that there has to be something to be said about a physician having more responsibility. He does make most of the decisions. He has spent a lot of time and money and sacrifice to get where he is, a lot more school. I think you have to take all of that into account. He's on call 24 hours a day."

This attitude reflected the missing element in these students' claim to professional status—the ability to stipulate an independent knowledge base. It also reflected the prominence they accorded to the hospital as the context of practice. There was no acknowledgment, as was the case with some university-trained nurses, of the extended role of nursing beyond the confines of the hospital. Nor was there any discussion of the larger requirements of health care. For these reasons, their willingness to acknowledge the physician's superior responsibility paralleled the medical argument.

Greater responsibility arose out of educational and moral considerations. Physicians had more education, had sacrificed more, and hence deserved more. However, the same considerations were not extended to nurses trained in universities at either the undergraduate or the graduate level. In other words, their longer educational tenure was not taken as an indication of a legitimate claim to authority over hospital-trained nurses.

Of course many of the university-trained students were also willing to grant a degree of authority to the doctor, but more often this grant was restricted to areas of clinical judgment. In other areas, they acknowledged that the doctor does in actual fact have more authority than the nurse, but they were less likely to concede the appropriateness of this authority. The distinction between a recognition of actual authority and the willingness to grant professional legitimacy to such authority is important in determining how well students' responses accord with the nursing argument.

Judy was just completing nursing school at the university and expressed much bitterness about the financial debt she had accumulated in doing so. In responding to the dying-patient situation, Judy's initial confidence in her own right to speak her mind fades with the realization that she is facing a situation where power is unequal.

> **Judy:** Being the person that I am and very forward, usually speaking my mind, when I get into that situation, when I feel comfortable in my role I think that I would probably say something to the patient.
>
> **Interviewer:** What do you think the consequences would be?
>
> **Judy:** Probably I'd lose my job. I don't know if I'd lose my job. Would I lose my job? If I lost my job, wait a second, that's a different story.

The interviewer responded by reporting the response Michael had given a few days earlier: "A medical student's response was: 'If a nurse did that, I would get her fired.' What would you do if you knew that was the consequence?" Judy then concluded, "I probably wouldn't say anything."

Other university-trained nurses saw Michael as arrogant and questioned his assumption that he could successfully fire the nurse. None of the university nurses, including Judy, indicated that they felt the doctor had any special professional authority in this matter, and all of them felt considerable tension as they recognized the conflict between their professional role on the one hand and their institutional role on the other.

The response of the hospital-trained nurses to this issue was somewhat different. They granted that the physician had the primary authority, but they were not willing to relinquish their own moral responsibility if the doctor should fail to act appropriately. A number of the students, during their hospital training, had encountered similar cases of dying patients and reluctant doctors. While they felt that, as students, it was not their place to counter the doctor, they also believed that, as nurses, they would have both a moral and a legal responsibility to do so if the circumstances seemed to require it. In contrast to Judy, these students were very comfortable in handling the issue and clearly had given it considerable thought. Unlike those arguing the case for the expanded autonomy of nursing on the grounds of superior knowledge, these students simply felt that there are times when the patient has a right to know. In their opinion, the issue became a moral one when the doctor failed to discharge his responsibility. The important questions seemed to be whether the patient had a right to know and whether the knowledge would have done more good than harm.

The response of the hospital-trained students was limited in a significant respect. Their ability to deal comfortably with the dying-patient issue arose from familiarity with the hospital setting. Yet this same familiarity made it difficult for them to view the practice of nursing in other contexts. They were not inclined to view professionalization as a structural issue relating not just to the authority of different professional groups, but also to the setting in which health care was delivered.

A number of medical students had similar difficulties addressing the basis for the professional status of both nursing and medicine. Some accepted the legitimacy of their own profession's dominance without question, but they were unable to provide a clear justification for it. There was a vague feeling that having sacrificed so much, they deserved a good deal in return, and there was also a strong sense that their education was preparing them for a unique social role. Yet when asked to explain some of the concrete links between their training and their eventual practical work as physicians, they had difficulty explaining the relevance of their coursework in the basic sciences. A number of students were unable to comprehend how their present study of the basic sciences related to their future work as doctors. For example, when Michael was asked to describe the relationship between the basic science courses that he was now taking and the curative function of the physician, he responded bluntly: "Well, there is almost none."

This response is significant when viewed in the context of the well-formulated arguments of both medicine and nursing. While these arguments differ from each other in important ways, they both articulate an essential connection between the scientific and theoretical knowledge required and the professional work of the practitioner. A number of students had trouble connecting their own work in scientific areas to their eventual professional status. This was especially the case with both the hospital-trained nursing students and medical students. The failure to understand this connection presents an additional obstacle for nursing's quest for autonomy. Those medical students who are unable to perceive the connection between their own training in basic science and their clinical role as physicians will be unlikely to perceive the connection that the nursing argument attempts to make between study in the social and behavioral sciences and the expanded function of nurses.

Moreover, to the extent that there is a failure to grasp the relationship between theory and practice among medical students, one argument for their own professional autonomy is undermined. Instead of justifying their own professional status on the basis of the unique importance of the biological and clinical sciences for clinical work, students were inclined to justify it on other grounds. Sometimes, they saw their status as resulting from their special intellectual endowments: "Well, I was interested in some form of service and had thought about nursing or social work. Fortunately I was born with some intelligence, and so I decided to enter medicine." Sometimes the justification of their future status was based on their willingness to work hard and sacrifice in pursuing their medical degrees. However, since neither intelligence nor sacrifice is unique to medicine, these are not especially strong grounds on which to justify the special status and rewards granted to members of the medical profession. Thus it is not only the insights of the nursing argument that escape some students, but those of the medical argument as well.

Brian and Ned, two medical students completing the first year of their program, had very different perceptions of this experience. They were interviewed together over a seven-week period devoted to exploring two conflicting views about the significance of the early part of medical education and its relation to professionalization. Brian believed that each of the components of medical education had an important functional value, and he was thereby convinced that the medical profession rested on a firm intellectual foundation. He was also very skeptical of nursing's claim to professional status. Ned was very skeptical of the value of his first year in medical school, believing that it had little relevance to medical practice. While he was willing to grant that there was a small functional relationship between the basic science courses and clinical practice, he looked upon most of the work in the first year as a kind of hazing, intended to produce humility and gratitude. He was also much more sympathetic than Brian to nursing's claim to professional status. While Brian and Ned differed radically in their beliefs about the intellectual foundations of medicine and nursing, neither was able to express a clear connection between the theoretical side of professional education and the practical side of professional work. While both agreed that a certain amount of the vocabulary learned in the first year of medical school would be useful later on, they perceived other connections very loosely. Brian was unable to find a justification for medicine's claim to a unique body of functionally relevant knowledge, and Ned was unable to find a similar justification for nursing.

Sometimes Brian, expressing his frustration with the grind of his first year in medical school, admitted that his faith that it all would add up to

252 Money, Power, and Health Care

something might be his "own justification for suffering through this year.... If I don't tell myself that there is something to come of it, then I wouldn't be able to get any work done." In other words, having rejected Ned's view that the first year's coursework is just a rite of passage, akin to the hazing of a fraternity, he needs the belief that there is a functional and intellectual justification. Because Ned largely rejects the significance of the first year's work in the basic sciences, he is more skeptical of the doctor's claim to a special status. However, this skepticism implies that when he argues for elevating the importance of nursing, he is doing so on the basis of a reduced standard.

Their differing perspectives are reflected in a segment of the interviews that begins with a discussion of the reasons for the high status and rewards of physicians and continues with a discussion of the comparative status of physicians and nurses. The interviewer has just asked why doctors have such high status and incomes.

> **Ned:** I think doctors have power over life and death, and they're shrouded in a mystique of a profession.
>
> **Brian:** They have the knowledge because people know that they have worked damn hard, like their whole life.... They have years of education at the finest schools, obtaining the most important knowledge as far as health and sickness goes, and I mean that sort of endows them with a certain mystique, that they are [of] the stature to withstand the system, to put up with the pressures, to learn the material, to master it, to be able to physically practice it, and that's pretty good. There are a lot of jobs you can get with a lot less education, and therefore it just seems they demand less dedication, and this profession demands a whole lot, you know one hundred percent.
>
> **Interviewer:** Those are two different perspectives . . . as I see it, but go ahead.
>
> **Ned:** One reason it is so difficult is to keep people out, to make it seem like it's so tough to be a doctor.
>
> **Brian:** It is tough to be a doctor.
>
> **Ned:** It is tough, but I think it's tougher than it has to be.
>
> **Interviewer:** The difference here is that Brian is saying there is a lot of training that goes into this, it is very hard work, it requires a heck of a lot of dedication, and that the rewards that come out of this work and dedication are in some way a reciprocity for it; that is, people realize the kind of work that goes into being a doctor and are willing to reciprocate that with a certain high status, higher income, and perhaps more authority. Ned is saying, well it's tougher than it needs to be, shrouded. . . .
>
> **Ned:** People think it needs to be tough. I'm agreeing with him, and my first thought was in addition to what he said.
>
> **Interviewer:** You're agreeing, but let me see if you're really agreeing with him. It seems to me that Brian is saying people think it's tough and it really is tough, and you're saying people think it's tough and it is, but needn't be.
>
> **Ned:** Okay, there is that difference.

Interviewer: Let me push those two responses. Let me try Brian's . . . first. There are other fields that are tough too, that require dedication, hard work, like for example, nursing. From what I understand, it's a tough job. But the status is clearly not the status of a physician, the income is not nearly what a physician's is. How would you explain that variation?

Brian: I think the difference is explained by first of all the level of training there is. . . . There is still more training that a physician has to have; he is endowed with greater responsibility, and alternatively the success or failure of any treatment or any patient outcome will fall most probably on his shoulders. For sure in the patient's mind if not in the legal sense. . . . Therefore, his accepting greater responsibility is sort of commensurate with higher status.

Interviewer: Would you agree?

Ned: I agree that this is the standard explanation. Frankly, the disparity in income I don't think can be fully accounted for. I don't think you can justify it. I mean nurses do an awful lot, at least in hospitals and intensive care units. They are the ones there with the patients all the time. They have a legal responsibility just like the doctor. They can be sued along with the hospital and the doctors.

Brian: They don't carry buzzers or beepers.

Ned: No, they're on call too.

Brian: When they are out on the weekend . . . and you hear a beep, the male that stands up is not a nurse, but a doctor. He doesn't have the right to say I'm not coming in. He's got to get to the office.

Ned: But nurses are under a lot of pressure to come in and fill in for other nurses. . . . They work really hard also. It's not the same as a doctor.

Brian: I think their work is more mechanical though. . . . You're never going to see a doctor making a bed, you're never going to see a doctor feeding a patient, and so in the patient's mind, the nurse sort of becomes their friend and the doctor just sort of pops in and out and that means that the minutes are like sacred.

While Ned wants to make a case for nurses, he is able to do so only on the grounds of hard work. He does not raise the possibility that nursing may, through its own body of knowledge, make a unique contribution to health care. This may not be surprising, given the question that the interviewer asked. However, when the question of nursing's knowledge was raised, Ned failed to address it, and Brian saw it as proof of his point.

Brian: I think that says it really clearly, the social sciences . . . is . . . a body of knowledge that I consider accessible to anyone with any talent as far as being able to read a book. I can teach anyone that body of knowledge. Could I teach anyone the sciences, the biological sciences? Probably not.

Ned was more skeptical of the professional claims of medicine, believing that the teaching of biological sciences is more difficult than it need be. However, while Ned was generally sympathetic to the claims of nursing and Brian was not, neither paid much attention to the notion that a grounding in the social sciences could provide nurses with a unique professional identity. The essence of Ned and Brian's dispute over the status of nurses rested on the question of how hard nurses worked. It also rested on how accessible they felt biology was as compared to the social sciences. It should be remembered, however, that neither student was certain of the nature of the relation between the study of the biological sciences and the practice of medicine.

The responses of Brian and Ned suggest not only that some future physicians may have difficulty understanding the argument for an expanded professional status for nursing but also that their understanding of medicine's claim for professional status may be more fragile than is commonly thought.

The inability to articulate a strong rationale for the courses in the basic science program reveals a serious deficiency in students' understanding of their own professional identity. When students are selected for medical school, their performance in the basic, premedical science courses and their scores on national medical admissions tests, which emphasize scientific achievement, are perceived to count more than most other aspects of their college work. The undergraduate transcript of a medical student is generally filled with courses in the natural and the biological sciences, with a minimum of courses in other areas. As important as the clinical aspect of medical training may be for the medical student, it is not this aspect of the program that constitutes the distinctive feature of a medical professional. Seasoned nurses, and especially well-trained nurse practitioners and physician assistants, are often more than the clinical equals of any new physician. Quite correctly, when the medical argument justifies the strong boundaries between medicine and other health care professions, training in the basic sciences is an essential component of that justification. However strong one's belief in the viability of the medical profession, and however much one may feel that physicians deserve their income and their status, the inability to identify a reasonable connection between the theoretical component of medical studies and the practical component of medical work leaves a gaping hole in one's faith. More important, it precludes the formation of certain opinions about the roles of other professionals in a reconstructed health care system.

NURSING IN THE CONTEXT OF A
RECONSTRUCTED HEALTH CARE SYSTEM

Theory, Practice, and Professional Status

The difficulty that many students have with the rationale for an enhanced conception of the nursing profession may be partly due to the present characteristics of health care and the way in which the public image of nursing is molded. It may also be due to some of the real and intractable requirements of health care itself. These two factors are related. Some of the medical students who were interviewed associated nurses' work with the routine and the mechanical. For Brian, the nurse was the person who made the bed and fed the patient. As he put it, "You're never going to see a doctor making a bed, you're never going to see a doctor feeding a patient." Of course this remark is exaggerated both because of the extent to which it overestimates the routine nature of the nurse's work and because of the implication that the physician's work is rarely routine or mechanical. Yet it does make a point about the nature of professional work and about the relations between professional groups: professional training provides a level of skill and know-how that enables the professional worker to address contingencies that otherwise would be unmanageable. Theoretical knowledge is useful when it expands the area of effective practice.

The hospital, as the site of practice, reinforces the medical argument more than the nursing one. Within a hospital, many routine tasks need to be performed. Patients need to be bathed and fed and to have their bedding changed. While these jobs are as important as the surgery that is performed or the medication that is prescribed, they do not require extended training.[8] Of course, there is other work that does entail extended education. Yet much of this work is performed under the jurisdiction of a physician. While some hospitals and clinics have begun to expand the role of their nursing staffs, the argument for nursing makes more sense in the context of an analysis of health care on a system level. In this analysis, the hospital becomes only one of the arenas in which services are delivered, and crisis intervention becomes only one of the services provided. As one of the university nursing students put it,

> I think that the training of the physician is really pertinent when you have someone who has slipped through all of the prevention and is acutely ill, and someone has to figure out what is wrong and what needs to be done to reverse the process, but that should be like the last resort. . . . The health care system is upside down in terms of its priorities, in that we are not preventing poor health. But in terms of taking care of acutely ill patients we have the best health care system in the world, but I don't think we should have as many acutely ill people as we do.

When one fails to consider an expanded context for health care delivery, certain aspects of nursing's argument become difficult to sustain. For example, the idea that nurses should be equal members of the health care team makes fine rhetorical sense. However, when asked who should captain the team, many nursing students assume that a hospital is the setting under consideration, which leads them to respond, often reluctantly, that the doctor should. Indeed, one of the reasons that the dying-patient example created so much hesitation, backtracking, and confusion may have been that it led the students to presuppose the hospital as the arena of decision making. One can certainly understand why, in this setting, a doctor would be reluctant to turn over certain kinds of authority to a nurse. While the nursing argument makes a rather radical distinction between a nursing and a medical judgment, there are times when the two are difficult to separate. Suppose that a patient had a 90-percent chance of dying. Suppose, too, that the physician thought that telling her she would die would increase the chances to 95 percent. Should the responsibility, having shifted once to the nurse because a final determination had been made, now shift back to the physician because there is yet a small chance for life? Who decides whether a decision is a medical one and therefore the doctor's to make, or a psychological or social one which should be made by a nurse? Should the nurse or the doctor decide where jurisdiction lies? Clearly a doctor who does not consult an experienced nurse in this situation would be silly, stupid, or incompetent, depending on the circumstances. To neglect the nurse's insights would be to ignore one of the most important sources of information a doctor has. Moreover, a physician who establishes a climate in which nurses are reluctant to voice opinions or to make suggestions should not be tolerated by the staff or the administration. This is a matter of human decency, but it is also a matter of professional competence. The doctor who contributes to a climate in which relevant information is not forthcoming diminishes clinical effectiveness. Yet within the hospital setting it is not easy to divide ultimate authority for the patient's treatment.

Limitations of the Hospital Setting

The hospital places certain limitations on even the most highly trained nurse—limitations that are not placed on the physician. Even when hospitals have provided expanded roles for nurses—for example, through the development of nurse practitioner programs—they usually maintain strong limitations on the rights and responsibilities of the nursing staff. For example, the usual restriction that allows only physicians to admit patients places an important limitation on the authority of the nurse.

This kind of limitation is illustrated in an interview that took place in a primary care unit of a teaching hospital. A graduate student in nursing, now training to be a nurse practitioner, was working with an 84-year-old woman who had arrived from a nursing home with stomach cramps. Both the graduate nursing student and her supervisor, a certified nurse practitioner, had read the x-rays and determined that the woman needed a simple enema. After reviewing the record from the nursing home, however, the nurses had some reservations about the level of care that the woman was receiving and even more concern about the nursing home physician. Given the age and weakened condition of the patient, they determined that it would be best if she could remain in the hospital overnight to be given the enema. But the decision was not theirs to make. It required the concurrence of the primary care unit's physician, who, they both felt, would find a needed enema to be medically uninteresting and therefore would likely turn down the request. Between the session with the patient and the meeting with the physician, the supervisor coached the student as she practiced the strategy that would shortly prove successful in convincing the physician to allow the patient to be admitted.

The doctor was initially reluctant to admit the woman to the hospital, noting that cases of impaction were not very interesting to staff physicians. The student gently reminded him of the age of the patient, of her generally fragile condition, and of the difference between the facilities of the nursing home and those of the hospital. In doing this she was implicitly challenging the basis on which the doctor was making his decision and asserting the relevance of social and environmental considerations. Despite the importance of the nurse's insights, and the willingness of the doctor to listen to her concerns and ultimately meet her request, he maintained control over the decision regarding admission. The three professionals were acting as a team, but it was clear to all that the doctor was its appointed captain.

Role of the Nurse under Competitive Approaches to Health Care

It is interesting to speculate about the effect that the new competitive models of health care might have on the role of nursing within hospitals. On the one hand, there are many roles that nurses can perform as well as physicians and at lower cost. Competition between hospitals may lead to a redefinition of the nurses' role within that setting, allowing nurses to exercise a wider range of professional skills under conditions of increased autonomy (Fagin 1978; 1982; Freund and Mitchell 1985; Gillis 1983). The primary care unit described above is an example of a movement in that direction. Except for admitting patients into the general hospital and prescribing medication, the nurse practitioners had taken over many of the tasks formerly assigned to physicians. On the other hand, the reduction in hospital census, coupled with a possible oversupply of physicians, may lead doctors to resume many of the activities that recently have been delegated to nurses in some places. While the hospital will likely remain a place where the role of the nurse is defined by the needs of the physician, recent changes in its organizational and financial structure will have significant repercussions for both nurses and doctors.

The danger that we see for nursing at present is that the demand for market efficiency will encourage the traditionally powerful medical profession to tighten control over potential alternative providers. One possible response to the demand for competition is for the medical profession to exert an even stronger influence over the definitions of the roles of its legitimate competitors. We can see this occurring, for example, in the insurance market, in which the question of who should be eligible for third-party payment is being debated. As markets tighten through the introduction of cost-saving mechanisms such as DRGs, and as competition increases through the spread of HMOs, we can expect attempts to increase the control and authority of the medical profession over other providers. Such increased control would cushion the effects of these innovations on individual doctors. The success of these efforts will depend, to some extent, on the degree to which nurses and other health care providers can convince law-making bodies that increasing their autonomy can effectively address important, unmet needs. As nursing moves to gain more professional autonomy, it may find that a strenuous effort will be required even to maintain its present status.

Nevertheless, the full implications of the nursing argument seem to call for a reconsideration of the traditional structures for health care delivery. If the concern for professional autonomy is to be realized, nurses will probably need to begin to experiment with the development of health care services and facilities outside of doctors' offices and hospitals. It is possible that nurses might begin to develop alternative sources of care on the neighborhood and community levels, where the nursing staff itself could own or manage the facilities and hire physicians as needed.[9] Nurse-controlled associations might even begin negotiating with hospitals for the allocation of nursing services. While speculation along these lines is outside the scope of this chapter, it is clear that the nursing argument calls for some changes in the system of health care delivery.

CONCLUSION

In this chapter we have examined the way in which different groups of students relate to issues of professional identity, and we have tried to take note of some of the ways in which students understand the foundation of professional authority. While we have not attempted to assess the merits of what we have called the well-formulated arguments for nursing and medicine, it is, of course, clear that such an assessment would be useful if the evolution of the field is to be guided intelligently. We believe that if new professionals are to participate in guiding this evolution, they need to learn to think critically about the social context of their work. It is important, for example, for students to understand that arguments about professional autonomy and identity are not just arguments about the merits of different individuals. They must understand that such arguments are first and foremost about the needs of the health care system and as such must be addressed on this level. While the students that we interviewed may not be representative of the majority of nursing or medical students, it is likely that the tendency to reduce issues of professional status to questions about the inclinations and merits of individuals is fairly widespread. If so, it would be helpful to provide students with material that can initiate a critical analysis of some of the systemic issues of health care.

While our purpose in developing this chapter has not been to evaluate the well-formulated arguments themselves, we cannot resist the temptation to say a few words about the nursing argument.

In these times there is a tendency to be skeptical of claims to professional status. At a time when hotel managers, funeral parlor directors, and insect exterminators clamor for professional recognition, such skepticism seems healthy and well deserved. Nevertheless, because we are concerned about the gaps created by specialization and because we believe that health care services are not well distributed in this country, we believe that there is considerable merit in the argument that nursing is putting forth.

It should also be recognized that there are many questions that remain to be answered. For example, while there is a general recognition that the social and behavioral sciences should play an important role in nursing education, it would not be accurate to leave the impression that the nature of this role is unproblematic. There are many different conceptions of the social sciences themselves and many opinions about just which aspects of social science are most useful for nurses. While it may not be wise to try to forge a solid consensus on this issue, there is certainly room for much discussion.

While the argument for professional status is persuasive in many respects, it is important not to forget that there are problems related to professionalization in general, and we would hope that nursing might be able to develop along lines that can minimize some of these difficulties. As nursing itself points out, the professionalization of medicine has resulted in narrowing the scope of many specialties and intensifying the division of labor. These tendencies do have the advantage of providing more adequate treatment for certain kinds of illness. However, they also have the disadvantage of creating greater distance between the doctor and the patient. Nursing will need to be even more concerned about the tendency toward specialization that is found in moves towards professionalization. Nurses, as one student put it, "do more than just mop the brow and wipe the fanny," yet there are times when mopping the brow and wiping the fanny need to be done. In other words, the range of activities required for patient care is wide and varied. Some are quite routine and would, by themselves, require little specialized training. Some are essentially medical and might best be supervised or initiated by physicians. Others require a great deal of understanding of social and cultural factors and do indeed suggest the need for the kind of education that the nursing argument is calling for.

The concern is not about the establishment and recognition of professional identity per se, but about the kind of professional identity that will be established. Nurses may well need to develop stronger professional recognition and to open up avenues of autonomy and control. However, they need to do this while maintaining the nontechnical, nurturing role that good health care requires.

NOTES

1. While the 1923 Goldmark report addressed the issue of university education for nursing as a means of upgrading professional nursing, its stress was on the educational needs of the leadership of the profession; see Committee for the Study of Nursing Education 1923.
2. The emphasis on prevention is not, by itself, new to nursing. It can be found in the writings of Florence Nightingale. What is new is the use of this goal to argue for a more autonomous status for the profession. See Nightingale 1859, 6, 75.
3. Fagin 1977 uses Nightingale's emphasis on nursing's role in promoting health to argue for an expanded role of nursing in primary health care.
4. For a 1983 Missouri court case in which the Supreme Court of Missouri "eliminated the requirement that a physician directly supervise nursing functions," see O'Neil 1984, especially p. 103. This was the first case in which the expanded role of nursing practice was upheld in a state supreme court.
5. Bates 1975 elaborates the territorial ramifications of this issue.
6. Physicians therefore developed significant influence over the training of nurses, and many were intent upon limiting this training to the most routine understanding of health care; e.g., "Nurses' Schools and Illegal Practice of Medicine" 1906 quoting, from a French source, the resolutions of the "Congress for the Suppression of Illegal Practice":
   1. Every attempt at initiative on the part of nurses . . . should be reproved by the physician and by the hospital administration. 2. The programs of nursing schools and the manuals employed should be limited strictly to the indispensable matters of instruction for those in their position, without going extensively into purely medical matters which give them a false notion as to their duties and lead them to substitute themselves for the physician. 3. The professional instruction of nurses should be entrusted exclusively to the physician, who only can judge what is necessary for them to know. . . . The maxims should certainly be borne in mind by the physician who has dealings with the nurse, as a matter of simple justice to her that she be not encouraged to take steps that are not in her province.
7. Among the exceptions was a 39-year-old, first-year medical student who had been associated with a number of radical causes. This student objected to the treatment that he felt was provided to poor people by the medical profession, noting that "in this country it seems to me that the paradigm of medical economics is your money or your life."
8. The clinical importance of this seemingly routine work for well-trained, experienced nurses may be seriously underestimated. These occasions can provide the nurse with a good opportunity to assess the patient's needs and

condition in a way different from a structured clinical interview and examination.
9. These hypothetical experiments would be examples of nurses moving outside of traditional facilities and institutions to develop ownership and administration of organizations that provide nursing services to other agencies and facilities. See Dayani and Holtmeier 1984.

REFERENCES

American Nurses' Association, Committee on Education. 1965. "American Nurses' Association's First Position on Education for Nursing." *American Journal of Nursing* 65 (December): 106–11.
Ashley, Jo Ann. 1976. *Hospitals, Paternalism, and the Role of the Nurse.* New York: Teachers College Press.
Bates, Barbara. 1975. "Physician and Nurse Practitioner: Conflict and Reward." *Annals of Internal Medicine* 82: 702–6.
Becker, Howard S., Blanche Geer, Everett C. Hughes, and Anselm L. Strauss. 1961. *Boys in White: Student Culture in Medical School.* Chicago: University of Chicago Press.
Bullough, Vern L., and Bonnie Bullough. 1978. *The Care of the Sick: The Emergence of Modern Nursing.* New York: Prodist.
Committee for the Study of Nursing Education (Josephine Goldmark, Secretary). 1923. *Nursing and Nursing Education in the United States.* New York: Macmillan.
Dayani, Elizabeth C., and Patricia A. Holtmeier. 1984. "Formula for Success: A Company of Nurse Entrepreneurs." *Nursing Economics* 2: 376–81.
"Equal Access to Care is Nursing's Challenge." 1985. *American Nurse* (February): 1.
Fagin, Claire M. 1977. "Nature and Scope of Nursing Practice in Meeting Primary Health Care Needs." In *Primary Care by Nurses: Sphere of Responsibility and Accountability,* ed. by American Academy of Nursing, 35–51. American Nurses' Association.
———. 1978. "Primary Care as an Academic Discipline." *Nursing Outlook* 26: 750–53.
———. 1982. "Nursing's Pivotal Role in Achieving Competition." In *From Accommodation to Self-Determination: Nursing's Role in the Development of Health Care Policy,* ed. by American Academy of Nursing. American Nurses' Association.
Fawcett, Jacqueline. 1984. *Analysis and Evaluation of Conceptual Models of Nursing.* Philadelphia: F. A. David.
Flexner, Abraham. 1910. *Medical Education in the United States and Canada.* New York: Carnegie Foundation for the Advancement of Teaching.
Freund, Cynthia M., and Jane Mitchell. 1985. "Multi-Institutional Systems: The New Arrangement." *Nursing Economics* 3: 24–32.
Gibson, Rosemary. 1984. "Nurse-Midwives and Competition: Testing an Assumption." *Nursing Economics* 2: 42–6.
Gilliss, Catherine L. 1983. "Collaborative Practice in the Hospital: What's in It for Nursing?" *Nursing Administration Quarterly* 7: 37–44.
Kalisch, Philip A., and Beatrice J. Kalisch. 1978. *The Advance of American Nursing.* Boston: Little, Brown.
Melosh, Barbara. 1982. *The Physician's Hand.* Philadelphia: Temple University Press.
Nightingale, Florence. 1860. *Notes on Nursing: What It Is and What It Is Not.* London: Harrison.

"Nurses' Schools and Illegal Practice of Medicine." 1906. *Journal of the American Medical Association* 47: 1835.

O'Neil, Eileen A. 1984. "A Gavel Falls for Nursing: *Sermchief v. Gonzales.*" *Nursing Economics* 2: 102–4.

Starr, Paul. 1982. *The Social Transformation of American Medicine: The Rise of a Sovereign Profession and the Making of a Vast Industry.* New York: Basic Books.

9

Thirty Years of Change in Medical Education, Money, and Power: Differing Effects on Generations of Physicians and Clinical Practice

Harold M. Swartz and Ann Barry Flood

Few would deny that physicians have played a central role in the medical care system in America and have helped to shape the ways in which medical care services are supplied, delivered, and reimbursed. Scholars of our system have often focused on the influence physicians have had at the national, state, and county levels through such powerful professional groups as the American Medical Association. The assumption often implicit in this focus is that physicians have a unified viewpoint regarding the appropriate methods of delivering and paying for medical services, and the roles that physicians should take in developing and using these methods. Scholars have neglected to study the differences between the perspectives of those physicians who have been in practice for years and those who have newly entered it. A generation gap among physicians is evidenced by their differing conceptions of the functions of the medical care system, expectations about their roles in it, and ability to adapt to changes. The impact of these generational differences is exacerbated by two recent trends: physicians are working much more closely with each other as the predominant mode of practice changes from individual practitioners (or small group) to large group practice; and physicians as a profession have a greatly increased need to respond formally and informally to many societal groups, ranging from consumers to the federal government.

We gratefully acknowledge research assistance from Geraldine Pawlik, Research Assistant, Medical Scholars Program, Colleges of Medicine and Law, University of Illinois.

In this chapter, we focus on the effects of changes in medical education and in the broad environment of the medical care system on the experiences and perspectives of physicians graduated during the period 1955
through 1985. This group encompasses physicians who are at the height of
their careers, as well as new physicians. We compare the educational experiences of physicians graduated 30 years apart and contrast their attitudes and expectations.

The past 30 years have also witnessed an enormous increase in the
complexity of arrangements for the delivery and reimbursement of medical care, and in the knowledge and technology available to those providing medical services. We examine the differences in the environment of the
medical profession, focusing on three themes: *money,* especially the sources
of reimbursement for medical services (for example, physicians' fees) and
of funds for medical education; *power,* especially factors and agents that influence the clinical decision-making process, the medical services provided,
and the types of patient treated; and *technology,* especially the knowledge
base and medical instrumentation available for diagnosing and treating patients. We explore these three themes with reference both to the environment of physicians specifically and to social changes generally, since broad
social changes influence the roles and status of physicians.

We emphasize the perceptions of the various groups now involved
in health care decisions: students seeking to become physicians, physicians,
other health professionals, patients and their families, policy makers, and
society in general. Altogether the changes we review in this chapter have
involved profound shifts in the power and technical capabilities of physicians, leading to significant differences in the perspectives of medical
graduates trained 30 years apart.

Generational differences continually interact with other factors in
the environment of medicine and are likely themselves to lead to further
changes in the medical care system. They therefore should be taken into
account by those who seek to understand the medical care system and to
plan rationally for changes in it. For example, the degree of influence of
organized medicine (whose leaders tend to be senior physicians) over the
profession as a whole (whose composition includes many younger physicians) must be interpreted in light of these differences between generations. Health policy researchers, policy makers, and members of the
medical profession, among others, would benefit from understanding
these changes in the medical care system and appreciating their impact. Finally, medical educators need to take into account the causes and implications of these changes if medical education is going to prepare new
physicians to cope with the environments in which they will practice clinical medicine.

ENHANCED EFFECT OF RECENT SOCIETAL CHANGES
ON THE MEDICAL PROFESSION

Recent societal changes in power and money (described more fully in chapter 2) have had an especially profound effect on physicians, for several reasons. Since the early part of the twentieth century, American physicians have enjoyed a high degree of professional autonomy due to the technical complexity of their profession, their professional and legal status, and the success of efforts by organized medicine to ensure that society accommodates their professional and economic interests (Freidson 1970a; 1970b; Starr 1982). For many years, as a consequence of this autonomy, the profession of medicine remained relatively insulated from many of the changes occurring in most other segments of society. For example, while there were attempts to change the delivery of health care to the elderly and the poor (through Medicare and Medicaid, respectively), these initial actions were not directed toward changing the clinical decision making or professional prerogatives of physicians. Physicians were not being held accountable to the public directly, but to the profession and its standards of performance.

When these barriers started to break down, physicians began to be confronted with the same forces affecting other parts of our society; their right to make unilateral, unquestioned decisions regarding the provision of care was challenged. Physicians viewed profound changes in their power and control over their work as an assault on the formerly sacrosanct area of professional decision making. For example, increased pressures to restrict physicians' autonomy and question the motives and judgments involved in clinical decisions often lead to considerable frustration for physicians.

This is especially true of senior physicians who were trained in and used to making unilateral clinical decisions with little or no knowledge about costs and little concern for choosing the cheapest methods. Training of physicians 30 years ago virtually ignored the complex set of nonmedical factors that influence clinical decision making today. Confronted with tools to apply and a patient in need, the physician was taught to expect to do everything possible to help the patient and to be the patient's advocate in seeing that care is performed in an appropriate and timely manner. When new actors and nonmedical interests, such as the catastrophic costs associated with some care, are introduced explicitly into the process, they restrict the clinical options. Physicians often feel that their reduced control over clinical practice compromises their professional imperative to provide all necessary care and to be the patient's advocate.

A second factor explaining the profound effect of recent changes on physicians has been the increase in the number of people being educated in American medical schools and, even more important, the advent of a general belief that our country has too many physicians, rather than too few. In the 1950s, government and private concerns focused on redressing an apparently insurmountable shortage of physicians. The attitudes and expectations of physicians educated during this period strongly reflected the opportunities and power associated with a "seller's market," which existed because of a perceived shortage of physicians. Since then, the number of graduates per class has more than doubled. Competition for patients has grown and has recently become particularly visible as governmental regulatory agencies have removed constraints on advertising by health provider groups and introduced legislation and programs designed to promote competition among providers. Coupled with these competitive pressures, several commissions have forecast a physician surplus within a few years, particularly for secondary care specialists (see reviews in Tarlov 1983a and Schofield 1984). As a consequence of these developments, the new graduate of today perceives more restricted professional career choices and opportunities to practice than did the graduate of 30 years ago. Table 9:1 summarizes the differing career choices confronting graduates in 1955 and 1985.

That young physicians might have difficulty in being accepted into a residency program, or in successfully practicing their preferred specialties, is a concept alien to most of the mature physicians currently in active practice. In 1955, new physicians felt that, no matter what career options they chose initially, there would always be ample opportunity to shift into general practice, because there would always be a high demand for practicing physicians. This belief inevitably had strong effects on the attitudes and choices of physicians. In the past, specialty training generally was chosen on the basis of the student's desires, and choices could be postponed until two or three years into a general residency (Becker et al. 1961; Roller and Pembrook 1983). Today's student must consider practice opportunities and financial rewards and must select a specialty when choosing a residency program, which is done during the senior year of medical school (Roller and Pembrook 1983; Wagoner 1986). This process can be very competitive in the 1980s, especially for residency programs that are quite selective, due to their prestige, type, location, or any combination of these factors. In addition to comparing students for residency positions on academic grounds (such as grades received during clerkships, scores on National Boards Part I, grades in basic sciences, and class standing), the programs usually interview each student and consider these interviews when ranking applicants (Wagoner, Suriano, and Stoner 1986). Since most medical schools have agreements with other medical schools to permit a student to receive credit for a four-to-eight-week clinical rotation, a student interested in a competitive residency program will often complete a clerkship at the medical

Table 9:1—Patterns of Career Choices and Clinical Practice for Medical Students

1955	1985
Residency Training and Specialties	
1. Significant number of students chose a general practice internship, which to a large extent determined career direction, mode of practice, and even location of practice.	Virtually all students took three- to five-year residencies, including those going into general practice.
2. General practice was not a "specialty." All types of internal medicine were considered to be specialties.	Emergence of several different routes to train for general medicine; all required three- to five-year residency training. (Sixty percent of all residents were in primary care specialties including internal medicine, family practice, general surgery, pediatrics, and obstetrics and gynecology.) Subspecialties required additional training and fellowships.
3. Limited types of specialties.	Large numbers of specialties and subspecialties (24 major specialty areas), with development of general specialties (e.g., general diagnostic radiology) and subsubspecialties (neuroradiology, cardiovascular radiology). Eighty-five percent of all practicing physicians were specialists.
4. Abundant number of residency positions. Less attractive positions were filled by graduates of foreign medical schools.	Increased competition for residency positions, particularly for selected specialties. Waiting lists for some programs. Increased pressure to train more primary care doctors and fewer subspecialists.
5. Students planning to specialize initially chose between a surgical and nonsurgical program. After two or three years, they decided on a subspecialty.	Students generally must decide on a specialty during their senior year. Some advanced specialties begin after two or three years of residency training and may select candidates during their senior year, prior to the "transitional" residency.
6. High student interest in making research an important component of career, but most medical schools and residency programs had only modest opportunities for formal research.	Reduced student interest in research careers but increased formal opportunities as indicated by emergence of formal M.D.-Ph.D. programs and formal requirements for research components in some medical schools and residencies.

Continued

Table 9:1—Continued.

1955	1985

Location/Organization of Practice

7. An apparently large number of options for clinical practice; numerous sites actively looking for physicians.

   General perception of impending physician surplus with possibility of severe restriction of options in the near future.

8. Clinical practice in a solo or in a two-partner setting with informal arrangements for sharing evening and weekend coverage. Some multiple-physician partnerships and very small groups, but involvement in larger groups a source of suspicion among colleagues.

   Group practice accepted and most popular practice arrangement for new physicians. Increasing acceptance of legitimacy of working for a for-profit or large health care organization. Growth in forms of group practice continues, but not as rapidly as in the early 1970s.

Postspecialty Education

9. Military service (via "doctors draft") a routine part of male students' plans, usually resulting in two years of intermediate responsibility after residency and before private practice.

   Military service not a general consideration (3.5 percent of residency positions were with the military).

10. Continuing medical education (CME) a voluntary academic pursuit.

    Many states had legislation that mandated physician participation in CME, in response to pressure to maintain physician competency.

References by row number: (1) Becker et al. (1962); Benson et al. (1985); Keith and Drew (1985). (1,4,5) Roller and Pembrook (1983). (2) Tarlov (1983b). (2,3,4,9) Wagoner (1986). (3) "Future Directions for Medical Education" (1982). (4,5) Wagoner, Suriano, and Stoner (1986). (6) *OSR Report* (1979); Petersdorf and Wilson (1982). (7,8) Tarlov (1983a). (8) Freshnock and Jensen (1981). (10) O'Reilly, Tifft, and DeLena (1982).

school where the residency program is located, to be better acquainted with the faculty and therefore better able to compete.

In the past, prospective physicians could usually afford to forego such measures, knowing that there would be a large demand for practitioners of any specialty. In addition, if physicians did find their practice less satisfying than anticipated, they were reassured by the beliefs that there was a seemingly infinite number of sites in which to set up a practice, and that they could easily alter their practice to a type for which there was an ample supply of patients. New physicians in 1955 were thereby unusually well shielded from making career decisions on the basis of economic necessity, and experienced little or no insecurity due to limited opportunity.

In 1985, the 1955 graduates, who often occupy influential positions in medicine, complain that the attitudes of today's graduates toward choices of practice are offensively pragmatic and based on financial considerations. At the same time, they acknowledge that their own attitudes and habits—which they regard as appropriately professional—are not well suited for today's competitive situation.

Technical changes in medicine have also affected the physician's role in the medical care system. During the past three decades, medicine has significantly expanded its ability to understand many diseases at a basic level, and to use this understanding to improve the health of patients. This increased ability to affect the course of a disease is a relatively new aspect of clinical medicine. From the beginning of this century to the 1950s, the major gains in health had been due to the development of antibiotics and to public health measures (for example, sewage disposal and water treatment), which were essentially unrelated to individual decisions. Many diseases that formerly could be treated only by palliative measures are now amenable to medical intervention (for example, cures of Hodgkin's disease and leukemia by chemotherapy, and the use of intravenous enzymes to reduce the effects of myocardial infarctions). Under development are new therapeutic techniques, such as genetic engineering to replace defective or missing genes and to treat tumors selectively by monoclonal antibodies; and new diagnostic techniques, such as magnetic resonance and positron emission tomography (PET scanning), which can detect and characterize early anatomic and metabolic changes associated with diseases. Technical progress in surgery and intensive care has accelerated during the past three decades, especially for complex procedures such as organ transplants and artificial replacements, open heart surgery and neonatal intensive care.

The increased effectiveness of medicine and the potential for even greater and more accelerated progress are exciting developments for providers, especially for the specialists in the fields affected. These developments, however, usually carry an expensive price tag and may not easily pass the cost-benefit examination required of an overall improvement to society. The attempts of third-party payers or government to restrict or slow down the development and use of new medical technology place pressure on provider and patient alike, but are particularly frustrating for the physician who has been in practice for some time and who has witnessed the changes in the efficacy of medical care.

CHANGES IN MONEY AND POWER AS THEY
AFFECT MEDICAL EDUCATION

The Process of Medical Education and Professionalization

In this section we examine the nature of medical education (summarized in Tables 9:2 and 9:3), emphasizing the features that contribute to the acclimation of students to the culture and knowledge of medicine, and contrasting the experience of physicians-in-training 30 years ago and today.[1] Medicine has long been used as a primary example to describe the features of a profession. Thirty years ago, theorists describing the professional model focused on such features as the long period of training needed to obtain the specialized knowledge and skills demanded of professionals and to learn the culture of appropriate professional conduct (Greenwood 1957; Gross 1958; Goode 1957). In this model, senior members of the profession were charged not only with the training of novices, but also with selecting students who could meet the demands of medicine (that is, those who could enter medical school) and of a specialty practice (that is, those who could obtain additional training in a residency and a license to practice). These features were designed to ensure that each practicing physician could control his or her own behavior. In this way, each professional acted as a miniature organization, managing his or her work as a physician while enjoying almost complete autonomy in decision making (Flood and Scott 1978). Rewards for physicians included not only personal pleasure in performing their services well, but also recognition, prestige, and financial success.

Later, critics challenged the sufficiency of these controls, and asserted that the physicians' work needed to be evaluated and sanctioned—if not by the profession through peer review mechanisms and organization controls (such as admission by peers into a group practice or hospital staff)—then by lay members of society (Freidson 1970b). We will return to these issues but will focus first on medical education as a process of acquiring the knowledge and culture of medicine. Even if the importance of medical education in determining physicians' attitudes and behaviors has been exaggerated, the effects of medical education—and the differences in those effects due to changes in medical education over 30 years—should be understood by those who seek to understand such behaviors and attitudes.

During the past 30 years, medical educators have increasingly discussed the nature of medical education and how to develop competent decision makers; the involvement of professional educators in the four years of pre-M.D. education increased during the same period. These efforts appear to have had relatively little influence on the fundamental methods of acquiring clinical skills and knowledge, perhaps due to the nature of clinical practice and the lack of change in the residency phase of medical edu-

Table 9:2—Changes in the Nature of the Medical School Programs and Training Sites

1955	1985

Basic Science Years (first two years)

1. Very traditional teaching content and format in basic sciences (large group lectures and many laboratories).	Less emphasis, with none at some schools, on traditional content and format for teaching basic sciences (virtually no laboratories in physiology and biochemistry) and widespread explicit consideration of clinical relevancy; (all schools offered at least some clinical preparation during the second year, ranging from 78 hours to 964 hours).

Clinical Science Years (second two years)

2. Authoritarian teaching by clinical preceptors and their designees.	Clinical training essentially unchanged in style and setting.
3. Clinical education had heavy emphasis on learning techniques and medical procedures.	Clinical education aimed more to teach clinical principles; much less emphasis on technical procedures.
4. Designed to produce a physician capable of independent practice after one year of internship.	Designed to prepare for graduate medical education lasting at least three years before independent practice.
5. Clinical education used "charity patients," with medical students having considerable authority and responsibility for their care. Little contact with private patients; clear two-level system of patient care.	Clinical education used mixture of patients. Almost all patients were to some degree "paying" or "private" patients (following advent of Medicare and Medicaid). Some schools relied heavily on private patients in community hospitals.
6. Clinical education occurred in few sites, was almost always in large urban areas, and was exclusively hospital-based. Most school hospitals delivered tertiary care and depended on referrals.	Clinical education occurred in multiple sites (including small urban and rural areas) and types of hospitals. Increased competition for tertiary care patients caused need to develop primary care and outpatient sites to obtain patients; these sites were also used for teaching.

Continued

Table 9:2—Continued.

1955	1985

General Features of Medical School Education

7. Little or no role of professional educators; little emphasis on innovative approaches to medical education.

   Prominent role of professional educators (although declining somewhat from the 1970s); considerable emphasis on innovative approaches, including new approaches to medical education, especially for the first two years (such as problem-based learning or tutorial style sessions).

8. Sociomedical teaching nonexistent or very limited and entirely optional.

   Sociomedical teaching increasingly common; (41 percent of schools offered such curriculums during the second year, ranging from 10 hours to 135 hours; 50 percent of medicine, 40 percent of pediatrics, and 40 percent of family practice chairpersons said medical sociology was formally taught to medical students and residents). Portions required at some schools.

9. Relatively few students enrolled.

   More students enrolled and more medical schools operating (100 percent increase in the number of medical students and 50 percent increase in the number of medical schools).

References by row number: (1–7) DeMuth and Granvall (1970). (1,8) Siegel (1986). (4,9) Schofield (1984). (5,6) Petersdorf and Wilson (1982); Beaty et al. (1986). (6) Perkoff (1986); Fordham (1979). (8) Webster (1971); Petersdorf and Feinstein (1981). (9) Wagoner (1986).

cation (which for most physicians now occupies a period as long as or longer than medical school).

Medical education clearly is practice-oriented rather than directed toward teaching the student how to generate new knowledge. Practicing medicine in a rational and scientific manner is preached as the primary goal, but pedagogy emphasizes the acquisition of specific facts and, to a lesser degree, the learning of clinical concepts and recipes for identifying and treating diseases. Little emphasis is placed on understanding the fundamental principles and processes of pathology and therapy.

In most medical schools, students spend the first two years learning basic medical sciences (anatomy, biochemistry, microbiology, pathology, pharmacology, and physiology) in a format similar to that followed by much of their premedical undergraduate education but with more concentrated and time-intensive study in and out of the classroom. The emphasis is on the acquisition of detailed knowledge (often referred to as "rote

Table 9:3—Changes in the Clinical (Physician) Faculty and the Power and Support of Academic Medicine

1955	1985
Faculty Interests	
1. Comparatively few full-time clinical faculty.	Large increase in full-time clinical faculty (300 percent increase in size of medical school faculties).
2. Full-time clinical faculty had fairly extensive teaching responsibilities with little or no requirement for producing revenue via patient care or research.	Clinical faculty had extensive responsibilities for producing revenue via patient care activities or externally funded research. (Only 7,000 of 38,000 hospital-based physicians listed themselves as primarily medical teachers.)
3. Moderate research orientation of faculty; tenure or salary largely independent of research activities or external grants; grants were less competitive and required less supervision by faculty.	Some faculty with strong research orientation; salaries often dependent on funds generated by successful research applications to federal and other external sources. (8,500 physicians classified themselves as primarily in research; 97 percent of faculty with M.D. only reported research activity, with 27 percent spending 50 percent or more of their time in research; 90 percent of faculty with M.D.-Ph.D. reported research, with 45 percent spending at least 50 percent of effort on research; 95 percent of Ph.D.-only faculty spent their time at research, 50 percent of them doing nothing else.).
Support for Faculty	
4. Salary level of academic physicians relatively low compared to that of practicing physicians.	Salary levels below but closer to that of practicing physicians; salary varies more by specialty; for M.D.s teaching in basic sciences, salary is considerably lower.
5. Salary dependent almost exclusively on base salary from medical school.	Salary arrangements varied from no base to a substantial base salary and with a varying percentage of patient fees retained beyond the base salary.
6. Sources for medical school budget largely from university/state funds with increasing dependence on research grants.	Increase of 500 percent in medical center budget, largely due to increase in dependence on patient fees and somewhat on grant support.

Continued

Table 9:3—Continued.

1955	1985
7. Considerable amount of teaching by voluntary faculty who were primarily in private practice and who donated time to teaching.	Role of voluntary faculty variable, generally reduced in academic centers but of considerable importance in community-based clinical teaching programs.

Power of Faculty

1955	1985
8. Relative power of faculty within medical school based primarily on relative clinical importance of the specialty.	Power of individual faculty members and departments often related to their success in generating funds via successful research grants or via patient care.
9. Authority of faculty and other physicians vis-à-vis patients very high, especially for charity patients.	Considerable decrease in formal authority vis-à-vis patients.
10. Authority of faculty and other physicians vis-à-vis nurses and other health professionals very high and unquestioned; few occupational groups involved.	Increased role and authority of other health professionals often discussed and sometimes implemented; increased number of types of other health professionals involved at all levels.
11. Relationship with hospital administrators usually based on complete authority of physicians for all "medical matters"; authority of hospital administrators limited to "hotel services"; hospital administrators were usually physicians.	Complex relationships with hospital administration varying for university-owned and community hospitals. Hospital administrators participated in decisions formerly considered to be strictly limited to the professional staff. Administrators are often specially trained in hospital administration and without an M.D.

References by row number: (1,4,11) Petersdorf and Wilson (1982). (1,6), Wagoner (1986). (2–5) Roller and Pembrook (1983). (2,3,8) Jonas (1978), 240–50. (3) Beaty et al. (1986). (3,6,7) Petersdorf (1982). (1,2,3,5,6) Petersdorf (1980). (3,4) Petersdorf (1981). (10) Tarlov (1983a). (11) Shortell (1983); Starr (1982).

memorization"). This emphasis is underscored by the type of detailed examinations, such as the National Board Examination Part I, used by most medical schools as a gate-keeping mechanism for entering the next phase of medical education. Emphasis on memorization is also generated to a great extent by the students themselves. Their concern is often expressed as a belief that failure to know a particular fact may someday result in their harming a patient.

Many medical schools attempt during these first two years to imbue the students with a spirit of scholarly inquiry (Funkenstein 1971). For most students, and in most schools, this effort is in vain because the students are overwhelmed by the magnitude of the subject matter that they are asked to master, by the anticipation of the responsibility they will have as physicians to apply the knowledge correctly, and by the emphasis on memorization. Opportunities to participate in more scholarly learning are often available through elective or supplemental activities, but most students are fully occupied with attempting to master the required curriculum. The effort required to absorb this seemingly overwhelming amount of material is a disconcerting shock to many medical students, most of whom are accustomed to being recognized for their outstanding undergraduate performance (Coombs and Blake 1971; Johnson 1983). This consternation is furthered by students' discovery that their classmates' academic records are as good as or better than their own.

Conflicting expectations and goals arise from the contrast between this type of education and that experienced by the basic science faculty (almost all of whom have Ph.D.s rather than M.D.s). This contrast between physicians and scientists tends to enhance the attitude of young physicians that their learning should be directed toward the acquisition of practical knowledge relevant to solving patients' physiological problems, and not toward basic principles, which they see as appropriate for performing basic research in science rather than medicine.

The clinical phase of medical school usually takes place in a hospital environment. Today, it often begins in the second or even the first year of medical school and may include outpatient care, but the main part of the clinical phase occurs in the hospital during the final two years of medical school, after the basic medical sciences phase. During this phase, the student clerks spend full time participating in the care of patients, as well as being responsible for attending lectures and rounds and reading related material. They are junior members of a team that generally includes residents with varying years of experience, and attending physicians. Typically, during the first year of the clinical phase of education, students rotate every six to eight weeks through a required set of clerkships that address the major branches of medicine: internal medicine, obstetrics and gynecology, pediatrics, psychiatry, and surgery. The second clinical year consists of additional clerkships in specialty branches of these subjects and in other areas of medicine.

In the clinical phase, teaching is based on the various patients in whose care the student participates. Although some formal lectures may occur, the overwhelmingly prevalent mode of learning is through the student's direct experiences with patients and involvement in medical teams' discussions of patients. Socialization includes learning facts about and at-

titudes toward patients and the practice of medicine; it takes place in a
mentor-pupil relationship in which more senior medical students, residents, and attending physicians supervise and serve as role models.

In the residency (taken by virtually all students today),[2] the same type
of clinical education continues, usually for a minimum of three years and
often for periods of up to seven years. The student's experiences as a resident are similar to those of the clinical phase of medical school but involve
taking on increasing responsibility and authority.

The extensive use of the apprenticeship mode involving the actual
treatment of patients is not new to medicine during the period we are
reviewing (although the financial dependence of medical schools on fees
from patients did increase significantly over this period). As Petersdorf and
Wilson (1982, 1155) remind us, however, not all professional education
uses this model for training: "The necessity of caring for patients is unique
to medical schools. A business school does not manage, a law faculty does
not prosecute, nor does an engineering school build bridges, but a medical faculty does practice medicine."

This unique emphasis on education by practical experience results
in an unusually effective professionalization. Except for the first two years
of a seven-to-nine-year process (medical school and residency), education
occurs in a small group with very structured lines of authority; the teachers
and role models of the students are almost exclusively physicians; and clinical education takes place not at the university but in teaching hospitals
and outpatient clinics, where physicians have long been dominant. These
factors act together to expose students widely and persuasively to the values
and expectations of older physicians in general and powerful faculty physicians in particular. When the values of these physicians differ from students' initial views, strong professional pressures on students can be a
cause of considerable stress and a source of conflict between the generations of physicians.

In addition to these factors, there has been a major change in the
character of clinical education of physicians during this period: a lessening of emphasis on clinical care of patients who are hospitalized for complex, specialized needs. In the 1950s, almost all clinical training was
hospital-based, usually in a tertiary care hospital that received its patients
by referral due to either the complexity of the cases or the patients' lack
of sufficient insurance to cover catastrophic medical costs. This setting and
the types of medical problem and patient encountered in it contrasted
sharply with the environment of the majority of practicing physicians, who
spent most of their time in ambulatory care settings, treating paying patients with less acute and less serious medical needs. Physicians often experienced a form of professional culture shock when they entered private
practice. A whole new set of interactions with patients and their families

had to be learned as one switched from passive, dependent charity patients to patients who were more directly responsible for the financing of their health care and who had different expectations regarding their treatment from physicians.

The clinical education of today's student is more varied in setting, because other tertiary care facilities draw complex patients away from the academic centers, because patients are more likely to have some form of insurance and therefore are financially attractive to other hospitals, and because academic centers need to have outpatient sites and additional community hospitals since they cannot depend upon referrals to obtain sufficient numbers of patients. Thus, there is often greater congruence between the educational experience and the typical medical practice of today's students. Nonetheless, the majority of academic physicians in university-owned hospitals continue to value more highly the treatment of tertiary care patients and the central importance of the academic-center hospital for preparing students to care for all medical exigencies they may encounter over the course of their careers. While there is more "clinic" experience in clinical education, there is still a gulf between what the faculty teaches as important clinical activities and what the majority of doctor-patient encounters actually entail.

Professionalization and Attitudes toward Patients

Medical education focuses on the diagnosis and treatment of an individual patient presenting with some medical complaint. There is a strong emphasis on the need to do everything possible to diagnose and treat the problem of that particular patient. Although today some discussions may occur about the larger aspects of providing medical care (for example, the problems of providing care to the uninsured, containing medical care costs, or identifying special health care needs of the elderly), the focus during clinical encounters necessarily remains on individual patients. Inevitably this emphasis becomes incorporated into the attitudes of most medical students and residents about the rights, duties, and appropriate focus of attention of physicians. The student is taught that each patient is different and that only with knowledge of the individual patient can one accurately and effectively carry out diagnostic and therapeutic procedures. Because each patient has specific medical needs fully understood only by the attending physician, the student learns that physicians require complete discretion to decide appropriate medical actions for a given patient. This discretionary authority over the medical care of patients brings with it responsibility for making appropriate decisions.

This traditional view of medicine portrays a profession in which clinical decisions are based solely on the health needs of the patient, and any

intrusion of economic concerns into medical decisions is considered highly undesirable. These attitudes encourage physicians to view the financial
rewards, prestige, and power traditionally enjoyed by physicians as for-
tunate but deserved byproducts of a process whose primary objective is the
responsible and wise provision of available care to patients. Lack of concern for economic aspects was reinforced for physicians trained in the
1950s by a system that assured them of high financial returns without needing to focus on profit.

The foregoing model of professional values was clearly predominant
in medical education 30 years ago. It remains strong today, especially for
senior academic physicians, who were trained in it and who have remained
relatively insulated from changes confronting the nonteaching physician.
Central assumptions of this model and its attendant attitudes and behaviors are being questioned today. Do or should physicians make judgments without considering their financial impact? Are high financial
rewards for physicians appropriate? Should the individual physician have
autonomous control over clinical decisions? That physicians in training are
among those raising these questions is another source of tension between
academic physicians trained 30 years ago and today's students.

A major change affecting the attitudes of medical students toward patients has been the shift of teaching patients from being charity cases to
paying clients (at least paying with government insurance) and from
providing care in large public hospitals to doing so in a variety of teaching hospitals. In 1955 medical students dealt primarily with charity patients, whose free care was justified in part by virtue of their being
"teaching material." The typical teaching hospital was a hospital whose patients were almost all publicly supported. Care took place in large, open
wards, and patients received only minimal amenities.

In 1985, by contrast, physicians in training provided care to a much
broader spectrum of patients, most of whom were similar to those they
would encounter in their practice. Moreover, most patients, including the
poor, had their hospitalization paid for by third-party payers and, as such,
were likely to expect to participate in the selection of clinical alternatives
and to be treated with dignity and respect. The large wards were gone even
from the large, public teaching hospitals; patients in teaching hospitals
were more diverse, including private as well as public patients, both of
whom could choose not to participate in the teaching programs.

In spite of these changes in the status of teaching patients, significant
differences do persist between the care of public patients and that of private patients. These differences arise because the extent to which clinical
decisions are supervised prior to their implementation varies (Jones 1984;
Flood 1985; Flood and Scott 1987). In hospitals or on wards that use a
"learn-by-doing" model, public patients are more likely to be treated by

teams of residents. In this situation the resident has almost exclusive responsibility to diagnose and treat the patient, and the faculty member and senior residents review the clinical decisions and orders that a resident has carried out. Private patients are more likely to be treated in hospitals or on wards where a "learn-by-example" model is followed. The attending physician takes a much more active role in caring for the patient; the resident learns by observing and participating in the decisions and having his or her decisions reviewed prior to their being implemented. Because these models differ, the care received by public and private patients can differ. Several studies have documented that patients in the more closely supervised teaching setting were likely to have better outcomes, fewer services, and lower costs (Flood 1985; Schroeder and O'Leary 1977; Martz and Ptakowski 1978; Garg et al. 1982; Boice and McGregor 1983; Jones 1984). Not all teaching hospitals are alike, and the type of setting in which new physicians are trained may influence both their attitudes toward patients and their relationships with senior physicians.

In summary, although the intent is seldom made explicit, medical education has been extraordinarily effective in professionalizing the student's attitudes and behavior, not only in regard to the classic professional values of the Hippocratic oath, but also with respect to doctor-patient and doctor-doctor relationships.

Types of Students Entering Medical School

Table 9:4 summarizes some of the expectations and demographic characteristics of students selected to attend medical school in the years 1955 and 1985. With a few notable exceptions, the differences are modest. In 1985 medical students were in general more diverse in their parental and educational backgrounds than in 1955 (Funkenstein 1971). White, upper-middle-class values and expectations still predominated, and most students (including women and minorities) tended to acquire these values (if they had not already had them when they entered medical school). One major change was the increased role of women in medicine (as in other aspects of society). The proportion of women medical students has increased significantly (from about 9 percent in 1963 to about 30 percent by 1985), though women still form a minority in the profession and are still disproportionately likely to choose primary practice over academic medicine or specialties (Eisenberg 1983; Benson et al. 1985; Iglehart 1986). Similarly, the proportion of minorities (that is, Afro-Americans, Hispanics, and Native Americans) increased from about 3 percent in 1955 to about 9 percent by 1985. Several studies of practices of minority physicians have reported that minorities are also disproportionately likely to choose primary care specialties, to set up practice in medically underserved areas,

**Table 9:4—Changes in Characteristics of Students
Entering Medical School**

1955	1985

Demographics of Students

1. Relatively homogeneous (white, upper-middle-class and male).

Significant variation in background of many students, especially an increase in numbers of female, minority, and older students. (In 1985, 33.9 percent of entering medical students were female; 8.5 percent were minority students.)

2. Background was usually a four-year bachelor's degree in biological and physical sciences; some students entered after three years of college.

More diversity in curriculums acceptable to qualify for entry to medical school; almost all students had at least a bachelor's degree; more students had advanced degrees.

3. Of first-year medical students, 70.6 percent had an undergraduate grade point average (GPA) between 2.6 and 3.5 (on 4.0 scale).

Almost 50 percent of entering first-year medical students had an undergraduate GPA above 3.6 (on a 4.0 scale).

Competition

4. Moderate competition for acceptance into medical school; 1.9 applicants for each first-year space in 1958.

Competition for first-year places peaked at 2.9 applicants per space in 1973 but then declined to 2.1 applicants per place.

5. Candidates applied to relatively few medical schools (3.6 per person).

Students applied to an average of 9.4 medical schools.

6. Better students were more concentrated at major private university medical schools.

Because of costs of medical education and few career advantages to the graduate of major private university schools, state schools and less prestigious medical schools competed successfully to attract better students.

Expectations for Career

7. Expected lifestyle consisted of long hours, professional autonomy, financial security, and concentration on practicing medicine. Expected prestige and respect from, and dominance over, other health professionals and patients.

Increased interest in a lifestyle with significant activities outside of medicine; less financial security; expected less deference from other health professionals and patients.

Continued

Table 9:4—Continued.

1955	1985
Support	
8. Virtually all students or their families paid for education directly; little governmental role in financing of students directly or through loans.	Majority of students received financial aid of some type, usually from the government. More common to graduate with significant debt. (In 1985, 87 percent of graduates were in debt at the end of medical school; the average indebtedness was about $30,000.)

References by row number: (1,8) Iglehart (1986). (1) Eisenberg (1983). (2) Purcell (1976). (3–5) Johnson (1983). (6) Petersdorf and Wilson (1982). (7) Frieman and Marder (1984). (8) "Consequences of the Student Loan Proposals" (1982).

and to treat public patients, even though most, in common with non-minorities, locate in medically well served areas and treat mostly private, paying patients (Keith et al. 1985; Penn et al. 1986). One explanation for the differences in career choices of women and minorities is that they experience discrimination in securing the most prestigious and lucrative positions. Another is that women and minorities entering medicine in the 1980s do not feel that they must adopt the roles and attitudes of white male physicians.

Another notable change over the past 30 years is in the expectations of all medical students regarding their future professional and personal lifestyles. In the past, one of the basic justifications of the power and economic advantages afforded to physicians has been the expectation that they center their lives on medical practice and work very hard at it. Even those physicians who did not conform to this norm tended to hide their lifestyle preferences from colleagues, and at least to pay lip service to the norm that physicians should devote virtually all of their energies toward the practice of medicine. Recently a combination of societal changes has made it more acceptable for physicians to embrace openly a lifestyle that does not center exclusively on the profession. In the 1980s part-time or shared residencies have been available. Leading medical journals have contained advertisements offering positions emphasizing lifestyles with considerable time for leisure or for nonclinical activities. These more diverse definitions of acceptable professional lifestyles, combined with the altered competitive environment of medical practice, contribute further to generational differences between the work ethic of new physicians and that of their colleagues who began 30 years ago.

Such changes in lifestyle are likely to lead to further changes in the economics and power of the profession. For example, in the past, the high income of physicians was due in part to their willingness to work a

60-to-80-hour week and the availability of enough patients to enable them to do so (Mechanic 1976). Similarly, some of the power and economic security of physicians derives from public acceptance and expectations of physicians' dedication to their profession and willingness to put in long hours. For example, patients and senior physicians alike expect physicians to visit their hospitalized patients on Saturdays and Sundays (Mechanic 1976; Freidson 1970b). Senior physicians today are often puzzled and disturbed when their younger colleagues, especially those still in training, are less willing than they are to work evenings and weekends. As these aspects of the daily work activities of physicians approach societal norms, the acceptance of physicians' claims to special status may decrease similarly.

Financing Medical Education

Medical education, especially during clinical training, is expensive. In recent years, the increase in the cost of medical education has accelerated. Tuition increases have outstripped the rate of inflation by a considerable margin. Society has deemed it acceptable and even desirable for medical students to assume a large burden in financing their education. This is due in part to the assumption (reasonable in light of past experience) that a graduate of medical school will enjoy a large and secure income. This assumption may no longer be warranted, at least for all physicians, for two reasons: new physicians today find their opportunities to have a high-paying practice limited by competition for patients in desirable geographic settings and financially rewarding specialty practices; and the selection of primary care specialties (like family practice), and practice sites that permit a more desirable lifestyle or offer less intense competition for patients, tends to result in lower salaries. On the other hand, there is some evidence that nonminority students who had a high level of indebtedness after medical school were disproportionately likely to choose a high-paying specialty (including general surgery) rather than primary care, apparently in an attempt to recoup their financial investments (see review in Iglehart 1986).

The methods students use to pay for medical education have also changed. In 1955 there were essentially no governmental loan programs directed to students in medical school. Students usually paid for their education with personal funds or loans. Governmental support was limited in availability and usually involved considerable obligation. Over the intervening 30 years, a variety of private and governmental programs have developed. In the 1980s, most expenses of medical education are financed by several types of financial aid, usually administered through medical schools, with much of the financial backing through governmental funds or government-guaranteed loans (Iglehart 1986). Some forms of student aid were tailored to encourage students to choose primary care specialties and to locate in specific communities, but such programs have achieved varying success (President's Commission 1983, 119–28). The prevailing attitude of the government toward financing medical education is reflected by the restructuring of programs to include other health professions and to limit subsidies to the economically disadvantaged. Perhaps signaling a new era, by 1985 guaranteed loans for students of health professions were under threat of being reduced or discontinued by the federal government (Iglehart 1986).

In 1955 residents were paid primarily by benefits (for example, room and board, uniforms, malpractice and health insurance coverage, vacation, and parking) plus a low salary from the hospital (approximately $600 per month in 1985 dollars for a beginning resident, based on American Medical Association 1969). An unmarried resident, having few free moments in which to spend money, could manage on this salary. (First-year residents were estimated to average over 70 hours per week in professional activities in a survey conducted in 1975 [Macy Foundation 1980, 118].) In 1983 first-year residents received similar benefits and a significantly higher salary (approximately $1,600 per month in 1985 dollars (Association of American Medical Colleges 1983, 7). This increase in salary for residents (which may seem even larger to the senior physician who remembers the salary in real dollars: $125 in 1955), coupled with a perceived less-professional work ethic in residents today, can be a cause of considerable grumbling among senior physicians.

When governmental financing programs arose to give patients who would have been "teaching material" in 1955 full access to the usual channels for medical care, the effect on the organization and financing of medical education was profound. Some formerly showcase teaching institutions became much less important as their patients went elsewhere. Other hospitals (initially large urban hospitals, later community hospitals of all types), which previously had little or no affiliation with medical schools and residency programs, became much more central to education.

However, the biggest change, from the viewpoint of the academic medical center, was the increased availability of income to the medical school and its faculty for rendering previously unreimbursed services. This income, combined with the research monies available through increased federal support, accelerated the transformation of medical schools into large, complex, academic medical centers that paid physicians full-time salaries. The patient fees earned by these academicians became another source of funding for residents. Because of the substantial financial benefits, medical schools and their faculties fairly readily accommodated the profound changes in the status of their teaching patients and the need to compete for patients. In many medical schools, the income from the professional fees of physicians in clinical departments, especially radiology and pathology, became one of the principal sources of financing (Petersdorf 1980; 1981; 1982; Petersdorf and Wilson 1982; Wagoner 1986).

The practice of cross-subsidization of medical education and research in teaching hospitals via patient fees has come under increasing attack as the government and other third-party payers have sought to reduce expenditures for hospital care in particular. There are increasing calls for explicit funding of patient care, medical education costs, and research (Iglehart 1986; Task Force on Academic Health Centers 1985).

In the original formulation of Medicare's Prospective Payment System, for example, teaching hospitals received payment for direct costs of medical education and an adjustment factor that was intended to compensate for indirect costs. Direct costs of medical education (such as resident salaries and fringe benefits, faculty salaries, and administrative costs) are relatively simple to identify and agree upon. Indirect costs of medical education in teaching hospitals are more difficult to identify and assess. They include the costs of developing and applying new medical technologies; conducting more precise diagnoses even when they may not affect therapy; pursuing false leads due to the inexperience of some residents; treating more complex, difficult diseases; caring for socially disadvantaged patients who may have few or no other alternative sources of treatment; and ensuring security and meeting the higher cost-of-living expenses encountered in inner-city and large metropolitan areas.

The Medicare adjustment rested not on any attempt to quantify these costs, but on the resident-to-bed ratio. Several scholars have argued that this method has resulted in inequities in compensating for teaching costs, resulting in either over- or underpayment to teaching hospitals (depending upon their true indirect costs). The Task Force on Academic Health Centers (1985), assuming that a restructuring of the financing of medical education is inevitable, has recommended explicit consideration of four factors: location (costs in inner cities being higher than in other areas), technological sophistication of services, social severity of patients, and disease severity of patients.

By the early 1980s then, medical schools and hospitals had adjusted to receiving payment for patients, and this income became a main source of support for teaching programs. In this instance there were few generational differences, as both new and senior physicians appeared to have accepted this type of financing of academic medicine as normal and desirable. Now, a reduction in the overall reimbursement for these patients and inadequate or inappropriate means to fund resident care pose grave threats to teaching programs that have based their financing on this source of income.

The Nature of Academic Physicians and Their Environment

Table 9:3 summarizes some of the principal differences in medical school faculty for 1955 and 1985. The nature and role of full-time medical school faculty changed dramatically over this period in almost every major respect. The changes include a great increase in the number of full-time faculty; increased research activities during the early part of the period and increased patient care during the latter part; and a greater role for research grants and patient fees in financing medical schools.

The role of "voluntary" faculty—physicians in private practice who participate in the clinical education of students or residents but who are not salaried by the school or program—has also undergone considerable changes during this period. In the 1950s these physicians played a major role in clinical teaching, volunteering on a regular basis to teach medical students at charity and university hospitals. Their rewards were the prestige of being associated with the medical school and the satisfaction of teaching students. With the advent of increased governmental reimbursement for physician services for the poor, more full-time and salaried faculty became involved, and the dependence upon voluntary faculty declined. Important exceptions to the decreased dependence on volunteer and part-time faculty occurred in some of the new medical schools of the 1960s and 1970s; these schools were often based in community hospitals rather than traditional academic medical centers and relied heavily on volunteer faculty. Currently, the availability and use of voluntary and part-time faculty for teaching medical students appears to be declining in both academic and community hospitals as the increased emphasis on competition makes physicians more concerned with economic efficiency and therefore less willing to volunteer their services.

The availability and attractiveness of academic medicine as a career have been in flux throughout this period and continue to change dramatically. Petersdorf and Wilson (1982) label the period immediately preceding the 30 years under review as the Biomedical Research Era. This era paved the way for medical schools to develop a strong research base and to attract physicians with a strong academic orientation. Career disruptions due to military service in wars provided further stimulus for many physicians to switch to academic medicine rather than to resume their private clinical practices.

Recent slowing of the growth of expenditures on research—and some actual decreases—have been widely discussed in academic medical circles, with a subsequent increase in concern about the viability of academic careers. This concern has been heightened by the increased need for medical school faculty to bring in funds to support their activities (often including support of their salaries), at the same time as academic medical centers are being faced with increasing competition for grants, students, and patients. On the other hand, the overall level of federal and private support for medical research is probably at or near an all-time high. Recently, formal programs leading to the dual degrees of Ph.D. and M.D. have experienced great increases in enrollment and have broadened the scope of Ph.D. fields available, creating the likelihood that graduates of these programs will become the dominant force in research-oriented academic medicine over the next 30 years. Such changes in the faculty can be expected to alter the professionalization of new physicians in the future, adding a new source of tension between generations of physicians.

MONEY, INSURANCE, AND PHYSICIANS' DECISION MAKING

Insurance has affected the delivery and reimbursement of medical services (and has been affected by them) in numerous ways. Throughout this book, and elsewhere in this chapter, we discuss the impact of the widespread availability of insurance and the enfranchisement of the poor and aged, as well as the different incentives built into the fee-for-service and prepaid modes of reimbursement. Here we briefly note other ways that health and risk insurance have affected the costs and services provided.

The increased availability of medical insurance has tended to increase physician fees. Reimbursement schedules for particular procedures set by insurance companies such as Blue Shield were intended to represent average and reasonable fees; therefore, some physicians were charging less than the rate of reimbursement. However, these reimbursement schedules effectively set the lower limit of fees, so that soon after their implementation, physicians previously charging less than the Blue Shield reimbursement level tended to raise their fees to match it. The reimbursement schedules did not establish an upper limit because patients would pay the difference out of pocket. Also, insurance companies often would pay above their regular levels if the physician could justify the necessity of charging more than the usual and prevailing fees.

The growing threat of malpractice during this period provided additional fuel to the rise in costs of medical care (Mechanic 1978). Defensive practices encourage high use of diagnostic procedures to provide documentation of care and to rule out long-shot diagnoses that might require treatment (Charles, Wilbert, and Kennedy 1984). Doctors disagree on whether defensive medicine as practiced is good medicine or unnecessary (Tancredi and Barondess 1978). Some argue that ruling out long shots is an important indicator of good clinical decision making. Others argue that the threat of malpractice can also provide physicians who feel uncertain about the medical necessity of a test with an excellent excuse to sidestep potentially difficult decisions. Mechanic (1978) suggests that the litigious nature of the American public, coupled with the clinical standards used in malpractice suits, presents even more perverse incentives to practice costly and potentially unnecessary medicine. He argues that the standards of practice used in malpractice suits are almost always based on process measures and ignore evidence of both the costs and effectiveness of the standard practice. Thus, the clinical standards applied in successful malpractice suits can lag behind research evidence, which has challenged the cost effectiveness of standard practice. These standards tend to encourage the use of expensive resources like the intensive care unit because such a high standard of care will not be questioned in the event of a malpractice suit.

The cost of malpractice insurance premiums has been another important factor. Malpractice insurance rates for physicians in some specialties in certain geographic areas have risen greatly, sometimes to levels as high as $100,000 per year (Sullivan 1985). At least until very recently, this increase has not presented a major financial problem to physicians because they could pass these costs directly to the patients through fees, again with the reimbursement coming primarily from third-party payers.

For a variety of reasons (including the availability of more paying patients, the reimbursement policies of hospitalization insurance, the tendency for hospital workers to receive higher wages, and the increasing complexity of technological aspects of health care), the costs of hospitalization grew very rapidly over the period under investigation (Scott and Flood 1987). This rapid growth in the cost of hospitalization has been an especially powerful factor in triggering reactions that have altered and, in some cases, reversed trends observed in the beginning of the period.

In summary, the economic changes in medicine during the past 30 years have been profound and complex. Initially the income available to physicians and academic medical centers increased dramatically as their main patient population changed from being "charity" patients to patients who paid fully through governmental insurance. During the same period the income available to academic medical centers through federal research support also increased substantially. Governmental and health insurance company policies have changed their goals to emphasize cost containment. The effect of these governmental policies has been profound because of the rapidity with which they have been applied, the sometimes contradictory results they have engendered, and their application to a health care system that had begun to adapt to the initial set of changes. As argued elsewhere in this chapter, the type of economic change that could occur, and its effects, are intimately related to changes in power relationships during the same period. For new physicians, the current situation is the norm, and, in view of all of the other adjustments that occur at their age and stage of professional development, the financial situation is not a dominating factor. For senior physicians, the magnitude and rapidity of these changes are very disconcerting; these doctors are often puzzled by the apparent lack of concern of their younger colleagues.

SHARED POWER AND CLINICAL DECISION MAKING: NEW ACTORS

Changes in power over clinical decisions, once the nearly exclusive province of the physician, have arisen from the entrance into the process of many interested parties, ranging from the patient (newly recognized as having values that can affect choices) to the groups paying for the cost of diagnosis and therapy. From the perspective of the physician in 1955, the prototypic decision-making unit was a solo practitioner, who almost unilaterally made all medical decisions regarding patients. There was, at best, a minimal direct involvement of the patient, but little or no involvement of others, even the patient's family. In contrast, decisions for treatment in 1985 often involve the significant participation of the patient and family; also considered are the policies and needs of the group practice with which the physician is associated, the hospital's resources and needs, peer groups who will review the appropriateness and quality of services during hospitalization, consumer groups, insurance companies who pay the bills, federal and state agencies that supervise the insurance agencies or pay directly, and legal restrictions and concerns over potential malpractice.

The Role of Patients in Decision Making

The greatly increased role of patients and their families in decision making reflects a number of recent changes in society. These include increased recognition of the rights of all individuals to be involved in decisions that affect them and, in particular, recognition of the rights of the poor and women. The right of patients to be properly informed of the risks of particular procedures clearly has a long-standing legal foundation. More important for explaining the increased role of patients, however, is a shift in general societal expectations that patients should be informed consumers; that is, they should receive full information about their disease and treatment procedures and alternatives.

Today there is still evidence of a gap between patients' and doctors' expectations of patients' rights to make decisions and be informed about their care (Faden et al. 1981; Cassileth et al. 1980; Wolinsky and Kurz 1984). Faden and her colleagues found that patients preferred detailed disclosure of risks and alternatives, while doctors reported that they were likely to disclose only risks with a high probability of occurrence and to provide little information about alternatives. Cassileth and her colleagues found marked differences among patients depending upon their age (younger patients wanted more information), although the majority of patients at all age levels wanted to participate in decisions.

Other elements in the increased role of the patient in decision making include the political and economic enfranchisement of the poor[3] (discussed earlier) and a dramatic increase in recognition of the rights and expectations of women to be involved in decisions affecting them. One focus of the women's movement has been on removing the patronizing aspects of health care for women with the goal of permitting women to be actively involved in decisions that affect their own bodies and health. Although some older physicians have adjusted incompletely or not at all to this expectation, the students entering the system in 1985 are generally more aware and responsive to the need to involve female patients in decisions.

The demystification of physicians and medical care today is very broadly based. In a survey conducted in 1984, two-thirds of Americans agreed that people are losing faith in their doctors (American Medical Association 1984). This trend needs to be considered in a larger context, however. Lipset and Schneider (1983, especially 48–49) describe the remarkable decrease in public confidence in business, professionals, and the government over the past 20 years. For medicine, the proportion of the public expressing confidence has declined from 72 percent in the middle 1960s to 37 percent in 1980 in the Harris polls—but medicine received the highest level of confidence of all occupations polled at both times!

Another factor that has increased patients' involvement in decisions affecting their health has been a general increase in individual awareness, concern, and knowledge about healthful habits and illness prevention (that is, wellness), as well as increased public knowledge of specific diseases. In general, patients are much better informed about their bodies and illness and are therefore in a much better position to request and understand details about alternatives for treatment. This interest has been fed by a variety of guides to medical self-care, including many written by physicians and medical schools, for example, *The Harvard Medical School Health Letter* and *The Columbia University College of Physicians and Surgeons Complete Home Medical Guide* (1985).

Finally, it should be noted that just as there are generational differences between younger and older patients in their awareness of and willingness to participate in decision making, there are also parallel generational differences in physicians' views of the expectations of patients. We are generally cognizant of the reluctance of some older physicians to have patients take an active role in the decisions affecting their health care. There is a less appreciated but parallel problem with some younger physicians who may fail to recognize that, for a significant

minority of patients (especially older ones), attempts to force them to participate fully in decision making may increase rather than decrease their
anxiety. One of the challenges to today's physicians of all ages is to be sufficiently responsive to the right of patients to be treated in a way consistent
with their own needs and expectations (Marzuk 1985).

The Role of the General Public in Decision Making

The general public has also become much more involved in decision
making in medicine, as discussed in some detail in Chapter 5, "Consumer
Sovereignty in a Competitive Market: Fact or Fiction?" The health consumers' movement was essentially nonexistent in 1955. In 1985 it was a
major presence in discussions about decision making at the community or
regional level (for example, consumer involvement in certificate-of-need
hearings is now mandated). The actual strength of the consumers' movement may be arguable, but even at the most conservative estimates of its
influence, the contrast with 30 years ago is very great indeed. In 1955 there
were no patient's rights statements in hospitals, no human subjects protection committees, no ombudsmen, and few case-law decisions or legislation
to protect the rights of patients to receive or refuse treatment.

In addition to specific public organizations spawned by the health
consumers' movement, there has been a general increase in public
knowledge of medical topics (Reeder 1972). In-depth media news coverage
of spectacular health care events (such as artificial heart transplants) has
become more common. The news media have also facilitated public involvement in general analyses of such health problems as the advantages
and disadvantages of coronary bypass operations and nonsurgical alternatives for treating breast cancer. This increased knowledge has put both the
general public and individual patients in a much better position to seek out
and understand the factors involved in decisions about health care. The
past 30 years have also seen a dramatic increase in the number and involvement of public interest groups focused on specific diseases such as multiple sclerosis and Alzheimer's disease. For some relatively rare diseases, the
result has been a level of awareness that sometimes equals or exceeds that
of physicians who do not frequently encounter those diseases.

The relative power of the physician has declined as more interested
parties have begun to be recognized as having the right to influence health
care. Although medical problems were previously considered to require
professional skills and knowledge to be understood, the increased sharing
of decision making is much less of an issue to new members of the profession today, who often actively support such changes rather than resist or
resent them.

The demystification of medical decisions has been enhanced by economic imperatives to reduce or contain the costs of medical care. The emergence of formal mechanisms to question the appropriateness of medical decisions (for example, professional review organizations) is the topic of the next subsection.

The Role of Medical Colleagues in Decision Making

The past 30 years have also witnessed an increase in the involvement of other physicians and physician groups (albeit usually via retrospective review) in decisions that at one time were strictly between individual practitioners and their patients. This increased involvement resulted in part from the movement toward group practice. Physicians in a large group practice are often subject to discipline or expulsion if their practice falls below group standards of productivity or of quality in clinical decision making.[4] This kind of professional discipline tends to be exercised more frequently and effectively than disciplinary measures from peer review organizations at the hospital or local governmental level, where dismissals, formal censures, and revocations of state licenses are rare.

At the hospital level, too, there has been an increased involvement of other physicians in decision making. Today, peer review is mandated in hospitals. While it may have little formal power to alter a physician's actions, such review does have an effect on the physician's perception of his or her independence and autonomy and has been demonstrated to affect behavior. For example, Wennberg and his colleagues (1977) noted the effectiveness of feedback by peers to modify atypical medical practice, and others have reported that dissemination of criteria to be reviewed by tissue review committees can lead to significant alterations in practice (Dyck et al. 1977). Concomitantly, national, professional, and academic groups have increased their attempts to influence the nature and quality of practice. Medical research has also placed additional constraints on the latitude of physicians' decisions to alter individual therapeutic regimens, as community physicians have increasingly enrolled their patients in cooperative trials, testing particular types of treatment and the efficacy of various diagnostic modalities. Some physicians have even advocated the necessity of using a random trial procedure in individual patients to determine which of several alternatives is most appropriate for a given patient (Guyatt et al. 1986). In addition, dissemination of the results of these studies, and the results of federally sponsored consensus conferences, has constrained the freedom of individual physicians to use treatments and procedures that have been shown to be less effective. A shift in lawsuits to a national standard of practice in malpractice cases has had a similar effect (Danzon 1982).

The Role of Other Health Care Professionals in Decision Making

In principle, the power relationships between physicians and other health professionals have also altered in the past 30 years. This issue in regard to nurses and physicians is considered in detail in Chapter 8, "The Other Face of Competition: Nursing's Struggle for Autonomy." Much of this change is more apparent than real. Actual involvement of nurses and various technical specialists (such as occupational or respiratory therapists) in clinical decision making occurs in relatively limited circumstances, if at all. The concept of the health care team can offer both advantages and disadvantages for professionals and patients alike, although the practice of allowing an equal voice in decision making to all health professionals, with the physician as captain of the team, has not been generally realized (Duncanis and Golin 1979). It has been successfully implemented more often in certain chronic care situations, such as in rehabilitation medicine or complex crisis care situations such as cases of child abuse. Primary medical care by physician assistants and nurse clinicians, under the supervision of physicians, has been more successful in increasing the involvement of other health professionals in the actual diagnosis and treatment of patients. Overall, however, the dominance of physicians over other health care professionals in clinical decision making has changed very little in the past 30 years, despite the rhetoric to the contrary and some very active attempts by health professional groups to alter the situation (Banta and Fox 1972; Beckhard 1972; Twaddle and Hessler 1977).

With hindsight, the failure of these attempts, particularly those to change general medical care, seems quite understandable. Physicians cannot be expected to transfer power voluntarily to other health professionals when none of the interested parties has sufficient or long-term incentives to begin or to continue such arrangements. The potential advantages to primary care physicians were of two types: the ability to extend their practice by employing health professionals to perform some of the patient care tasks, and the ability to retain the more interesting tasks or patients. The first type, to be advantageous to the physician, required that the other health professionals' salaries and the resources they consumed be lower than the fees they generated and that the fees generated accrue to the physician (at least indirectly through a professional corporation). The second type, to be advantageous to the physician and to the medical profession in general, required that there be sufficient patients to keep everyone employed and that the physician's role in patient care be sufficiently stimulating (which includes being not only challenged medically but also rewarded in terms of stimulating patient interaction).

In an era of a perceived glut of physicians, the medical profession is reluctant to welcome additional actors to care for patients. Third-party, fee-for-service payers had originally accommodated the physician's desires by paying a relatively high rate of reimbursement for services performed by other health professionals. Thus the savings were not passed along to the consumer; the costs were borne by the insurance companies, who passed along high insurance rates to their clients. For public third-party payers, however, this arrangement was less than satisfactory, since high governmental expenditures on health care had become an important issue, and the public was less willing to see the economic advantages of hiring other health professionals passed to physicians instead of to the public. New demands for billing of services by other health professionals at lower rates, increased competition for patients, and the increased popularity of prepaid services have reduced the economic advantages for physicians and helped to slow, and in some cases reverse, the trends toward using other health professionals. The major exceptions (such as nurse midwives and nurse practitioners) are usually in organizational settings such as hospitals or prepaid health care clinics, where there is an economic advantage or power benefit from the change. More extensive changes may occur in the future, if economic concerns to reduce the cost of labor and the declining power of individual physicians alter power and economic incentives within such organizations as prepaid plans.

The Role of Fiscal Intermediaries and Government in Decision Making

Thirty years ago, insurance companies usually were passive payers of physician and hospital bills. Any questioning of the legitimacy of charges was directed at the patient, not the physician. That is, an insurance company might question whether a particular procedure was covered by the patient's policy but would not question whether the procedure was indicated medically, or whether it could have been accomplished at lower cost by alternative means. Very recently, insurance companies and other fiscal intermediaries have been adopting a variety of strategies to reduce unnecessary procedures and hospitalizations. The strategies include requiring second opinions prior to surgery; using capitation payments for specified services, thereby shifting the incentive to economize to providers; and refusing to pay for certain procedures unless performed on an outpatient basis.

Many of these actions by third-party payers began in response to the potential financial gains from such policies in an era of competition and rate setting. These early efforts were hesitant, often accommodating the professional and financial interests of physicians. Early corrective actions were limited to attempts by insurers to avoid cost-increasing incentives. For example, insurers tried to eliminate incentives to hospitalize in order to have the patient's insurance pay for laboratory services, simple surgical procedures, or x-ray procedures that otherwise would require out-of-pocket payment from patients.

Now the emphasis has shifted toward specific and deliberate attempts to decrease costs by increasing economic incentives for patients to choose low-cost physicians or by placing physicians at financial risk. In some cases, physicians have been offered financial rewards to use less costly alternatives (*Blue Shield Bulletin* 1982). As it became apparent that fiscal intermediaries (often led by the federal government) have the power and social sanction to make changes that alter the practice of medicine, they have become increasingly active. Public sanctioning of significant changes is illustrated by the recent enactment of the Prospective Payment System for Medicare, and by the shift in rhetoric to describe the government's mandate to caregivers to provide "adequate" care to the poor and elderly of the nation instead of equal care (President's Commission 1983). The muted, ineffectual, and often divisive response of physicians to these profound changes provides strong evidence of the decrease in the power of physicians.

Concern has been expressed that the recent changes can affect the quality of care (Davis 1979; Wyszewianski, Wheeler, and Donabedian 1982; Turk 1985; Freeman and Kirkmann-Liff 1982). Davis argues that Medicare may fail to provide for all necessary care. Wyszewianski and his colleagues have analyzed the potential effects of recent policy changes that reflect market-oriented cost-containment strategies in medical care; they concluded that such attempts are likely to diminish quality, primarily by inducing underutilization of medical services. Federally funded programs involving prepaid experiments to care for Medicaid and Medicare patients have had a history plagued with abuses and inefficiencies. Much of the reduction in costs to Medicaid programs appears to have been achieved by reducing levels of reimbursement for services, types of service covered, and eligibility of patients, rather than by increasing productivity or efficiency (McDevitt and Buczko 1985; Holahan 1985; Haynes 1985). However, others claim that only "fat" and inefficient production will be threatened by properly administered changes in policies for reimbursement (Galblum and Trieger 1982; Salkever et al. 1976; Fuller, Patera, and Koziol 1977).

While there is disagreement about the desirability of the changes, there is general agreement that they are likely to affect clinical practices significantly. This consequence represents a significant change from the ground rules under which Medicare and Medicaid were established. Then, great care was taken to preserve the existing fee-for-service organization of health care services for these entitled populations. This arrangement was considered essential to secure the acceptance and cooperation of organized medicine. As it has become apparent that the professional autonomy of physicians has decreased, the federal government has demonstrated an increased capability and willingness to make rule changes that alter practice. In turn, as these new policies are implemented without generating effective opposition, the ability and willingness of the government to make further changes are increased.

A recent trend that also affects clinical practices is the incorporation of the fiscal intermediaries into organizations that deliver health care. The most common mode has been for the health care organization essentially to take over the role of the fiscal intermediaries, as in the prepaid health plans in which the organization or group of physicians takes on responsibility for the total health care costs as well as health care delivery. The opposite will probably also be more common; that is, units starting out as fiscal intermediaries will become providers to deliver health care. Perhaps presaging this change, some fiscal intermediaries, such as state Medicaid plans and Blue Cross plans, have been encouraging capitation-based organizations to care for their populations. The next step, the direct involvement of insurers in health care delivery, seems likely. This movement toward integration of various components of the health care delivery system is discussed in some detail in Chapter 4, "Integration as a Provider Response to Shrinking Health Care Dollars."

The Role of Group Practice in Decision Making

The shift in the dominant type of practice, from solo or two- or three-person partnerships to group practice, has also affected the power and status of physicians. In 1955, solo practice was the norm. For most physicians in practice, and for medical students, the idea of group practice was considered antithetical to the proper role and proper practice of physicians, even though a small percentage of physicians did join group practices (Becker et al. 1961). Fifty-five years ago the American Medical Association endorsed group practice for the first time, emphasizing its potential for containing office costs; the acceptable motivation to join group practice was to reduce overhead costs, and not to alter the practice of medicine (Committee on the Costs of Medical Care 1932). Consequently, those physicians who joined other physicians in some form of partnership or association still tended to have a considerable degree of autonomy and authority. For a group practice to exist in an environment in which solo practice was the clear norm, the directors of the group practice had to be careful to avoid any indications of constraints on the professional prerogatives of physicians.

The early success of large group practices (including the prepaid Kaiser group) in attracting physicians was based in part on the appeal of being able to practice medicine while "administrators" took care of

bureaucratic and financial matters, such as billing for the services and supplies. These administrators were perceived to exercise little or no power
over clinical practice, limiting their domain to nonmedical aspects of the
business, including billing for clinical services delivered.

The norm has now shifted to group practice; it is believed that group
practice promotes better quality of care than solo practice (Freshnook and
Jenson 1981, Tarlov 1983a).[5] Group practice, particularly in large groups,
also offers a competitive edge in attracting patients and bidding for contracts with state and private preferred provider arrangements (Saward and
Gallagher 1983). This shift toward group practice has particularly profound implications for the power relationships of physicians. The autonomy and authority of physicians are much more apt to be circumscribed
in a group practice, especially one that is part of a large organization
administered by nonphysicians. At the same time, the ability of group practices to influence and control physician behavior has increased because of
the decrease of attractive and financially secure options for solo practice.
For today's new physicians, group practice is an option that must be considered seriously; for some of their senior colleagues, group practice will
always be an object of suspicion and, at best, a necessary evil.

The Role of Hospital Administration in Decision Making

During this 30-year period, hospitals have increased their power and ability
to influence clinical decision making. The hospital during the early part
of this period was described as the doctor's workshop, in which the doctor
practiced freely (Somers and Somers 1967). Describing the physician's role
in the first half of this century, Guest (1972, 286) wrote:

> Professional independence was reinforced by the fact that for many years the
> hospital was not the center of the physician's practice. The center of his prac-
> tice was his home and that of his patient. Unlike employees of the growing
> factory and business organizations he took no orders from agents of any or-
> ganization; he was responsible only to his patients, and this responsibility was
> supported by traditions going as far back as Hippocrates. It was assumed that
> only his independence to care for the welfare of his patients was the overrid-
> ing consideration. Unheard of was a suggestion that any form of organization-
> al bureaucracy would intervene between himself and his patient.

Despite voluminous building activity and expansion of hospitals as
a result of Hill-Burton funds, during the late 1950s and early 1960s occupancy rates in most hospitals were very high, and physicians were concerned about their patients having access to hospital beds. Nonetheless,
hospitals did not use this scarcity of resources to gain power over doctors,
presumably because of the prevailing consensus regarding the dominance
of physicians in health care. Indeed, hospitals were intent on garnering

special medical resources, such as new medical technology and facilities, to attract doctors to bring their patients to the hospital.

As hospitals became the repository of sophisticated and expensive technology that an individual physician or a group could not duplicate in a private office, doctors and hospitals became more interdependent (Guest 1972). The hospital administration was charged with hiring and supervising its employees and with management of their work as well as with raising capital and acquiring technology. Oversight of clinical functions was nevertheless left to the medical staff organization rather than to the hospital administration (Roemer and Friedman 1971). In general, the physicians associated with each hospital regulated admitting privileges to that hospital. Decisions on admissions usually followed rules that, at least in principle, lacked significant political or economic bases, although there were instances in which individual physicians or physician groups used admissions to control other physicians whom they viewed as potential economic threats. Today, however, this "dual authority" model has been replaced by a more sophisticated collaboration which has been described as a "shared authority" model (Shortell 1983).

Major changes in hospital use have been another factor affecting the power of hospitals to influence clinical practice. First, beginning in the 1970s, a considerable overcapacity developed in hospitals, largely as the result of federal initiatives begun 30 years ago (especially the Hill-Burton Act). Second, throughout the 30-year period there has been a general trend to reduce length of stay for many diagnostic categories (Wood 1984; U.S. Congress 1986, 490–98). Most recently, the impact of Medicare's Prospective Payment System has caused a marked and nearly universal additional reduction in length of stay for most diagnostic categories and has increased excess capacity (that is, most hospitals have experienced lower occupancy rates).

All of these trends have affected hospital-doctor relationships during the past 30 years. Excess capacity has again made hospitals more dependent on physicians to fill their beds and therefore increased the relative power of physicians over hospitals, although the perceived increase in the number of physicians may moderate the leverage of physicians in this regard. At the same time, with Medicare prepayments for each type of patient stipulated in advance and independent of services consumed, the hospital now has a strong incentive to regulate physician behavior in order to minimize costs. Heretofore, such incentives were limited to the few hospitals offering prepaid health plans in a group practice setting. At present, these incentives apply only to prepaid plans and Medicare patients, but these populations represent a sizable proportion of patients in most hospitals. Moreover, it now seems probable that additional types of patient will come under prospective reimbursement (that is, through

Medicaid, private insurance, and preferred provider organizations). The simplicity of organizational arrangements and federal regulations further dictate procedures that affect the services delivered to all patients rather than only to patients on a given insurance plan. The need and power to affect clinical decisions is likely to force a much closer collaboration between hospital administrators and physicians, however reluctantly and suspiciously they may view each other's interests (Glandon and Morrisey 1986).

The ability of hospitals to influence physician behavior is augmented by the various changes acting to decrease the relative autonomy of physicians and by physicians' increased involvement in organizational settings in which they had to modify their behavior in order to function successfully in the group. Therefore, it seems likely that hospitals will be successful in inducing physicians to respond to the hospitals' fiscal needs. Hospitals now can influence physician behavior by dealing directly with the group practice to which physicians belong; however, the size and subsequent power of the group potentially provide increased bargaining power over the hospital as well.

It is not at all clear how this complex set of new economic and authority relationships between physicians and hospitals will evolve over the next few years. The cohesiveness of physician attitudes may be a major factor in this evolution; it seems likely that today's newly trained physicians will be much more amenable to an increase in the relative authority of the hospital.

The Role of Health Care Corporations in Decision Making

One of the most important current changes in health care organizations is the trend away from independent, freestanding enterprises toward some mode of multiinstitutional collaboration. Hospitals and clinics are seeking ways to integrate both vertically (such as linking to insurance programs, nursing homes, and pharmacies) and horizontally (with a variety of collaborative arrangements linking similar organizations).[6] These linkages are appearing in both profit and nonprofit institutions. Although investor-owned systems are larger and growing somewhat faster than nonprofit systems, they are facing increasingly significant competition from the nonprofit sector and some belated growth in academic centers (Ermann and Gabel 1985; Derzon, Lewin, and Watt 1981; Zuckerman 1979; Levitan 1979). Today the distinctions are blurred between the goals and orientations of nonprofit and profit organizations, with regard to providing services in a particular community. This is especially true when the organization is a member of a multiinstitutional corporation and when the corporate-level management exercises strong power to set policies. Nevertheless, it is important to note that the medical staff organizations of multiinstitutional arrangements have remained relatively unaffected by policy decisions at a corporate level and that medical staff members continue to have important control over change (Glandon and Morrisey 1986). As Levitan (1979, 874) argues,

> Each hospital in a multiple hospital system takes on an identity of its own. Its medical staff makes demands for an array of services that permits the hospital to be a full-service institution. Physician independence is characteristic of American medicine, making it extremely difficult to organize clinical services for a multiple hospital system so that more sophisticated services are not duplicated. While it may be possible to limit service facilities on a regional basis by withholding resources, such a policy will put the governing body and management of the multiple hospital system under tremendous pressure from the medical staff.

Although there are many predictions of an increasing role of investor-owned corporate medicine in the health care delivery system (for example, Starr 1982), it is not yet clear that this development is inevitable or that it will continue its current directions. Some of the early growth of the multiinstitutional corporations was by the acquisition of existing small, for-profit hospitals that were owned by physicians and were financially vulnerable. Because the supply of these institutions is limited, the rate of such acquisitions is apt to slow. As the rules of reimbursement change toward fixed prepayment, and as other cost-restraining measures are implemented, the value of the institutions owned by large corporations may decrease. Evidence comparing investor-owned chains of hospitals to nonprofit hospitals suggests that the higher profits in investor-owned hospitals derive from more aggressive pricing practices rather than from more efficient production of services, and that neither type of hospital has a clear-cut advantage in the ability to adapt to cost-based reimbursement (Watt et al. 1986). On the other hand, the for-profit hospitals and multiinstitutional corporations have access to capital sources and management expertise that are limited or unavailable to single or nonprofit health care institutions (Ermann and Gabel 1985), and the need for these resources may increase. The recent volatile actions of corporations (to diversify, to close facilities or reduce capacity, and to acquire vertical or horizontal linkages to other organizations) reflect the prevailing uncertainty.

The prospect of a prominent role for corporate medicine—which is perceived to be associated with increased emphasis on minimizing costs to the organization and maximizing returns rather than on providing appropriate care—is extremely alarming to many physicians, especially those who entered the system 30 years ago.[7] Now physicians are confronted not only with the explicit involvement of profit in clinical decision making, but also with the potential that physicians will be employees in the full sense, working for health care corporations.

RECOMMENDATIONS FOR MEDICAL EDUCATION

Medical education should enable students to understand both the current state of the medical care system and the forces that are shaping it. These goals did not exist in the traditional medical education system of 30 years ago; today medical schools and examining boards have increasingly recognized their importance and implemented some curricular changes to begin to address them. Of course, the depth and details of the approach and the extent to which all students are exposed to the curriculum vary markedly from school to school (Petersdorf and Feinstein 1981; Siegel 1986).

The following sections provide a brief sketch of our concept of the general directions and the methods needed to provide an education to prepare medical students better for functioning in today's system and in the future. We consider the education needed by physicians who will practice medicine during the next 30 years or more and by those who will be the teachers of medicine during the same period.

Education of Future Clinical Practitioners

We describe here the curricular approach of the University of Illinois College of Medicine at Urbana-Champaign. It assumes that successfully educating future practitioners to understand interactions between society and the health care system requires a curriculum designed to form the necessary knowledge base in appropriate sociomedical disciplines and to demonstrate the applicability of these concepts to the practice of high-quality medicine.

The first goal is to provide a thorough understanding of the relevance of sociomedical disciplines to the health care system and the practice of good medicine.[8] The students begin with an introductory course in sociomedicine, in which they learn basic theories relevant to the study of medicine and receive an overview of the evidence on which these theories rest. This course is an intense series of lectures from faculty who hold joint appointments in their respective disciplinary departments as well as in the Medical Humanities and Social Sciences Program of the College of Medicine. Several practicums, such as participation in self-help groups for patients and field trips to public hospitals and health facilities in jails, are included as a component of the course. Finally, each student must prepare, under faculty supervision, a paper on a sociomedical topic and present a short summary of the paper to faculty and other students. Where appropriate, the student is encouraged to focus on the detailed modifications necessary to apply the theory to a specific disease or problem. In addition to providing a practical experience in professional writing and speaking, such an in-depth study assists the student in learning the complexities and depth of the sociomedical disciplines and how to apply them to medicine. The student's discovery of the extent, sophistication, and shortcomings of existing knowledge lead to a more realistic appreciation of how these disciplines bear on clinical medicine.

This course is designed to be taken before the first or second year of medical education, so that the student can apply these concepts and theories throughout his or her education. Advanced students from other disciplines are also encouraged to take the course, and in practice we usually have medical students from all four years participating. This contact with nonmedical students and older medical students is an unusual experience during medical school training and exposes our students to a variety of viewpoints and attitudes.

The second goal is to introduce clinical applications of sociomedicine. During the second year, a weekly seminar series introduces some of the clinical applications, such as how physicians can influence patient compliance and enhance quality of life. In addition, the student is introduced to the roles and responsibilities of the physician other than direct patient care and to the roles and responsibilities of other health professionals. This series is used as a forum to discuss and learn about recent and future changes in our health care system; factors to be considered in determining appropriate actions to take in a health care setting; and the importance of the differences in training, attitudes, and perspectives among doctors, patients, administrators, and society.

We and others have found that it is difficult to keep the attention of even the most dedicated students on sociomedical studies when they are simultaneously attempting to learn the basic biomedical subjects that are the traditional base of medicine. Therefore, at least for the near future, it seems inevitable that sociomedical studies should be isolated from the traditional biomedical core of medicine in order to be effective. Our approach has been to place the bulk of this teaching in an intensive summer course, during which the students have no other courses in the medical curriculum. It is essential that the teaching be done by well-qualified faculty who can demonstrate expertise in both a sociomedical discipline and in their clinical applications; such faculty are few. One approach, which we have found to be reasonably successful, is to educate university faculty from disciplines such as economics, sociology, philosophy, and law in relevant aspects of clinical medicine, and to educate physicians in sociomedical subjects, in an ongoing seminar series attended by both university faculty and appropriate academic and clinical physicians. (This book is one outcome of the seminar.)

A second important component of our approach is to have some direct involvement of physicians in the teaching of the course. They provide medical students with an explicit validation of the relevance of the sociomedical disciplines and of the perspectives of the university-based faculty. It is desirable to provide ongoing sociomedical education to practicing physicians involved in medical education. It is essential that those physicians participating in the sociomedical curriculum be sensitive to the general approach of the sociomedical teaching program.

A third important element of the teaching is to use readings that are drawn, in part, from publications addressed to physicians. We have found that articles in such journals as the *New England Journal of Medicine* and *Journal of the American Medical Association* have been particularly helpful in this regard, because of their high quality and the recognition and acceptability that come from publication in a prestigious journal read by clinical and academic physicians alike.

As indicated below, a very desirable fourth element would be to have the overall teaching program in these areas led by faculty who have medical training as well as extensive formal credentials in one of the sociomedical disciplines, especially at the doctoral level. The availability of such individuals currently is limited, but as discussed below, efforts are under way to redress this scarcity.

Finally, the clinical faculty involved in all aspects of medical education, both at the medical school and residency levels, need to become sufficiently versed in these subjects to incorporate relevant aspects into their teaching and to discuss the implications of sociomedical issues for the care of particular patients. The education of the clinical faculty in this respect is likely to be the most difficult part of the implementation of a sociomedical educational program. Perhaps the most effective force to motivate physicians to learn and understand these subjects is the impact that societal changes are having on the practice of medicine.

Education of a New Type of Academic Physician

The above discussion leads naturally to a consideration of how to develop new leaders in academic medicine who will teach and perform the research needed to improve the interactions between society and medicine. It seems clear that mere interest in these issues will not be sufficient. Successful educators and leaders need to have a sophisticated knowledge base in one or more of the sociomedical disciplines, as well as an awareness of the relevance of their knowledge to clinical medicine. There seems to be no simple and short way to provide such knowledge to physicians. The most effective way appears to be via the usual advanced educational route, in formal educational programs that use existing university and medical expertise. Here, as in most areas of scholarly endeavor, it seems desirable and perhaps essential that educators and leaders have expertise in research as well as in teaching. It follows, therefore, that these individuals need to be educated at a level equivalent to the Ph.D., in order to learn the research methodology and advanced concepts of the discipline they will combine with medicine. To have a complex understanding of the physicians' perspective, and to have maximum credibility for clinicians and medical students, they also need to earn an M.D.

The recent development of M.D.-Ph.D. programs in leading universities should facilitate the education of such individuals. Although most of the existing large M.D.-Ph.D. programs have concentrated on combining the M.D. with a Ph.D. in biomedical disciplines, programs are developing that allow students to earn a Ph.D. in disciplines such as anthropology, economics, health care policy, and sociology. There are also a few formal programs in which a student can combine law and medicine. The relatively few physicians who have doctoral-level education in sociomedical subjects already are playing significant roles in the health care system—by publishing in professional journals and holding teaching positions in academic medical centers, for example.

Our program is currently the most varied, and perhaps the largest, M.D.-Ph.D. program to offer a Ph.D. in a sociomedical discipline (we also offer M.D.-Ph.D.s in other biomedical and scientific disciplines). We describe it briefly in the appendix, with the hope that this approach may be a useful prototype for other programs.

CONCLUSIONS AND IMPLICATIONS

Based on our examination of the changes in medical education, power, and money over a 30-year span and their effects on clinical practice, we conclude that:

There have been significant changes in the medical care system and in the broader environment in which clinical practice and medical education occur. In particular, changes in power, especially the addition of new actors, and shifts in the political, social, and economic environments, have created extensive and effective challenges to the physician's once nearly exclusive authority to make clinical decisions.

These changes have helped to produce generational gaps in the attitudes and perspectives of physicians trained 30 years ago and those currently undergoing training. They differ in their views of the functions and place of medicine within society and of the roles and responsibilities of physicians. (There are other important system factors, such as type of specialty or involvement in teaching and research, that can also lead to differences in attitudes and perspectives among physicians.)

The attitudes and perspectives of each generational group have been internalized during professionalization, the foundation for which is laid during the years in medical school and residency training. Physicians trained 30 years ago have attitudes and perspectives that were more or less consonant with the medical care system and societal expectations of that period but are discordant in several important ways with the current events shaping our system.

Powerful positions within the profession tend to be held by physicians of the older generation. Thus, the official statements of professional organizations and the academic leaders of medicine may not always fully represent the attitudes and perspectives of new physicians. Health policy researchers and policy makers should understand the intraprofessional dynamics that result from these different perspectives in order to forecast and influence the future of clinical practice and the roles of physicians in the medical care system.

Freidson (1970b) and others (such as Mechanic 1985) have argued that the dominance and protected position, and hence the power, of physicians in society rest as much on their perceived duty to provide services in their clients' best interests as on their technical prowess and skills, if not more so. Therefore, to maintain professional dominance, physicians must exercise effective peer oversight with regard to moral as well as technical criteria. The divisions among physicians and the lack of a coherent voice may prevent the profession from maintaining its current position within the medical care system, further reducing the power of physicians and altering their roles as decision makers and producers of clinical services.

We have attempted not to take sides in indicating which generation has "better" attitudes and perspectives. We have suggested that new physicians fit into the contemporary medical care system more readily, being more prepared to accept the reduced power and the explicit consideration of economic and social interests in clinical decision making. Such attitudes may lead to fundamental changes in the physician's role vis-à-vis the patient, changes whereby the physician becomes an expert adviser with a clearly recognized economic interest rather than a professional whose decisions are directed entirely in the patient's best interests.

We have stressed the need for health policy analysts and activists to understand the extent and causes of the recent changes in the environment and perspectives of the medical profession. We also wish to emphasize the implications for physicians themselves. The consequences of a failure of the profession to understand and take into account the implications of trends may result in physicians' losing more control over their own work and work settings. Perhaps such changes are desirable, but they are not necessarily inevitable. Medicine should play an active role, along with society, in developing a system that serves our health care needs well.

During the 30-year period we examine, medical education has evolved in response to the availability and sources of funding for medical education, the forms of reimbursement for patient care services, and other societal changes. These responses to change have rarely been deliberately directed toward influencing or explaining the attitudes and perspectives of physicians under training or in practice. Indeed, the current environment for medical education still does little to prepare the physician for fundamental challenges to his or her power and authority, or for successful adaptation to basic restructuring of the medical care system. The physician trained today may be as ill-equipped to handle future changes as was the physician trained 30 years ago.

Medical education should provide medical students with an understanding of the extent and causes of changes in the medical care system and in the relationships between medicine and society. In addition, physicians should be trained so that, to continue to practice according to prevailing standards, they must keep abreast of changes not only in medical technology but also in the social and political factors affecting the provision of medical care services.

APPENDIX

The Medical Scholars Program (MSP), the nation's most diverse, and possibly its largest, dual M.D.-Ph.D.[9] degree program, began in 1978 at the University of Illinois at Urbana-Champaign (UIUC), the main campus of the University of Illinois. The UIUC is generally regarded as among the top ten research universities in the United States. The MSP is a joint effort of the Graduate College, the College of Medicine, and the College of Law, and its policy committee is composed of faculty and administrators representing the more than 30 participating academic units.

Students in the MSP pursue the Ph.D. degree in their respective departments in the Graduate College or in the College of Law. The policy at UIUC is that MSP students earn two genuine degrees, requiring study of sufficient time and depth to achieve an excellent research education and an excellent clinical education. Each student typically spends seven to eight years completing the two degrees. The graduate departments and the College of Medicine have cooperated in designing flexible curriculums, permitting each MSP student to plan an individualized and integrated program of study in both disciplines. Several activities, including a monthly seminar series and an annual conference, are designed to bring the students together from their diverse fields and to provide the impetus for stimulating exchange across disciplines. Thus, they learn to work with, and respect the perspectives and expertise of, persons in other disciplines related broadly to medicine. Students in the MSP are exposed to faculty, other professionals, and fellow students actively engaged in research and training in the sociomedical disciplines, as well as in the traditional bio-medical sciences and other fields not traditionally linked to medicine such as physics, engineering, computer science, and nutritional science. The setting and program are designed to provide unusual and, we believe, invaluable opportunities for students to learn the broad context of medicine and the differing disciplinary perspectives of medicine today and in the future.

In 1986 there were about 100 students enrolled in the MSP. Of these, approximately 25 percent were enrolled in sociomedical programs, that is, in programs with the departments of anthropology, business administration, clinical psychology, communications research, educational policy studies, health and safety studies, history, law, philosophy, physiological psychology, political science, social work, and sociology. The MSP can admit approximately 25 new students annually. Eventually, the program is expected to have about 175 active students enrolled in any given year, about 25 percent of whom can be expected to be in the sociomedical programs.

The effect on students of the interdisciplinary program, and the sociomedical disciplines in particular, is strengthened by three unusual features of the College of Medicine at UIUC. First, the college has a large interdisciplinary sociomedical program, the Medical Humanities and Social Sciences Program, which directs several required courses in sociomedical topics. Thus, the medical students (MSP and non-MSP) at Urbana-Champaign are exposed to sociomedical curriculums throughout their medical training as well as through the MSP program and its students. The second unusual feature of the college is the nature of the student body. Most MSP students have completed at least one year toward their nonmedical degree before starting in the medical curriculum at UIUC. The first year class in medicine consists of approximately 130 students, of whom at least 80 percent are pursuing the M.D. alone. After the first year of instruction in medicine, about 25 students remain at the Urbana-Champaign College of Medicine for their clinical sciences and clerkship experiences. The small size of each class in the second through fourth years of medical education, coupled with the large proportion in each class who are MSP students (60 percent of the second-year class in 1986 and projected to approach 100 percent eventually), yield a student body with an unusually varied background and a scholarly orientation.

Finally, we expect the majority of MSP students to become academic physicians, who will eventually be the leaders in medicine who can understand, and will educate their students to take into account, the many factors that affect the medical care system. These three features taken together present an unusual opportunity for the College of Medicine at UIUC to influence the attitudes of all of its students about medicine and its broad environment.

NOTES

1. Our description of medical students' and young physicians' perceptions of the environment is based primarily on: (1) personal experiences of one of the authors (H.M.S. began medical school in 1955 and has been involved in various aspects of medical practice since then and in medical school administration since 1970); (2) published reports describing medical students circa late 1950s, e.g., Merton et al. 1957, Fox 1959, Becker et al. 1961, Becker, Geer, and Miller 1972; (3) informal interviews with physicians engaged in clinical practice, especially members of the University of Illinois College of Medicine Class of 1959, and with faculty members of medical schools; (4) informal interviews with current medical students, especially those at the University of Illinois College of Medicine at Urbana-Champaign; and (5) other reference material.

2. Thirty years ago, the first year of residency was called an internship and virtually all students completed at least this initial phase of residency. Since that time, the length of post–medical school training has increased so that even physicians planning to enter family practice (termed general practice 30 years ago) complete a three-year residency (see Table 9:1).

3. It is, of course, a subject of considerable debate whether the current trends in the funding of Medicaid and other health programs for the poor may result in the reestablishment of the two-tiered system of the 1950s, in which the care of the poor was associated with fewer rights and privileges and an inadequate economic return for their health care. Because of changes that have occurred in society's expectations of the rights of the poor, it seems unlikely that there will be a complete return to the full two-tiered system. In that system the poor could receive medical care at a very restricted number of sites, and experienced infringement of their rights to adequate care, to participate in decisions, and to be protected by human subjects review of experimental care or peer review of substandard care.

4. For example, the head of a large multispecialty practice group indicated that new physicians have a trial period of 6 to 24 months, during which time the medical administration determines whether their level and style of practice are consistent with those of the group. If it is not, they are dropped from the group and must leave the area (because physicians joining the group must sign an agreement not to set up another practice in the community for at least five years after departing from the group).

5. See Freidson 1970b and Palmer and Reilly 1979 for a review of evidence supporting claims that group practice promotes quality; see Luft 1981, especially chap. 12, for a review of the effects of group practice on physicians.

6. See chapter 4 for a more extensive discussion of this subject.

7. See recent editorials in prominent medical journals, for example, Stern and Epstein 1985; Cunningham 1983; Bromberg 1983; and Shore and Levinson 1985.

8. The sociomedical divisions included in our program are cultural anthropology, economics, educational policy, health administration, health policy, health and safety studies, health services research, history, law, linguistics, philosophy, political science, psychology, sociology, and social work.

9. Some students are working toward the J.D., M.B.A., or M.S.W. instead of the Ph.D.

REFERENCES

American Medical Association. 1969. "Directory of Approved Internships and Residencies." *Journal of the American Medical Association* 210: 1–30.

———. 1984. *Physician Opinion on Health Care Issues: 1984.* Chicago: Survey and Opinion Research.

Association of American Medical Colleges. 1983. *COTH Survey of House Staff Stipends, Benefits, and Funding 1982.* Washington, DC: The Association.

Banta, D. H., and R. C. Fox. 1972. "Role Strains of a Health Care Team in a Poverty Community: The Columbia Point Experience." *Social Science and Medicine* 6: 697–722.

Beaty, H. N., D. Babbott, E. J. Higgins, P. Jolly, and G. S. Levey. 1986. "Research Activities of Faculty in Academic Departments of Medicine." *Annals of Internal Medicine* 104: 90–97.

Becker, H. S., B. Geer, E. C. Hughes, and A. L. Strauss. 1961. *Boys in White: Student Culture in Medical School.* Chicago: University of Chicago Press.

Becker, H. S., B. Geer, and S. J. Miller, 1972. "Medical Education." In *Handbook of Medical Sociology,* ed. by H. Freeman, S. Levine, and L. Reeder. Englewood Cliffs, NJ: Prentice-Hall.

Beckhard, R. 1972. "Organizational Issues in Team Delivery of Comprehensive Health Care." *Milbank Memorial Fund Quarterly/Health and Society* 50: 287–316.

Benson, M. C., L. Linn, N. Ward, K. B. Wells, R. H. Brook, and B. Leake. 1985. "Career Orientations of Medical and Pediatric Residents." *Medical Care* 23: 1256–64.

Bloom, Samuel W. 1971. "The Medical Center as a Social System." In *Psychosocial Aspects of Medical Training,* ed. by Robert H. Coombs and C. E. Vincent, 429–48. Springfield, IL: Charles C. Thomas.

Blue Shield Bulletin, Office Surgery Incentive Pilot Program. 1982. Durham, NC: Blue Shield.

Boice, John L., and Maurice McGregor. 1983. "Effect of Residents' Use of Laboratory Tests on Hospital Costs." *Journal of Medical Education* 58: 61–64.

Bromberg, Michael D. 1983. "The Medical-Industrial Complex: Our National Defense." *New England Journal of Medicine* 309: 1314–15.

Cassileth, B. R., R. V. Zupkis, K. Sutton-Smith, and V. March. 1980. "Information and Participation Preferences among Cancer Patients." *Annals of Internal Medicine* 92: 832–36.

"Changes in Hours Worked by Physicians." 1984. *American Journal of Public Health* 74.

Charles, S. C., J. R. Wilbert, and E. C. Kennedy. 1984. "Physicians' Self-Reports of Reactions to Malpractice Litigation." *American Journal of Psychiatry* 141: 563–65.

Committee on the Costs of Medical Care. 1932. *Health Care for the American People.* Committee on the Costs of Medical Care, Publication No. 28. Chicago: University of Chicago Press. Reprint ed. Washington, DC: U.S. Government Printing Office, 1970.

"Consequences of the Student Loan Proposals in the Administration's Fiscal 1983 Budget." 1982. *Journal of Medical Education* 57: 418–19.

Coombs, Robert H., and Boyle P. Blake. 1971. "The Transition to Medical School: Expectations versus Realities." In *Psychosocial Aspects of Medical Training,* ed. by Robert H. Coombs and C. E. Vincent, 91–109. Springfield, IL: Charles C. Thomas.

Coombs, Robert H., and C. E. Vincent, eds. 1971. *Psychosocial Aspects of Medical Training.* Springfield, IL: Charles C. Thomas.

Cunningham, R. M., Jr. 1983. "Entrepreneurialism in Medicine." *New England Journal of Medicine* 309: 1313–14.

Danzon, P. M. 1982. *The Frequency and Severity of Medical Malpractice Claims.* RAND Publication Series. Santa Monica, CA: RAND Corporation.

Davis, Karen. 1979. "Equal Treatment and Unequal Benefits: The Medicare Program." In *Health, Illness, and Medicine: A Reader in Medical Sociology,* ed. by G. L. Albrect and P. C. Higgins, 384–415. Chicago: Rand McNally.

DeMuth, G. R., and J. A. Granvall. 1970. "The Questionnaire and Its Analysis." In *The Medical School Curriculum,* ed. by William N. Hubbard, Jr., J. A. Granvall, and G. R. DeMuth, 15–29. Washington, DC: American Association of Medical Colleges.

Derzon, R., L. S. Lewin, and J. M. Watt. 1981. "Not-for-Profit Chains Share in Multihospital System Boom." *Hospitals:* 65–71.

Ducanis, A. J., and G. Annek. 1979. *The Interdisciplinary Health Care Team: A Handbook.* Germantown, MD: Aspen Systems.

Dyck, F. J., F. A. Murphy, J. K. Murphy, D. A. Road, M. S. Boyd, E. Osborne, D. De Vlieger, B. Korchinski, C. Ripley, A. T. Bromley, and P. B. Innes. 1977. "Effect of Surveillance on the Number of Hysterectomies in the Province of Saskatchewan." *New England Journal of Medicine* 296: 1326.

Eisenberg, C. A. 1983. "Women as Physicians." *Journal of Medical Education* 58: 534–41.

Enthoven, A. C. 1980. *Health Plan: The Only Practical Solution to the Soaring Cost of Medical Care.* Menlo Park, CA: Addison-Wesley.

Ermann, D., and J. Gabel. 1985. "The Changing Face of American Health Care: Multihospital Systems, Emergency Centers, and Surgery Centers." *Medical Care* 23: 401–20.

Faden, Ruth R., C. Becker, C. Lewis, J. Freeman, and A. I. Faden. 1981. "Disclosure of Information to Patients in Medical Care." *Medical Care* 19: 718–33.

Flood, Ann Barry. 1985. "The Effects of Teaching on Patient Care and Costs in Hospitals." Paper presented at the Annual Meeting of the American Public Health Association, Washington, DC, November.

Flood, Ann Barry, and W. Richard Scott. 1978. "Professional Power and Professional Effectiveness: The Power of the Surgical Staff and the Quality of Surgical Care in Hospitals." *Journal of Health and Social Behavior* 19: 240–54.

Flood, Ann Barry, W. Richard Scott, and Associates. 1987. *Hospital Structure and Performance.* Baltimore, MD: Johns Hopkins University Press.

Fordham, Christopher C. 1979. "Changing Medical Education—The New Schools." *New England Journal of Medicine* 301: 719–20.

Fox, Renee C. 1959. *Experiment Perilous.* Glencoe, IL: Free Press.

Freeman, H. E., and B. L. Kirkman-Liff. 1985. "Health Care under AHCCCS: An Examination of Arizona's Alternative to Medicaid." *Health Services Research* 20: 245–66.

Freidson, Eliot. 1970a. *Professional Dominance.* Chicago: Aldine.

———. 1970b. *Profession of Medicine: A Study of the Sociology of Applied Knowledge.* New York: Dodd, Mead.

Freshnock, L. J., and L. E. Jensen. 1981. "The Changing Structure of Medical Group Practice in the United States, 1969 to 1980." *Journal of the American Medical Association* 245: 2173–76.

Frieman, M. P., and W. D. Marder. 1984. "Changes in the Hours Worked by Physicians, 1970–1980." *American Journal of Public Health* 74: 1348–52.

Fuller, N. A., M. W. Patera, and K. Koziol. 1977. "Medicaid Utilization of Services in a Prepaid Group Practice Health Plan." *Medical Care* 15: 705–37.

Funkenstein, Daniel H. 1971. "Medical Students, Medical Schools, and Society during Three Eras." In *Psychosocial Aspects of Medical Training*, ed. by Robert H. Coombs and C. E. Vincent, 229–81. Springfield, IL: Charles C. Thomas.

"Future Directions for Medical Education." 1982. *Journal of the American Medical Association* 248: 3225–39.

Galblum, T. M., and S. Trieger. 1982. "Demonstration of Alternative Delivery Systems under Medicare and Medicaid." *Health Care Financing Review* 3: 1–11.

Garg, Mohan I., Mournir Elkhatib, Warren M. Kleinberg, and Jack L. Mulligan. 1982. "Reimbursing for Residency Training: How Many Times?" *Medical Care* 20: 719–26.

Glandon, G. L., and M. A. Morrisey. 1986. "Redefining the Hospital-Physician Relationship under Prospective Payment." *Inquiry* 23: 166–75.

Goode, William J. 1957. "Community within a Community: The Professions." *American Sociological Review* 22: 194–200.

Gray, Bradford H., ed. 1983. *The New Health Care for Profit: Doctors and Hospitals in a Competitive Environment.* Washington, DC: National Academy Press.

Greenwood, Ernest. 1957. "Attributes of a Profession." *Social Work* 2: 45–55.

Gross, E. 1958. *Work and Society.* New York: Thomas Y. Crowell.

Guest, Robert H. 1972. "The Role of the Doctor in Institutional Management." In *Organization Research on Health Institutions,* ed. by Basil S. Georgopoulos. Ann Arbor, MI: University of Michigan Press.

Guyatt, G., D. Suckett, D. W. Taylor, J. Chong, R. Roberts, and S. Pagsley. 1986. "Determining Optimal Therapy—Randomized Trials in Individual Patients." *New England Journal of Medicine* 314: 889–92.

Haynes, P. L. 1985. *Evaluating State Medicaid Reforms.* Washington, DC: American Enterprise Institute.

Holahan, J. 1985. "The Effects of the 1981 Omnibus Reconciliation Act on Medicaid Spending." Working Paper No. 333-0-03. Washington, DC: Urban Institute.

Iglehart, J. K. 1986. "Federal Support of Health Manpower Education." *New England Journal of Medicine* 314: 324–28.

Johnson, D. G. 1983. *U.S. Medical Students 1950–2000.* Washington, DC: Association of American Medical Colleges.

Jonas, Steven. 1978. *Medical Mystery: The Training of Doctors in the United States.* New York: Norton.

Jones, Katherine R. 1984. "The Influence of the Attending Physician on Indirect Graduate Medical Education Costs." *Journal of Medical Education* 59: 789–98.

Keith, S. N., R. M. Bell, A. G. Swanson, and A. P. William. 1985. "Effects of Affirmative Action in Medical Schools: A Study of the Class of 1975." *New England Journal of Medicine* 313: 1519–25.

Levitan, M. S. 1979. "Multiple Hospital Systems and the Teaching Hospital." *Journal of Medical Education* 54: 870–75.

Lipset, Seymour Martin, and William Schneider. 1983. *The Confidence Gap: Business, Labor, and Government in the Public Mind.* New York: The Free Press.

Luft, Harold S. 1981. *Health Maintenance Organizations: Dimensions of Performance.* New York: Wiley.

Macy Foundation. 1980. *Graduate Medical Education: Present and Prospective: A Call for Action.* New York: Macy Foundation.

Martz, E. Wayne, and Richard Ptakowski. 1978. "Educational Costs to Hospitalized Patients." *Journal of Medical Education* 53: 383–86.

Marzuk, Peter M. 1985. "The Right Kind of Paternalism." *New England Journal of Medicine* 313: 1474–76.

McDevitt, R., and W. Buczko. 1985. "Medicaid Program Characteristics and Their Consequences for Program Spending." *Health Care Financing Review* 7: 3–29.

Mechanic, David. 1976. *The Growth of Bureaucratic Medicine.* New York: Wiley.

———. 1978. "The Medical Malpractice Dilemma." In *Medical Sociology*, 503–15. 2d ed. New York: Free Press.

———. 1985. "Public Perceptions of Medicine." *New England Journal of Medicine* 312: 181–83.

Merton, R., G. Reader, and P. Kendall, eds. 1957. *The Student Physician.* Cambridge, MA: Harvard University Press.

O'Reilly, Patrick, Charles P. Tifft, and Charlene DeLena. 1982. "Continuing Medical Education: 1960's to the Present." *Journal of Medical Education* 57: 819–26.

OSR Report. 1979. 3 (2).

Palmer, R. H., and M. C. Reilly. 1979. "Individual and Institutional Variables which May Serve as Indicators of Quality of Medical Care." *Medical Care* 17: 693–717.

Panel on the General Professional Education of the Physician (GPEP). 1984. *Physicians for the Twenty-First Century.* Washington, DC: Association of American Medical Colleges.

Penn, N. E., P. J. Russell, H. J. Simon, T. C. Jacob, C. Stafford, E. Castro, J. Cisneros, and M. Bush. 1986. "Affirmative Action at Work: A Survey of Graduates of the University of California, San Diego Medical School." *American Journal of Public Health* 76: 1144–46.

Perkoff, G. T. 1986. "Teaching Clinical Medicine in the Ambulatory Setting: An Idea Whose Time May Have Finally Come." *New England Journal of Medicine* 314: 27–31.

Petersdorf, R. G. 1980. "The Evolution of Departments of Medicine." *New England Journal of Medicine* 303: 489–96.

———. 1981. "Academic Medicine: No Longer Threadbare or Genteel." *New England Journal of Medicine* 304: 841–43.

———. 1982. "Some Perturbations in Medicine: An Interview with Robert G. Petersdorf." *Journal of the American Medical Association* 248: 2098–2101.

———. 1984. "Managing the Revolution in Medical Care." *Journal of Medical Education* 59: 79–90.

Petersdorf, R. G., and A. R. Feinstein. 1981. "An Informal Appraisal of the Current Status of 'Medical Sociology.'" *Journal of the American Medical Association* 245: 943–50.

Petersdorf, R. G., and M. P. Wilson. 1982. "The Four Horsemen of the Apocalypse: Study of Academic Medical Center Governance." *Journal of the American Medical Association* 247: 1153–61.

President's Commission for the Study of Ethical Problems in Medicine and Biomedical and Behavioral Research. 1983. *Securing Access to Health Care: The Ethical Implications of Differences in the Availability of Health Services.* Washington, DC: U.S. Government Printing Office.

Purcell, E. F., ed. 1976. *Recent Trends in Medical Education.* New York: Macy Foundation.

Reeder, Leo G. 1972. "The Patient-Client as a Consumer: Some Observations on the Changing Professional-Client Relationship." *Journal of Health and Social Behavior* 13: 406–12.

Roemer, Milton I., and Jay W. Friedman. 1971. *Doctors in Hospitals: Medical Staff Organization and Hospital Performance.* Baltimore: Johns Hopkins University Press.

Roller, A. C., and L. Pembrook, eds. 1983. *The Pfizer Guide: Medical Career Opportu-*

    nities. New Canaan, CT: Mark Powley.
Salkever, D. S., P. S. German, S. Shapiro, R. Horky, and E. A. Skinner. 1976. "Epi-
    sodes of Illness and Access to Care in the Inner City: A Comparison of HMO
    and Non-HMO Populations." *Health Services Research* 11: 252–70.
Saward, E. W., and E. K. Gallagher. 1983. "Reflections on Change in Medical Prac-
    tice: The Current Trend to Large-Scale Medical Organizations." *Journal of the
    American Medical Association* 250: 2820–25.
Schofield, J. R. 1984. *New and Expanded Medical Schools, Midcentury to the 1980's.* San
    Francisco: Jossey-Bass.
Schroeder, Steven A., and Dennis S. O'Leary. 1977. "Differences in Laboratory Use
    and Length of Stay between University and Community Hospitals." *Journal
    of Medical Education* 52: 418–20.
Scott, W. Richard, and Ann Barry Flood. 1987. "Costs and Quality of Care in Hospi-
    tals: A Review of the Literature." In *Hospital Structure and Performance,* Ann
    Barry Flood, W. Richard Scott, and Associates. Baltimore, MD: Johns Hop-
    kins University Press. Preprinted in *Medical Care Review* 41 (1984): 213–61.
Shore, Miles F., and Harry Levinson. 1985. "On Business and Medicine." *New En-
    gland Journal of Medicine* 313: 319–21.
Shortell, Stephen M. 1983. "Physician Involvement in Hospital Decision Making."
    In *The New Health Care for Profit: Doctors and Hospitals in a New Competitive En-
    vironment,* ed. by Bradford H. Gray, 73–101. Washington, DC: National Acade-
    my Press.
Siegel, I. 1986. "Second Year Teaching Programs." Paper prepared for Subcommit-
    tee of Educational Policy Committee. College of Medicine at Urbana, Univer-
    sity of Illinois, May 2.
Somers, Herman M., and Ann R. Somers. 1967. *Medicare and the Hospitals.* Washing-
    ton, DC: Brookings Institution.
Starr, Paul. 1982. *The Social Transformation of American Medicine: The Rise of a Sover-
    eign Profession and the Making of a Vast Industry.* New York: Basic Books.
Stern, Robert S., and A. M. Epstein. 1985. "Institutional Responses to Prospective
    Payment Based on Diagnosis-Related Groups." *New England Journal of Medi-
    cine* 312: 621–27.
Sullivan, R. 1985. "Cuomo's Plan for Malpractice Rates." *New York Times* April 12.
Tancredi, L. R., and Barondess, J. A. 1978. "The Problem of Defensive Medicine."
    In *Health Care: Regulation, Economics, Ethics, Practice,* ed. by P. H. Abelson,
    37–40. Washington, DC: American Association for the Advancement of
    Science.
Tarlov, A. H. 1983a. "Shattuck Lecture—The Increasing Supply of Physicians, the
    Changing Structure of the Health Services System, and the Future Practice
    of Medicine." *New England Journal of Medicine* 308: 1235–44.
———. 1983b. "Consequences of the Rising Number of Physicians and of Growth
    of Subspecialization in Internal Medicine." In *Academic Medicine: Present and
    Future,* ed. by J. Z. Bowers and E. E. King, 106–21. North Tarrytown, NY:
    Rockefeller Archive Center.
Task Force on Academic Health Centers. 1985. *The Future of Teaching Hospitals.*
    Report III. New York: Commonwealth Fund.
Turk, E. 1985. "Arizona's Alternative to Medicaid—Model or Muddle?" *The New Phy-
    sician* (July/August): 11–20.
Twaddle, A. C., and R. M. Hessler. 1977. "New Health Workers." In *A Sociology of
    Health,* 202–16. Saint Louis: Mosby.

U.S. Congress, Senate Special Committee on Aging. 1985. *Quality of Care under Medicare's Prospective Payment System, II.* Appendix. 99th Cong., 1st Sess., Ser. Nos. 99-9, 10, 11.

Wagoner, N. E. 1986. "Preparing for a Residency is a Four Year Process." (Student booklet.) Cincinnati: University of Cincinnati College of Medicine.

Wagoner, N. E., J. R. Suriano, and J. A. Stoner. 1986. "Factors Used by Program Directors to Select Residents." *Journal of Medical Education* 61: 10-21.

Watt, M. J., R. A. Derzon, S. C. Renn, C. J. Schramm, J. S. Hahn, and G. D. Pillari. 1986. "The Comparative Economic Performance of Investor-Owned Chains and Not-for-Profit Hospitals." *New England Journal of Medicine* 314: 89-96.

Webster, Thomas G. 1971. "The Behavioral Sciences in Medical Education and Practice." In *Psychosocial Aspects of Medical Training*, ed. by Robert H. Coombs and C. E. Vincent, 285-348. Springfield, IL: Charles C. Thomas.

Weeks, Lewis E., and Howard J. Berman. 1985. *Shapers of American Health Care Policy: An Oral History.* Ann Arbor, MI: Health Administration Press.

Wennberg, J. E., L. Blowers, P. Parker, and A. M. Gittelsohn. 1977. "Changes in Tonsillectomy Rates Associated with Feedback and Review." *Pediatrics* 59: 821-26.

Wolinsky, Fredric D., and Richard S. Kurz. 1984. "How the Public Chooses and Views Hospitals." *Hospital & Health Services Administration* 29: 58-67.

Wood, Ann P. 1984. "Hospital Occupancy Down, Physicians Adapting to DRGs." *Internal Medicine News* 17: 1, i34, i42-44.

Wyszewianski, Leon, John R. C. Wheeler, and Avedis Donabedian. 1982. "Market-Oriented Cost-Containment Strategies and Quality of Care." *Milbank Memorial Fund Quarterly* 60: 518-50.

Zuckerman, H. S., and Lewis E. Weeks. 1979. *Multi-institutional Systems: Their Promise and Performance.* Chicago: Hospital Research and Educational Trust.

Index

For compiling the index with diligence, care, and speed, the editors are grateful to Gregory
Flentje, Michael Cantor, and Stephen Borodkin, research assistants to the Faculty Seminar
on Medicine and Society at the University of Illinois at Urbana-Champaign.

About the Editors

EVAN M. MELHADO is Associate Professor in the Departments of History and Chemistry and a member of the Program on Science, Technology, and Society at the University of Illinois at Urbana-Champaign. He also holds a concurrent appointment in the University of Illinois College of Medicine at Urbana. He obtained his Ph.D. in history from Princeton University, and he has specialized in the history of science and medicine. He has helped design and teach the summer medicine and society course in the College of Medicine at Urbana and has long been involved in the governance of the Medical Scholars Program. His research interests include the history of the physical sciences in the 18th and 19th centuries and of medicine and health care in the 19th and 20th centuries.

WALTER FEINBERG was formerly director of the Medicine and Society Faculty Development Seminar in the University of Illinois College of Medicine at Urbana and is Professor of Educational Policy Studies at the University of Illinois at Urbana-Champaign. He also holds a joint appointment in the Unit for Criticism and Interpretive Theory. He obtained a Ph.D. in philosophy from Boston University. His research interests include issues of equity and professional education as related to the growth and distribution of knowledge and authority.

HAROLD M. SWARTZ is Professor of Medicine at the University of Illinois College of Medicine at Urbana, and Professor of Physiology and Biophysics in the School of Life Sciences and an Affiliate of the Institute of Environmental Studies at the University of Illinois at Urbana-Champaign. He holds M.P.H., M.D., and Ph.D. degrees. His professional expertise is in radiation biology and biophysics, fields in which he has published extensively and continues an active program of laboratory research. He was a principal investigator for the project sponsored by the University of Illinois College of Medicine and the National Institutes of Health on Curriculum Development in Environmental Health and principal investigator for the Cost-Containment Project at the University of Illinois College of Medicine sponsored by the National Fund for Medical Education. He has been extensively involved in the design, development, and guidance of the Medical Scholars Program.